D1211607

12/10

UNAIDS
The First 10 Years

1996–2006

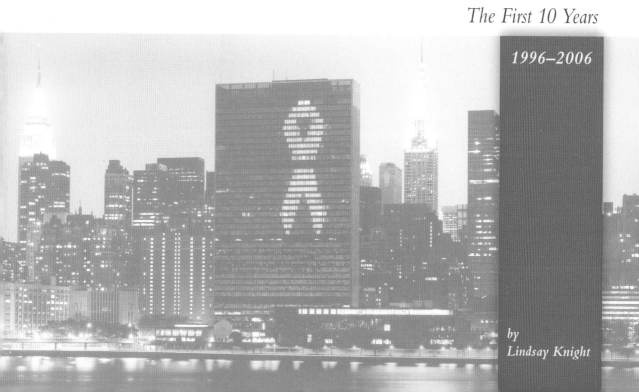

by
Lindsay Knight

Acknowledgements:

Initial concept and development: Julia Cleves

Research, additional writing and section on Malawi: Katya Halil

Additional research, writing and sections on Côte d'Ivoire, Haiti, Kenya and Ukraine: Froeks Kamminga

Photo editor: Sue Steward

Assistance with picture research: Manuel Da Quinta

Design: Lon Rahn and Nathalie Gouiran

Production: Andrea Verwohlt

Editor: Kath Davies

Proofreading assistance: AvisAnne Julien

History Reference Group

Elhadj As Sy: Director, Partnerships and External Relations, UNAIDS

Richard Burzynski: Executive Director, International Council of AIDS Service Organizations

Rob Moodie: Chair of Global Health, Nossal Institute for Global Health, University of Melbourne

Kim Nichols: Co-Executive Director, African Services Committee

Peter Piot: Executive Director, UNAIDS

Jeffrey Sturchio: Vice-President, External Affairs, Merck & Co, Inc

Debrework Zewdie: Director, Global HIV/AIDS Programme, World Bank

Internal Reference Group

Alistair Craik

Achmat Dangor

Siddharth Dube

Elisabeth Manipoud Figueroa

Timothy Martineau

Elizabeth Parker

Ben Plumley

Keith Wynn

Front page photo UNAIDS/R. Bowman

HIV estimates used in UNAIDS the first 10 years

The precise numbers of people living with HIV, people who have been newly infected or who have died of AIDS are not known. Achieving 100% certainty about the numbers of people living with HIV globally, for example, would require testing every person in the world for HIV every year—which is logistically impossible and pose ethical problems. But we can estimate those numbers by using other sources of data.

The availability and quality of these data have been improving over the ten years covered in this book. For this reason the best estimates of the historic trend in HIV based on current knowledge of the epidemic, have been used for this book. These estimates differ from what was published at the time, but are consistent with current knowledge of the development and of the spread of the HIV epidemic.

Contents

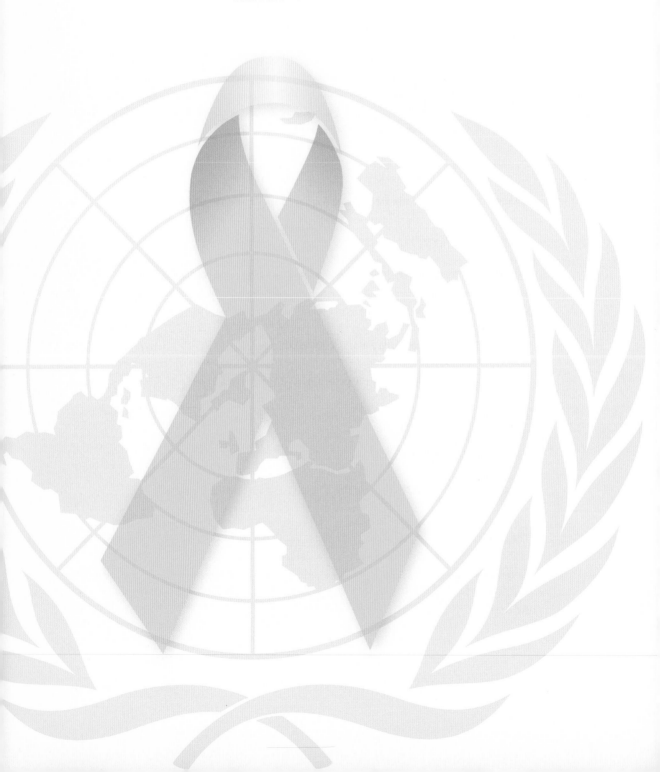

This book is in memory of Julia Cleves; a woman who had vision, humour, prodigious stamina and who was endlessly kind. These attributes and her contribution to international AIDS, health and development work will be remembered by many – and greatly missed by those fortunate to have worked with her.

UNAIDS History: Preface

This is the history of a relatively young organization – UNAIDS, launched in 1996 to strengthen the way in which the United Nations (UN) was responding to AIDS, one of the worst pandemics the world has ever known. By 1996, some 15 years since a few cases of the new condition were first reported in a scientific publication, over four million people had died from AIDS, several million were living with HIV and the future predictions were dire.

This book relates the struggles and achievements of the institution, and the contribution it has made to the progress, however slow and faltering at times, in the battle against one of the greatest threats humankind has faced. It also attempts to explain the innovative nature of UNAIDS – a joint programme that has brought together a number of cosponsoring UN organizations (originally six, now 10). Only a special UN programme was deemed capable by its creators of 'orchestrating a global response to a fast-growing epidemic of a feared and stigmatized disease whose roots and ramifications extend into virtually all aspects of society[1]'.

However, due to limitations of space, this is mainly a history of the UNAIDS Secretariat; the readers should not expect a full account of the 10 UNAIDS Cosponsors' and other partners' involvement in the fight against AIDS. Although, as the book reveals, partnership with individuals and organizations from all sectors of society is, and always has been, key to the work of UNAIDS.

So, largely a history of an institution and its staff, the book is structured according to the Programme's decision-making cycles: its central chapters each span a two-year period because UNAIDS develops its budget and workplan every biennium. Thus, the biennial chapters represent a significant and specific period in the life of the organization: every two years, UNAIDS staff, building on the work and lessons of previous years, critically review strategies, initiatives and partners to help contain AIDS. Every two years, UNAIDS staff have a specific set of concerns and priorities in their attempt to multiply the number of fronts on which the battle against AIDS is fought. Not only do the chapters represent a specific phase in the history of the organization, they also describe paradigm shifts and global progress made in the AIDS response.

Each chapter describes the efforts that UNAIDS and its partners were making on many fronts – advocacy, fundraising, prevention, treatment and suchlike, and describes the fruits and failures of UN and global efforts. As such, every chapter weaves in the many different themes and areas of work that together make up the full multisectoral effort and that are at the heart of UNAIDS' mandate. The themes addressed in this book include access to HIV treatment; advocating politicians to make AIDS a national priority; fighting stigma; working with partners to significantly raise the funding for AIDS and supporting countries and donors to use these monies effectively; coordinating the actions of the many AIDS actors; promoting implementation of effective programmes and technical support in countries; and renewing the focus on women's vulnerability and prevention.

At the heart of this history are the stories of many people and their efforts. More than 150 men and women were interviewed; the book is largely based on their accounts. Clearly these are subjective, we do not pretend to have any absolute truths. But we do hope we have provided a multifaceted account of the history of UNAIDS based on multiple subjective views. These most importantly include those of people living with HIV, whose contribution is vital to effective work on AIDS.

Although the history plots progress on many levels through the work of UNAIDS and its partners, ultimately it highlights the many challenges the world still faces if this deadly pandemic is to be reversed.

[1] *Report of the Committee of Cosponsoring Organizations of the Joint and Cosponsored United Nations Programme on HIV/AIDS.* E/1995/71,19 May 1995.

6

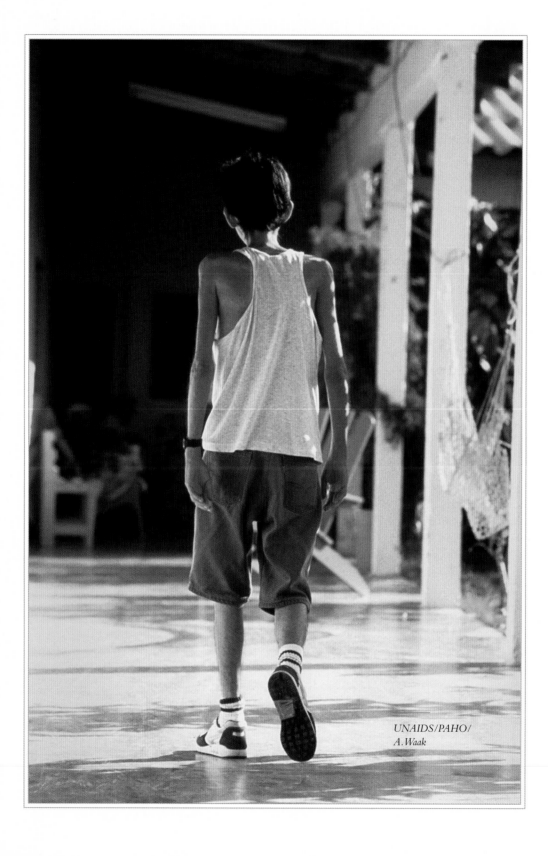

UNAIDS/PAHO/
A. Waak

Chapter 1:

The beginning of the AIDS epidemic and the United Nations response, 1981–1993

The early days

No one could have imagined that a few cases of rare diseases damaging the immune system would herald a pandemic that has killed more than all those who died in battle during the whole of the twentieth century.

On 1 January 1996, UNAIDS – the Joint United Nations Programme on HIV/AIDS – opened for business. This was 15 years after the first published report of AIDS cases, 15 years during which most of the world's leaders, in all sectors of society, had displayed a staggering indifference to the growing challenge of this new epidemic.

UNAIDS and the World Health Organization (WHO) estimated in 1996 that more than 4.6 million people had died from AIDS since the beginning of the epidemic and that over 20.1 million were then living with the virus that leads to AIDS. The majority of those infected (over 15 million) lived in sub-Saharan Africa, followed by more than 31.8 million in Asia, 1 million in Latin America and the Caribbean and about 1.5 million in North America and Western and Central Europe[1].

On 5 June 1981, the United States (US) Centers for Disease Control and Prevention's (CDC) *Morbidity and Mortality Weekly Report* described some rare pneumonias seen in five gay men and 'the possibility of a cellular-immune dysfunction related to a common exposure that predisposes individuals to opportunistic infections such as pneumocytosis and candidiasis'. No one then could have imagined that a few cases of rare diseases damaging the immune system would herald a pandemic that has killed more than all those who died in battle during the whole of the twentieth century. Similar cases had been seen by doctors in the main gay communities of the United States of America (USA), in New York City and California, during the previous three to four years. A new syndrome was named, 'gay-related immunodeficiency syndrome', or GRID. But because similar cases appeared over the next year among people who were not gay men – women, injecting drug users and at least one child – in 1982 the CDC adopted the term AIDS, Acquired Immune Deficiency Syndrome. Doctors in Belgium and Paris reading the June 1981 report realized that they had treated similar conditions since the mid-1970s, mainly in Africans from the equatorial region or Europeans who had visited this area[2].

MMWR

Weekly

June 5, 1981 / 30(21);1-3

Epidemiologic Notes and Reports

Pneumocystis Pneumonia --- Los Angeles

In the period October 1980-May 1981, 5 young men, all active homosexuals, were treated for biopsy-confirmed *Pneumocystis carinii* pneumonia at 3 different hospitals in Los Angeles, California. Two of the patients died. All 5 patients had laboratory-confirmed previous or current cytomegalovirus (CMV) infection and candidal mucosal infection. Case reports of these patients follow.

Patient 1: A previously healthy 33-year-old man developed *P. carinii* pneumonia and oral mucosal candidiasis in March 1981 after a 2-month history of fever associated with elevated liver enzymes, leukopenia, and CMV viruria. The serum complement-fixation CMV titer in October 1980 was 256; in may 1981 it was 32.* The patient's condition deteriorated despite courses of treatment with trimethoprim-sulfamethoxazole (TMP/SMX), pentamidine, and acyclovir. He died May 3, and postmortem examination showed residual *P. carinii* and CMV pneumonia, but no evidence of neoplasia.

Patient 2: A previously healthy 30-year-old man developed *p. carinii* pneumonia in April 1981 after history of fever each day of elevated liver-function tests, CMV viruria, and titer of 16 and a convalescent-phase features of his illness included of intravenous

---

[1] UNAIDS/WHO *2007 AIDS epidemic update*, November 2007.

[2] Iliffe J (2007). *The African AIDS Epidemic*. A history. Oxford, James Currey.

8

At about the same time, doctors working in various African countries were treating patients with very similar symptoms. In 1983, a team from the Ugandan Ministry of Health investigated a new disease – known as 'Slim' because patients rapidly lost weight – in the Lake Victoria fishing village of Kasensero, and concluded that it was AIDS. Also in 1983, a team of American and European scientists, led by Peter Piot (now UNAIDS Executive Director and who had been to the hospital years earlier, investigating the first outbreak of Ebola), visited the capital of Zaire, Kinshasha, and, in a single hospital, found dozens of patients dying from AIDS.

"In 1976, there were hardly any young adults there except for traffic accidents in orthopaedic wards", Piot told a reporter. "Suddenly I walked in and saw all these young men and women, emaciated, dying"[3]. His colleague Joseph McCormick wrote: 'Some developed such exquisitely sore mouths and tongues that they were unable to eat. Those who could manage a few bites of food were suddenly stricken by cramps and disgorged a copious amount of diarrhoea. Their skin would break out in massive, generalized eruptions. … When the infection didn't consist of voracious yeast cells [as in cryptococcal meningitis], there were many other parasites ready to eat the brain alive. None of the victims could comprehend in any way what was happening to them or why. And we? All we could do was watch in horror, our roles as physicians reduced to scrupulous observers and accurate recorders of documentation. Our one hope was that if we could understand the processes we were observing, someone, somewhere, might find a solution'[4].

Significantly, as many women as men were among these Kinshasa patients; it was clear that transmission was taking place through heterosexual as well as homosexual contact. Soon, AIDS cases were also identified in Congo, Rwanda, Tanzania and Zambia. The team quickly wrote a paper about the Zairian cases and submitted it to the prestigious *Lancet*, which initially rejected it but then published it in 1984[5]. In these early years of the epidemic, many scientists refused to believe that AIDS was a heterosexual problem; they also dismissed concerns about its potential to become a global pandemic as unnecessarily alarmist.

Yet soon, cases were being reported in every region of the world, in most European countries as well as Australia, New Zealand, and parts of Latin America.

A slow response

From the beginning, people with AIDS were stigmatized. Many came from marginalized populations – gay men, injecting drug users, sex workers, Haitians living in the USA and haemophiliacs. Many religious groups believed the illness was God's vengeance on anybody who was sexually promiscuous or behaved in an 'unnatural' fashion. Famously, the President of the USA, Ronald Reagan, made no pronouncement on AIDS until 1986. In most of Africa,

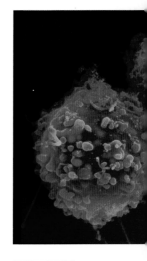

The Human Immunodeficiency Virus was identified in 1983 as the cause of AIDS.
UNAIDS

---

[3] Malan R (2001). 'AIDS in Africa: in search of the truth'. *Rolling Stone*, 22 November.
[4] McCormick J, Fosher-Hoch S (1996). *Level 4: Virus Hunters of the CDC.* New York, Barnes and Noble Books.
[5] Piot P, Quinn TC, Taelman H, Feinsod FM, Minlangu KB, Wobin O, Mbendi N, Mazebo P, Ndangi K, Stevens W et al.(1984) 'Acquired immunodeficiency syndrome in a heterosexual population in Zaire'. *The Lancet*, 2(8394), 14 July.

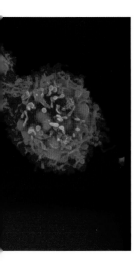

AIDS was also treated as a 'disease of the Other'[6] – foreigners, whites, sex workers, long-distance truck drivers, migrants and city dwellers.

The epidemic has always been fuelled by ignorance and fear. But, as McCormick had hoped, there were scientists who recognized the urgent need to discover the cause and then a cure and a vaccine. In 1983 and 1984, Luc Montagnier at the Pasteur Institute in France, and Robert Gallo at the National Institutes of Health (NIH) in the USA, identified a new virus as a possible cause of AIDS; this is what is now known as the Human Immunodeficiency Virus (HIV). It was generally agreed that the main routes of transmission were blood and semen.

The history of the early years of AIDS, in the developed world as well as in developing nations, is a story of wasted time and opportunities, of failure of leadership, of denial and discrimination. Politicians across the globe feared associating themselves and their countries with death and sex and, for many years, only a trickle of funding was made available for research into AIDS, let alone for care and support for those people living with the condition.

In middle- and low-income countries, AIDS was seen as yet another major health problem facing governments with poor health services and a lack of resources. It would be some time before the impact of the epidemic on societies and economies would be widely discussed, or even accepted, by governments already under other pressures, or before it was taken as seriously as other diseases, such as malaria and diarrhoea that killed so many young children.

The history of the early years of AIDS, in the developed world as well as in developing nations, is a story of wasted time and opportunities, of failure of leadership, of denial and discrimination.

The nature of the virus meant that the extent and impact of AIDS, unlike other pandemics such as the Black Death or Spanish Flu, remained hidden. It is now clear that doctors in western Africa were seeing patients with HIV as early as the 1970s and a few cases from even earlier have been identified. For most people who are HIV positive there is a time lag of several years between infection and the development of AIDS-related symptoms that lead to death. This 'silent' epidemic made it easier for leaders to remain silent in their response, even while scientists and activists were publishing ever more disturbing statistics and projections. The result was that by 2005, around 60 million people had been infected with HIV, and AIDS has killed nearly 25 million since 1981[7].

In the industrialized countries where the disease was first identified, there was little domestic political pressure to address the issue and, in fact, a great deal of pressure to avoid recognizing it at all[8]. Public fear and panic about this new disease, about which they knew little, meant that countries harked back to the judgemental and stigmatizing reactions seen in earlier times to other pandemics. Many countries introduced compulsory HIV testing for people entering the country or for particular groups such as students[9]. Some countries also refused entry to people known to be HIV positive, and still do today.

---

[6] Carael M (2007). 'Face à la mondialisation du sida. Vingt ans d'interventions et de controverses', in Philippe Denis and Charles Becker (eds), *L'épidémie du sida en Afrique subsaharienne. Regards historiens*. Louvain-la-Neuve et Paris, Academia Bruylant et Karthala.

[7] UNAIDS/WHO estimates, November 2007.

[8] Soni A K (1998). From GPA to UNAIDS: Examining the Evolution of the UN Response to AIDS. Essay presented to the Committee on Degrees in Social Studies for a BA Honors degree, Harvard, November.

[9] Sabatier R (1989). *AIDS and the Third World*. London, Panos Books.

At the same time that these restrictive measures were being introduced, denial of the disease's existence was widespread. Piot recalled[10] waiting, sometime in the mid-1980s, with another AIDS expert, Frank Plummer from Canada's University of Manitoba, for nearly a day in the office of the Kenyan Minister of Health while officials debated whether or not to expel the two because they had talked to reporters about AIDS in Africa. In 1985, Zaire refused to give the *New York Times* journalist, Larry Altman, a visa to report on AIDS, and the Government of Kenya confiscated copies of the *International Herald Tribune* containing his article, as leaders denied the severity of their AIDS problem. That same year, the Zambian press secretary denied Altman's request for an interview with President Kenneth Kaunda. A year later, however, Kaunda announced that he had lost his son to AIDS; three years later he became one of the first African leaders to speak out on the need to combat the epidemic.

The activists

The AIDS activist movement, starting in North America, spread to Europe and Latin America and eventually, over several years, to every region of the world. Activists put the rest of society to shame in the early years of AIDS. Not only were they powerful advocates for more funding, better care and treatment, further research, and commitment from leaders, they also pioneered ways of caring for people with HIV. These included providing support through 'buddying', advising on nutrition and treating the opportunistic diseases commonly experienced by positive people.

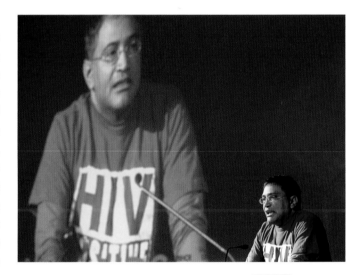

South African AIDS activist and founder of the Treatment Action Campaign, Zackie Achmat.
UNAIDS/P.Virot

New York's Gay Men's Health Crisis, founded in 1981, was the world's first AIDS service organization and is still a powerful force. The Terrence Higgins Trust was the first AIDS organization in the United Kingdom (UK), established in 1983. In France, AIDES was founded in 1984 and is now one of the largest community-based organizations tackling HIV. The AIDS Coalition to Unleash Power (ACT UP) started in 1987 in the USA, and was committed to direct action against an indifferent (if not hostile) government; it campaigns for better access to drugs and an end to AIDS-related discrimination. In Brazil, gay activists successfully advocated the adoption of the first government AIDS programme in 1983 in São Paolo State[11].

---

[10] Altman L K (1999). 'The doctor's world: in Africa, a deadly silence about AIDS is lifting'. *New York Times*, 13 July.
[11] Berkman A, Parker R et al. (2005). 'A critical analysis of the Brazilian response to HIV/AIDS: lessons learned for controlling and mitigating the epidemic in developing countries'. *American Journal of Public Health*, 95 (7), July.

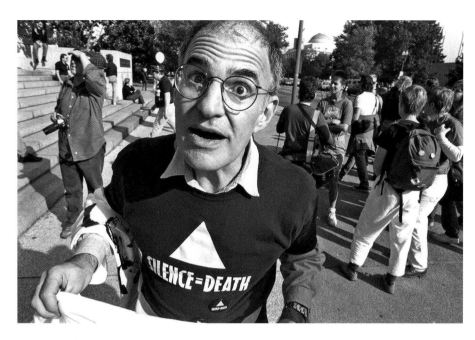

AIDS activist and writer Larry Kramer at an ACT UP rally in 1987
Marc Geller

In the North, especially in the USA, the activists were mainly gay men, often living with HIV. They refused to see themselves as 'victims' and fought for their rights, a result of the stigmatization and discrimination they faced every day. As early as 1983, the US National Association of People with AIDS, a not-for-profit advocacy organization, released a mission statement: 'We condemn attempts to label us as "victims", a term which implies defeat, and we are only occasionally "patients", a term which implies passivity, helplessness and dependence upon the care of others. We are "People with AIDS"'. The statement included a list of recommendations for health care providers and others on treating people with AIDS which became known as the Denver Principles.

The Global Network of People living with HIV/AIDS (GNP+) was started in 1986 by Dietmar Bolle, an HIV specialist nurse who was HIV positive (until 1992 it was known as the International Steering Committee of People with HIV/AIDS). Bolle aimed to empower people living with HIV and to help them share their personal experiences. Regional networks of people living with HIV were established on every continent, and although those in low income countries are often underresourced compared with their rich counterparts in the North, they have combined powerful advocacy with providing care and support services.

Activist and self-help organizations appeared in the South some years after their emergence in the developed world, partly because of more limited resources. In Uganda, in 1987, following her husband's death from AIDS, Noerine Kaleeba set up The AIDS Support Organisation (TASO) with a group of friends also personally affected by AIDS. Her own heart-breaking experience revealed the need to support the families caring for people with HIV, to educate the community, including health care workers, about the disease and

12

in so doing, to combat stigma and discrimination. TASO has become a role model for similar organizations around the world, spreading its philosophy of 'Living positively with AIDS'.

As Kaleeba explained, '… at that time the public health messages were saying "Beware of AIDS, AIDS kills."… There were no messages for people who were already infected. What was implied was that people who were already infected should die and get it over with. We adopted the slogan of "living positively with AIDS" in direct defiance of that perception. We emphasised *living* rather than *dying* with AIDS. For us it was the quality rather than the quantity of life which was important'[12].

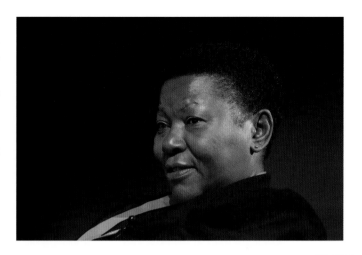

AIDS activist Noerine Kaleeba who founded The AIDS Support Organisation in Uganda.
UNAIDS/P.Virot

Elhadj As Sy, who worked in Senegal for ENDA Tiers Monde, a nongovernmental organization on environment and development, and is now Director of Partnerships and External Relations at UNAIDS, co-founded[13] the African Network of AIDS Service Organizations. He recalled that in those days, when few resources were available and stigma was rife, poor African communities displayed 'a good sense of solidarity, supporting each other, spending their last cent and taking care of their loved ones travelling miles and miles for treatment, whatever they thought could help. There were times when I'd say to myself "Why did we need an epidemic like HIV/AIDS to see this?"'

For Zackie Achmat, his and others' early activism around AIDS in South Africa was partly about equality for gay people, and partly because, in the apartheid era, in the mid-1980s, the HIV test was being used for discriminatory purposes. He explained: "It [the test] was being used against Malawian miners to try and exclude people from employment. It became very clear … that what HIV was going to do was … to utilize or reinforce existing inequalities. It became very clear to me at the outset that HIV was going to be a human rights issue".

---

[12] Kaleeba N with Ray S and Willmore B (1991). *We miss you all. Noerine Kaleeba: AIDS in the family.* Harare, Women and AIDS Support Network.

[13] The following people contributed to the creation of the Network: Mazuwa Banda, then Chair of the Southern African Network of AIDS Organizations, and now with WHO; Hakima Himmich, then Chair of the Association Marocaine de Lutte Contre le Sida, and Convener of the Northern African Network of AIDS Service Organizations; and Richard Burzynski, of the International Council of AIDS Service Organizations (ICASO). As Sy was also supported by two colleagues from ENDA – Tiers Monde, Abdelkader Bacha, now with the International HIV/AIDS Alliance, and Moustapha Gueye, now with UNDP.

The United Nations response to the AIDS epidemic

The United Nations (UN) was as slow to respond to this new global challenge as many of its Member States. WHO was clearly the natural UN 'home' for work on AIDS with its mandate on maintaining global health. Cases had been reported to WHO annually since 1981 but only one person in the organization was working in the area of sexually transmitted infections in the early 1980s[14]. The agency's first official acknowledgement of the new disease was to call a meeting in Denmark in October 1983 to assess the European situation; it summoned another meeting in Geneva at the end of 1983 to consider the global AIDS problem. Here WHO's role was defined primarily as one of monitoring developments.

An internal WHO memo noted in 1983 that the organization did not need to be involved in AIDS because the condition 'is being well taken care of by some of the richest countries in the world where there is the manpower and the know-how and where most of the patients are to be found'[15].

WHO's Director-General, Halfdan Mahler, later admitted that denial had been a major cause of WHO's delayed response to AIDS: "I know that many people at first refused to believe that a crisis was upon us. I know because I was one of them"[16].

In 1985, the first International Conference on AIDS was held in Atlanta, Georgia, USA, organized by the CDC and cosponsored by WHO and the US Department of Health. By this time, 17,000 cases of AIDS had been reported, more than 80% of them in the USA, but there was mounting evidence of cases in many African countries. Yet the focus was very much on the Western world and only three Africans attended – doctors Kapita, Odio and Pangu. Even these three might not have attended were it not for the American physician Jonathan Mann and the Belgian doctor Peter Piot, who were working with them in Zaire on Projet Sida (the first international collaboration on AIDS in Africa) and saw the conference as an important opportunity to debate AIDS in Africa.

The doctors' expectations for the conference were not met. Some participants aggressively refused to accept that HIV could be transmitted through heterosexual intercourse. "In a non-scientific way they were saying … these men must be closet gays, and transmission from women to men is impossible", Piot recalled. Other participants presented estimates of incidence in African countries that Piot knew from his own experience were wildly exaggerated.

Far more disturbing were the cultural ignorance and personal abuse displayed – an American journalist asked one African doctor whether it was true that AIDS could spread because

[14] Berridge V (1996). *AIDS in the UK. The Making of Policy, 1981–1994*. Oxford, Oxford University Press.
[15] Soni (1998).
[16] Speech to final plenary session of the Fourth International Conference on AIDS, Stockholm, July 1988.

14

Africans had sex with monkeys. The African scientists were appalled. Scepticism and denial among African leaders were reinforced when it became clear that the exaggerated estimates presented at the conference were wrong. Peter Piot had been amazed as he watched 'some of the world's most prominent scientists' presenting estimates of HIV in Africa 'that were absolutely stratospheric, off the charts.' He ' knew from firsthand experience that the numbers presented here were gross overestimations.'[17]

In 1986, five years after the first CDC Note on AIDS cases, WHO's Executive Board requested its Director-General to seek funding to develop activities on AIDS. By this time, it was hard to deny that AIDS was an international threat to global health. At the World Health Assembly in May, the Ugandan Minister of Health declared that his country had AIDS, and asked WHO for help; other African countries followed suit[18].

Wealthy donor countries inevitably chose WHO, the UN agency designated to combat globally endemic threats and facilitate the sharing of medical knowledge among Member States, as their 'middleman' in providing assistance. Donor nations also chose the route of multilateral rather than bilateral assistance because they did not yet have specific international programmes of their own.

As Mahler explained at an informal meeting on AIDS during the World Health Assembly in 1987: 'A number of major bilateral donors have stated clearly that their bilateral efforts to combat AIDS have been constrained by political sensitivities and inadequate knowledge, expertise, experience and financial and human resources … That is why they have decided to complement WHO's Programme and centrally-funded activities'[19].

So the Control Programme on AIDS was set up within WHO in 1986, and Mann, by then one of the world's leading experts on the epidemic, was appointed its Director from his post as Director of Projet Sida in Zaire. Mann had warned that 'one to several million Africans may already be infected'[20].

The first few months of the new Programme saw major efforts to raise money from donors (like most of WHO's new programmes, the Control Programme on AIDS did not receive money from WHO's core budget) and to increase public awareness about the disease and its impact. Mann was a persuasive advocate and he succeeded in convincing a sceptical Mahler of the scale of the challenge. In August 1986, Mahler announced: 'We stand nakedly in front of a pandemic as mortal as any pandemic there has ever been. In the same spirit that WHO addressed smallpox eradication, WHO will dedicate its energy, commitment and creativity to the even more urgent, difficult and complex task of global

In August 1986, Mahler announced: 'We stand nakedly in front of a pandemic as mortal as any pandemic there has ever been'.

[17] Behrman G (2004). *The Invisible People*. New York, Free Press.
[18] Berridge (1996).
[19] WHO GPA (1992). *Report of the External Review of the World Health Organization Global Programme on AIDS*. Geneva, WHO GPA, January.
[20] Iliffe (2007).

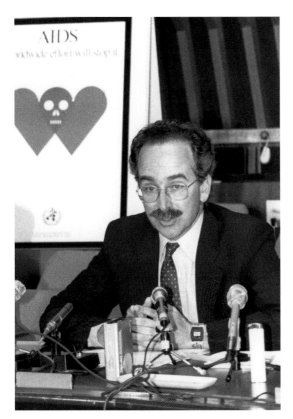

Jonathan Mann, the first Director of WHO's Global Programme on AIDS
WHO/T.Farkas

AIDS prevention'. In December that year, he announced at a press conference in New York that AIDS presented 'an unprecedented challenge to public health'.

The Control Programme on AIDS was renamed the Special Programme on AIDS in February 1987. In January 1988, it became the Global Programme on AIDS (GPA), in recognition of the fact that this was neither a temporary nor a short-term emergency. In 1987, the UN General Assembly had designated WHO as the 'lead agency' in the global response to AIDS; GPA was to provide leadership and coordinate the joint efforts of the UN agencies.

In the same year, Mann had published the Global AIDS Strategy; it was based on three objectives – to prevent HIV infection, reduce the personal and social impact of HIV infection and mobilize and unify national and international efforts against AIDS.

Under Mann's directorship, GPA never addressed AIDS solely as a medical problem. When, in late 1987, the Director-General of WHO addressed the UN General Assembly on the issue of AIDS, the first time a disease had been discussed in that forum, he described the impact of AIDS as 'social, economic, demographic, cultural and political'. It brought forth a resolution that acknowledged the 'pandemic proportions' of AIDS, demanded a 'coordinated response' by the UN system and confirmed that WHO would 'direct and coordinate the urgent global battle'.

From his experience of working in Zaire, Mann strongly believed in the need to work with partners, such as nongovernmental organizations and networks of people living with HIV, nationally and internationally. He supported their work, helping to establish the International Council of AIDS Service Organizations (ICASO) and GNP+.

Nina Ferencic, a social scientist with a background in communication research, monitoring and evaluation, joined GPA as a consultant. She recalled the challenge posed by countries' denial of the epidemic, and the need to encourage them to talk about sexuality openly. "This was a time when we had to get countries to realise that this is a local epidemic, that it is a national issue, and that it didn't matter whether it came from a neighbouring country, and that stigmatising specific groups of people will not improve the response".

A human rights perspective on AIDS was key to GPA's work. 'If we do not protect the human rights of those who are infected, we will endanger the success of our efforts, national and international, to control AIDS', Mann stressed to the meeting of Participating Parties in April 1988[21]. Although GPA had played a major role in dispelling some of the myths around the casual transmission of HIV, many countries had passed repressive and discriminatory legislation on AIDS. The President of the German Federal Court of Justice announced that it might become necessary to tattoo or quarantine seropositive people but this was never enacted. In Germany, all applicants for extended residency permits in Bavaria were required to undergo HIV tests. In China and India, HIV testing was mandatory for all foreigners entering for over one year and all returning citizens. The US Senate voted unanimously to mandate HIV tests for all individuals applying for legal immigration. Many countries in South and South-East Asia copied these examples[22].

Some 81 countries developed anti-AIDS immigration laws[23]. Mann and his colleagues at GPA saw the urgency of advocating a different approach, not only because these laws contravened human rights conventions but also because they were ineffective in halting the progress of HIV. GPA used the existing body of human rights law 'to pressure and cajole their member states to adopt practices that ensure public health'[24].

Piot believes that Mann's contribution, especially on taking a human rights perspective on the epidemic, cannot be overstated[25]. Without Mann as leader of GPA, he said, a much more repressive approach might have been taken, perhaps using quarantine, an idea that had many supporters, especially in the early years of the epidemic.

'GPA … took on the role of global AIDS advocate … [it] spoke with clear, consistent scientific advice in order to dispel myths and encourage socially just responses'[26].

GPA was successful in attracting funding; between 1987 and 1990 donors' commitment increased from just over US$ 30 million to US$ 90 million, at a time when many donor states were questioning the appropriateness of multilateral or bilateral funding. Interestingly, given the debates to come in future years over harmonization, the UK decided to channel funds through GPA because it was felt countries would not be able to cope with 'invasions of donors'[27].

The bulk of GPA's funding was spent on country activities. A major priority was working with countries to assist in the creation of national AIDS programmes; GPA took a proactive role in aiming to ensure country responses were adequate as well as dealing with many urgent requests for guidance. GPA staff and a large number of consultants

"If we do not protect the human rights of those who are infected, we will endanger the success of our efforts, national and international, to control AIDS".

---

[21] WHO GPA (1992).
[22] Soni (1998).
[23] Ibid.
[24] Ibid.
[25] Behrman (2004).
[26] Soni (1998).
[27] Interview with UK civil servant, 1988, in Berridge (1996).

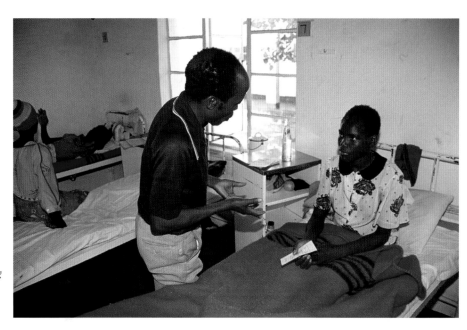

A Zimbabwean woman being told she is HIV positive. UNAIDS/Michel Szulc-Kryzanowski

were sent out to work with countries. By 1988, GPA was providing direct financial support to more than 130 states.

However, some of GPA's donors, especially the USA, were becoming more critical of its operations and spending. This switch in attitude also sprang from a change in the culture of development; the end of the Cold War had coincided with an economic recession in the industrialized West. Both these factors led to an overall reduction in overseas development assistance. The late 1980s also saw the beginning of a movement critical of the UN, and calls for its reform.

The difficulties with donors were exacerbated when Hiroshi Nakajima replaced Mahler as WHO's Director-General in 1988. Nakajima insisted on strict observance of protocol in relation to Member States and WHO's powerful regional offices. He believed that the development and distribution of effective drugs was the key to encouraging international public health[28]. His own reserved personal style contrasted sharply with Mann's ability to grab the headlines. Nakajima tried to limit Mann's personal power and scope, and to scale back GPA, which, by that time, had become the largest and wealthiest WHO programme in history. A WHO official, quoted in a *New York Times* article[29], said that Nakajima felt that too much attention was being paid to AIDS, compared with other diseases. Yet, by 1990, WHO stated that up to five million people were living with HIV[30].

In March 1990, Mann resigned. Michael Merson, previously WHO's Head of the Control of Diarrhoeal Diseases, was appointed acting Head of GPA, then confirmed as its Director

---

[28] Interview with Hiroshi Nakajima in *Health Horizons*, 1988.
[29] Hilt P J (1990). 'Leader in UN's battle on AIDS resigns in dispute over strategy'. *New York Times*, 17 March.
[30] WHO GPA (1990). *Progress Report* 6. Geneva, WHO GPA, May.

in May 1990. He was an experienced UN bureaucrat and during his five years' tenure he worked hard to increase global funding for AIDS and to improve the management of GPA. However, following Mann's departure, there was considerable demoralization among the staff and growing concern among the major donors that GPA was not the most effective instrument or mechanism to combat the epidemic.

In 1991, GPA's income from donors declined for the first time, as did total bilateral and multilateral contributions for AIDS prevention and care in the developing world[31].

During the later years of GPA, donors and some staff were concerned that WHO/GPA was taking too medical an approach to the AIDS epidemic. Merson disagreed: "We appreciated the importance of involving multiple sectors in the national response. There were people who wanted their agencies to be more prominent in the pandemic and to have more money, and one way to do that was to accuse WHO of being more medicalised". GPA staff tried hard to take a multisectoral stance but, as part of WHO, they inevitably had to work with ministries of health that were wary that multisectoralism would take power and money away from them. The concept of multisectoralism was accepted by countries but rarely put into operation; for example, other ministries such as education, interior and justice, defence or finance, were hardly ever involved in AIDS activities and interventions[32]. Two obvious exceptions were Thailand and Uganda; in the early 1990s both had strong multisectoral responses led by the heads of government in Thailand and of state in Uganda, and strongly supported by GPA.

Another major criticism of GPA was that it took the 'one-size-fits-all' blueprint to countries when developing national AIDS plans. Such a standardized approach did not meet the need for culturally sensitive plans and programmes. As development experts Tony Barnett and Alan Whiteside have written, GPA was 'medically and epidemiologically driven and adopted a short-term and conceptually limited fire-fighting perspective based on experience of other more explosive and shorter-wave infectious disease outbreaks'[33]. 'The WHO adopted a series of "Short- and Medium-Term programmes" in a laudable effort to contain the spread of the epidemic. These packages were all more or less the same as they were manufactured and exported from Geneva to the countries of Africa, Asia and Latin America'[34]. It has also been said that many of the national plans were copies of each other because GPA staff were overwhelmed and 'couldn't cope with the money coming through the system'[35].

Merson explained that beginning in 1992, GPA did start to work with a number of countries in preparing their second medium-term plans, which were more country specific.

Another major criticism of GPA was that it took the 'one-size-fits-all' blueprint to countries when developing national AIDS plans. Such a standardized approach did not meet the need for culturally sensitive plans and programmes.

---

[31] Jönsson C (1996). 'From "lead agency" to "integrated programming": the global response to AIDS in the Third World', in Helge Ole Bergeson and Georg Parmann (eds), *Green Globe Yearbook 1996*. Oxford, Oxford University Press.

[32] WHO GPA (1992).

[33] Barnett A, Whiteside A (2002). *AIDS in the Twenty-First Century: Disease and Globalization*. New York, Palgrave Macmillan.

[34] Ibid.

[35] Interview with former WHO staff member, quoted in Berridge (1996).

GPA's fate was sealed in 1989 when it was decided to instigate an external review of its work, initiated partly (as explained by David Nabarro, who became Chief of Health at the UK Department for International Development [DFID] in 1990) because the donors were concerned about the infighting between WHO and other agencies, especially the United Nations Development Programme (UNDP), United Nations Children's Fund (UNICEF) and the World Bank. This was mirrored at country level where ministries of health were fighting to maintain leadership on AIDS and other ministries were opposing them.

In her foreword to the review, the Management Committee's chair, Bernadette Olowo-Freers, wrote: 'We came to the conclusion that although other diseases, both past and present, share common features with AIDS, no other disease presents the same threat to public health and challenge to science. Its unique status derives from the combination of a number of characteristics:

- the fact that at least 75% of HIV transmission is through sexual intercourse, and that sexual behaviour is difficult to change and even to talk about; moral and religious judgements have restricted a range of interventions, from public information and education in schools to condom promotion

- the fact that although not all those infected with HIV have developed AIDS, the disease is invariably fatal

- the fact that AIDS primarily affects young adults in their reproductive and economically productive years, with serious consequences for families and communities

- the fact that, although no country is safe from AIDS, rates of infection are increasing faster in the low-income countries, undermining the developmental and health gains of the past two decades – especially those in child health and life expectancy'.

The final report, published in January 1992, highlighted GPA's farsightedness and vision; it had been instrumental in defining AIDS as a global problem requiring international solidarity. According to the authors of the report, GPA provided effective advocacy and information exchange at global and national levels.

'Unusually for a relatively cautious organization, WHO made a huge effort to raise public awareness about the epidemic'[36]. The Programme played a critical role in combating discrimination and promoting human rights, and in ensuring that AIDS was perceived as a multidimensional and multisectoral issue. Finally, the report noted GPA's rapid operational response. The spread of the epidemic 'was paralleled by the growth of GPA – a growth unprecedented for any programme in WHO's history'[37].

[36] Ibid.
[37] Ibid.

But the report also criticized the 'inefficiency of coordination between different UN agencies', noting that 'UN agencies have not systematically charted information or coordinated the development of their AIDS policies and programmes' and, at country level, 'duplication of effort and territorial rivalries threaten to weaken the global response to AIDS'. Some UN agencies had developed unilateral programmes and activities that duplicated those of GPA and other agencies.

Various possible structures for improving collaboration were discussed in the report but, in true UN fashion, it recommended that the Management Committee of the Global Programme set up a Working Group to consider the structuring of UN collaboration. Thus began the tortuous process that would result in the establishment of UNAIDS.

In April 1992, the GPA's Management Committee's Working Group submitted its report, as requested. It asserted the 'necessity to establish a much broader participation in national action than is currently the case'[38] and urged that the coordination of international HIV/AIDS programming be improved. It added: 'One of the most important lessons ... has been that no single agency is capable of responding to the totality of the problems posed by AIDS; and, as never before, a cooperative effort, which is broadly based but guided by a shared sense of purpose, is essential'.

GPA suggested a yearly forum open to all stakeholders to coordinate efforts, but the donor agencies were not satisfied with this proposal. Furthermore, as Nils Kastberg, then a Swedish diplomat, explained, he and his other Nordic counterparts believed that the Member States should assume responsibility for improving coordination, and "for not having exercised proper governance". He led his country's delegation to the GPA's Management Committee at the end of 1992. "We were looking at a broader set of stakeholders, perhaps, for the first time, broader than the UN – people living with HIV, NGOs, advocacy groups."

Kastberg proposed an alternative to the forum: a Task Force representing all the key stakeholders, which was approved. There were 12 members – three from donor countries (the Netherlands, Sweden and the USA), three from low-income countries (Bulgaria, India and Sudan), three from UN agencies (the World Bank, WHO and UNDP) and three from civil society organizations (the Netherlands-based AIDS Coordination Group, GNP+, with headquarters in the UK, and ENDA Tiers Monde from Senegal). The networks of people living with HIV pushed hard for a place, and their representatives mobilized the networks for their support over the next few months.

'One of the most important lessons ... has been that no single agency is capable of responding to the totality of the problems posed by AIDS; and, as never before, a co-operative effort, which is broadly based but guided by a shared sense of purpose, is essential'.

---

[38] GPA Management Committee (1992). *Report of the Ad Hoc Working Group of the GPA Management Committee*, GPA/GMC(8)/92.5. Geneva, WHO, 24 April.

The Task Force's main priority was to design a new body for coordinating the work of the UN on AIDS. Its terms of reference included: encouraging the exchange of information; providing a focal point at global level for addressing coordination issues and concerns; actively promoting coordinated implementation of policies and programmes; identifying coordination issues among external support agencies of urgent concern at various levels; and organizing special meetings on key issues.

Kastberg always firmly believed in the need for a joint, cosponsored programme: "I had to insist on this throughout the process or otherwise the other agencies would have washed their hands of it, saying that it is WHO's responsibility. It was clear that what we needed would be something that would be viewed as something that had the ownership of a broad set of UN agencies".

In March 1993, Nabarro called a meeting in London of donors involved with work on AIDS and Kastberg presented the Task Force's thinking on a new joint and cosponsored programme. He advocated a relatively strong Secretariat joined to the different Cosponsors and, recalls Hans Moerkerk (a diplomat from the Netherlands Ministry of Foreign Affairs and at that time Chair of the GPA Management Committee and a member of the Committee's Task Force on HIV/AIDS Coordination), "we agreed more or less".

Two months after this meeting, in May, the Canadians surprised everyone by tabling a formal proposal for a joint and cosponsored programme on HIV at the World Health Assembly – much along the lines of the current structure of UNAIDS. Some fine diplomacy was needed with WHO, who were apparently 'up in arms'[39] at the Canadian proposal. Thus it was reformulated as a request to the WHO Director-General to work out a proposal for a joint and cosponsored programme, in close consultation with UNICEF, UNDP, the United Nations Population Fund (UNFPA), the United Nations Educational, Scientific and Cultural Organization (UNESCO) and the World Bank. These agencies were selected because they were members of the GPA Management Committee at the time. There is a view that WHO probably thought they would be able to retain management – and thus control – of the new Programme, as had happened with other programmes cosponsored by multiple UN system agencies such as the Special Programme for Research and Training in Tropical Diseases.

Kastberg admits that the Canadian proposal was made a little earlier than he would have wished, but it was in line with the Task Force's own recommendations and it was a "nice way" of saying firmly that GPA would have to close.

During 1993, the Task Force met several times to discuss the form of the new Programme. At the same time, WHO and the other five agencies were working on their proposal. As

[39] Jönsson (1996).

the UN agencies could not reach agreement on a single approach, three options were proposed, involving different balances between the Secretariat and the Cosponsors. Debate over different approaches to the new Programme was heated, with UNICEF supporting a small Secretariat for exchange of information, UNDP supporting a middle option and donors generally supporting the option of a strong Secretariat.

"We faced ... threats from all the heads of agencies", recalls Moerkerk. Kastberg agrees that "it was not easy. It was also a question of getting Member States engaged. We made clear that what we wanted at the global level was one voice around where is the pandemic, what is happening, what are the main avenues for treatment, what are the numbers we're talking about. It was clear that the Secretariat should have a normative strength".

Eventually, in October 1993, the UN Secretary-General convened a meeting of the executive heads of the six agencies and expressed his support for option (A), the option preferred by the Task Force and the most far reaching in terms of reform, giving the Programme a high level of coordinating control over the Cosponsors. It proposed a unified Secretariat, headed by a director and governed by a Programme Coordinating Board (PCB) consisting of representatives from donor governments, recipient governments, nongovernmental organizations and the Cosponsors.

"It was clear that what we needed would be something that would be viewed as something that had the ownership of a broad set of UN agencies".

In general, the donors were satisfied with the decision, although Moerkerk explained that "we in the Task Force wanted the new programme to be a funding agency, like the Global Fund is now, but UNICEF, UNDP and the World Bank were too powerful and would not allow it to be more than a coordinating and advocacy organization".

So when WHO published the requested study on the new Programme in December 1993, it stated that 'a consensus was reached among the secretariats of five of the organizations in favour of option A'. The World Bank required more information at this point. Despite some scepticism, the Executive Board of WHO endorsed the plan for the new Programme in January 1994 and requested endorsement from the Economic and Social Council (ECOSOC)[40] as well. The final decision would be made during 1994. Significantly, GPA did not renew the contracts of any staff beyond December 1995.

Given the reluctance of the Cosponsors, especially WHO, to agree to such a programme, the period of time between the formation of the initial idea and agreement on the structure was fairly brief. The view of several involved at the time was that the cospon-

---

[40] ECOSOC serves as the central forum for discussing international economic and social issues, and for formulating policy recommendations addressed to Member States and the UN system. It is responsible for promoting higher standards of living, full employment and economic and social progress. ECOSOC was established under the UN Charter as the principal organ to coordinate economic, social and related work of the 14 UN specialized agencies, 10 functional commissions and five regional commissions. It also receives reports from 11 UN funds and programmes.

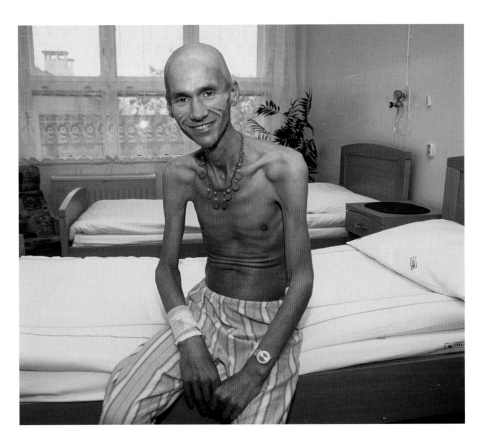

With growing rates of HIV in countries around the world, specialist clinics like this one in the Czech Republic began to be set up. UNAIDS/Liba Taylor

soring agencies had little choice: 'The donors offered the agencies the following choice: "either we will pull out funding altogether and we fund bilaterally, or, if you want us to continue to fund multilaterally, you will get together and [work through] a cosponsored agency"' [41].

Susan Holck had joined GPA when Merson took over as its Director and is now Director, General Management, WHO: "the push for [UNAIDS] certainly did not come from the UN agencies. The push came from the donors, who were fed up with having to individually respond to requests for funding from each of these different agencies, fed up with the lack of coordination, and fed up with WHO's inability to really be operational at country level".

Moerkerk was Chair of the GPA Management Committee from mid-1994 until its demise and a member of the Task Force on HIV/AIDS Coordination. In his opinion, "the lack of collaboration between UN agencies was indeed a major problem … in the UN there is

---

[41] Soni (1998).

not a strong tradition of collaboration. ... [Another problem] was the fact that GPA was never financed through WHO's regular core budget. It could have continued as a WHO programme otherwise. GPA did a wonderful job, let's not forget that".

There is also a view that donors wanted to cut back on, and have more control over, their funding on AIDS to abandon the large Programme they had helped to build – that is, GPA. Certainly some hoped that the new Programme might pave the way for UN reform – a cheaper, more flexible body, more rooted at country level and more accountable to donors.

Interagency rivalries and the behaviour of some WHO staff undoubtedly provided ammunition to those supporting the demise of GPA. Rob Moodie, who had been a consultant to GPA (and the first Director of Country Support at UNAIDS) recalled that after Mann left, WHO's approach was, "let's keep AIDS in the health sector" and "let's ignore the other UN agencies". Former UNICEF staff such as Deputy Executive Director Richard Jolly said that in the 1980s WHO resented UNICEF's work on AIDS education and social mobilization; "they were saying, 'Hands off' our territory". Yet in September 1990, when there was a World Summit on Children to set goals for children's health by the year 2000, Merson really pushed for a goal on children and AIDS, and UNICEF Executive Director Jim Grant categorically refused to include any mention of AIDS in the targets.

Nabarro noted that interagency rivalries and disagreements reflected "a fairly major tension on the ground" that he had experienced when working in Uganda in the 1980s. "It was very interesting", said Nabarro, "to see then, in the mid- to late-80s, and to recall now 20 years later, how profound was the ideological split. Some agencies said, 'we must deal with HIV/AIDS as a communicable disease. The control of everything, including how to communicate about HIV to societies and how to handle the resources, should be with people who have qualifications in public health and epidemiology, and the ministry of health'. Others said, 'HIV and AIDS are societal issues; responses have to take account of cultural context, sexual practice, reality and denial, the status of women and education of girls'. Even then, in the mid- to late-80s, we saw the elements of discord about the handling of HIV that has lasted for 10 to 15 years".

Jolly is very clear about UNICEF's attitude towards the new Programme. "The UNICEF position was positive towards collaboration ... [but] negative or at the very least extremely cautious [about] coordination ... but we did recognize the need to work together."

Discord between the UN agencies – and between some of the donors – would certainly complicate the establishment of UNAIDS during 1994 and 1995, and its operating capacity for several years thereafter. Yet the AIDS pandemic was spreading and the numbers of cases rising. UNAIDS/WHO would later estimate that in 1993 there were about three million new HIV infections and more than 14 million people living with HIV – the vast majority, more than 10 million, in sub-Saharan Africa – followed by nearly 980 000 in South and South-East Asia[42].

Kastberg agrees that all the players involved in the demise of GPA and the birth of UNAIDS could be accused of ignoring the spread of the pandemic. "I would say you can never hit the bells sufficiently strongly around HIV and AIDS issues. But I think we have to recognize that most of the development community and the health community, even, felt at the time: 'Why are we putting so much emphasis on AIDS at a time when many more kids are dying of malaria, of diarrhoea, of all sorts of things, and not AIDS?' So lip-service was [paid] to HIV and AIDS issues but [there was] not a true engagement". True engagement by these communities was a major target for UNAIDS over many years.

---

[42] UNAIDS/WHO *2007 AIDS epidemic update*, November 2007.

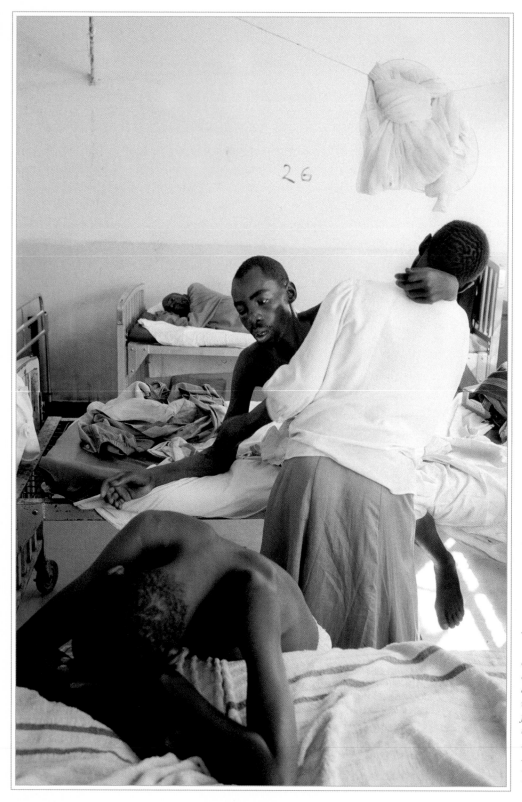

The fast-growing epidemic was a major global challenge. People with HIV were filling wards like this one in Homa Bay hospital, Kenya.
Getty/
Tom Stoddart

Chapter 2:

The development and difficult birth of UNAIDS, 1994–1995

UNAIDS/World Health Organization (WHO) estimate that in 1993 there were more than 13 million people living with HIV worldwide and that over half a million people had died from AIDS that year[1]. However, at this time, there was no single accepted source of reference for data on the epidemic. Global expenditure on AIDS was US$ 224 million in 1993, and US$ 292 million in 1996[2].

'Only a special United Nations system programme is capable of orchestrating a global response to a fast-growing epidemic of a feared and stigmatized disease whose roots and ramifications extend into virtually all aspects of society …'.

The importance of the new United Nations Programme was emphasized in a report from the Committee of Cosponsoring Organizations (CCO) to the United Nations Economic and Social Council (ECOSOC)[3] outlining features of the new Programme about the AIDS epidemic:

'… Because of its urgency and magnitude, because of its complex socioeconomic and cultural roots, because of the denial and complacency still surrounding HIV and the hidden or taboo behaviours through which it spreads, because of the discrimination and human rights violations faced by the people affected … in short, only a special United Nations system programme is capable of orchestrating a global response to a fast-growing epidemic of a feared and stigmatized disease whose roots and ramifications extend into virtually all aspects of society …'.

While the document revealed a deep understanding of the challenge AIDS represented to the world, the unity needed to create the Programme it envisaged was particularly difficult to achieve. Over a period of two years, from January 1994 to December 1995, the form and function of UNAIDS gradually emerged, even as agencies and donors disagreed over its size and objectives, and concerned observers and staff wondered whether it was 'simply an exercise in rearranging the organizational furniture'[4].

In the same article, British activist Robin Gorna commented: 'in theory it sounds wonderful but a lot of us are cynical because we don't believe they can pull it off'.

Nils Kastberg, the Swedish diplomat who chaired the Task Force that was midwife to the new 'child', agreed it was not easy to 'pull off' the establishment of this new organization.

---

[1] UNAIDS/WHO *2007 AIDS epidemic update*, November 2007.
[2] Mann J, Tarantola D, Netter T (eds) (1992). *AIDS in the World.* Cambridge, MA, Harvard University Press; Mann J, Tarantola D (eds) (1996). *AIDS in the World II.* Cary, NC, Oxford University Press.
[3] UN Economic and Social Council (1995). Paper E/1995/71,19 May, paragraphs 20–21.
[4] Balter M (1994). 'UN readies new global AIDS plan'. *Science*, 266, 25 November.

One cannot overestimate the importance of the fact that some of the six UN cosponsoring agencies did not want a new body and certainly not one that would coordinate or, as they might see it, control their activities. As Kastberg explained, the UN's Member States also had to be engaged in developing an understanding that "in terms of AIDS, UNAIDS had to draw on the best of its Cosponsors to represent a common position that established to the world, 'This is where we stand on HIV/AIDS'".

Kastberg was concerned about widening the involvement among agencies and donors beyond those people immediately engaged in the task of developing UNAIDS. At that time, AIDS was, he explained, very much "a specialization of the few, it was using a jargon very few knew". This was an issue that "intimidated" many of the senior staff within governments, UN agencies and nongovernmental organizations.

During the first three months of 1994, an interagency working group met several times and, with the exception of the World Bank, developed a consensus on the structure and function of the new Programme. In the lead-up to the meeting of ECOSOC in July that would endorse UNAIDS, disagreements between agencies over the size and structure of the new programme continued from the previous year, 'a number of agencies originally argued for the lightest of mechanisms, with the emphasis strictly on coordination rather than implementation'[5]. WHO continued to maintain that the new Programme would be 'administered and located in WHO'[6].

According to Jim Sherry, then Chief of the Health Promotion Unit at the United Nations Children's Fund (UNICEF) (who often stood in for its Director, Jim Grant, at the meetings about the new Programme), UNICEF was prepared to accept a cosponsored programme but not if WHO insisted on being 'primus inter pares' or 'first among equals' – that is, explained Sherry, it was "… they were really going to be driving the show".

The donors were equally in dispute over the form of the new Programme. The UK, explained David Nabarro, then Chief of Health at the Department for International Development (DFID), "wanted a programme that focused on the need for 'clear and relevant outcomes and high-level coordination to ensure that the international system focused on these outcomes, advocacy for the outcomes and monitoring of their achievement, with a small strategic Secretariat'. The UK preferred to see improvements in the operation of existing institutions rather than the establishment of a new body with executive authority at country level. But other governments wanted an agency with strong field presence. There was – as is not unusual – a battle about this".

Paul De Lay, who was a senior technical adviser for the United States Agency for International Development (USAID) in 1994, recalled: "We felt very strongly at USAID that to rip out the budgets and the implementation side was a mistake, while other major donors felt very

[5] Leather S (2001). *Historical Background to the Establishment of the Joint United Nations Programme on HIV/AIDS* (unpublished).
[6] WHO (1994). Press Release, 21 January. Geneva,WHO.

strongly that UNAIDS by not being an implementing agency at country level would do a better job coordinating the other UN agencies and leveraging increased commitment".

Hans Moerkerk, from the Netherlands Ministry of Foreign Affairs, was disappointed "… that the final outcome was not a very strong mandate for UNAIDS. … I was in favour of a funding agency, so that they had power. Money is power … collaborating and coordinating is not enough". From its inception, the fact that UNAIDS was not a funding agency would indeed create problems with countries.

Economic and Social Council endorsement of the Joint Programme

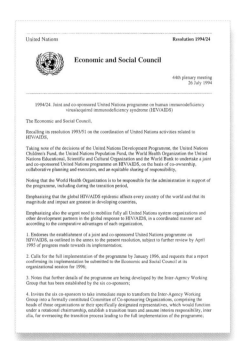

On 26 July 1994, ECOSOC formally endorsed the establishment of the new Joint Programme created by Resolution 1994/24.

On 26 July 1994, ECOSOC formally endorsed the establishment of the new Joint Programme created by Resolution 1994/24. Six programme objectives were listed:

- to provide global leadership in response to the epidemic

- to achieve and promote global consensus on policy and programme approaches

- to strengthen the capacity to monitor trends and ensure that appropriate and effective policies and strategies are implemented at country level

- to strengthen the capacity of national governments to develop comprehensive national strategies and implement effective HIV/AIDS activities

- to promote broad-based political and social mobilization to prevent and respond to HIV/AIDS

- to advocate greater political commitment at global and country levels including the mobilization and allocation of adequate resources.

The resolution stressed the 'vital' importance of cosponsorship by the six agencies in undertaking the Joint Programme 'on the basis of co-ownership, collaborative planning and execution, and an equitable sharing of responsibility'. Given the earlier interagency wrangling and the UN's history of poor collaboration among its agencies, there might reasonably have been some doubt about the chance of the resolution being implemented:

'The Cosponsors will share responsibility for the development of the programme, contribute equally to its strategic direction and receive from it policy and technical guidance relating to the implementation of their HIV/AIDS activities. In this way, the programme will also serve to harmonize the HIV/AIDS activities of the Cosponsors'.

The resolution also stressed that priority should be given to the Programme's activities at country level, and urged the six to initiate country-level programme activities as soon as possible.

From the outset, and for many years to come, there would be a lack of clarity about the role of the Secretariat and about how exactly the Cosponsors would work with the Secretariat. This created confusion among staff, governments, nongovernmental organizations and others who worked with UNAIDS. It also exacerbated the existing tensions between the cosponsoring agencies and the Secretariat.

Kastberg explained his vision: "What we would be creating at the central level [i.e. the Secretariat] would be a big department on HIV that was part of WHO, part of UNICEF, part of the United Nations Development Programme (UNDP), of the United Nations Population Fund (UNFPA), of the United Nations Educational, Scientific and Cultural Organization (UNESCO) and the World Bank. We knew it was a difficult construction but we thought it was better to construct it that way and then make sure the Member States would follow up on the boards of the Cosponsors to make sure they would act as good Cosponsors of UNAIDS. [But] they didn't in general and I think Member States were not sufficiently strong in ensuring consistency of [the Secretariat's] approaches in Geneva and New York".

Several years later, in the spring of 2000, when Kathleen Cravero joined UNAIDS as Deputy Executive Director, the concept of the Secretariat was still not fully understood. She recalled that the idea of UNAIDS as a Secretariat did not always come easily to staff members, whereas she felt the aggravation was worth the final result.

"The idea of a Secretariat, of being a Secretariat, was not doing things ourselves but getting other organizations to do things. The really euphoric moments of seeing this diverse group of agencies around a table come together around a contentious issue – the moments when everybody dropped their institutional mandates and their self-interest in a solid, constructive way behind an important issue – was enormously satisfying. For me, it was worth many months of aggravation, to see that happen. But that's what being a Secretariat is about. Unfortunately, many people in the Secretariat didn't really understand the essence of this role and when they figured it out they didn't really want to be part of a Secretariat".

Back in the summer of 1994, ECOSOC had laid out a timetable to ensure that the new Joint Programme would be operational no later than 1 January 1996. The interagency working group of the six agencies, established in 1993 to develop the plans for the new Programme, was formalized as the CCO, composed of the heads of the six agencies and charged with interim responsibility for overseeing the transition to full implementation of the Joint Programme. This committee was a compromise, explains Kastberg, "not necessarily a good idea … but to engage the heads of the UN agencies, the Cosponsors, and in part to ensure

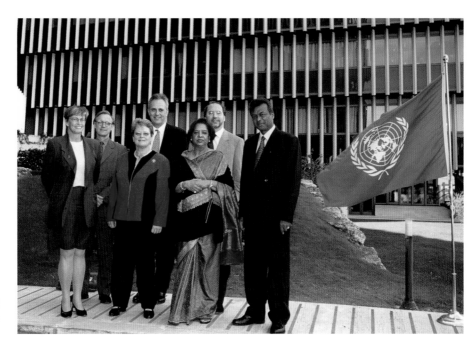

*15th meeting of the
UNAIDS
Committee of Cosponsoring
Organizations, Rome, Italy,
April 2000.
UNAIDS*

that at least the UN wouldn't be fighting in the Programme Coordinating Board and that what went to [this board] had been formally agreed upon".

Following the ECOSOC resolution in July 1994, the CCO was required to start searching for a Director as soon as possible, through an open, wide-ranging search process; the appointment would then be made by the UN Secretary-General, Boutros Boutros-Ghali.

The bureaucratic and legalistic process intensified. The CCO met for the first time in September 1994 and a transition team was established, with staff members from the six agencies, to work on the new Programme's structure, budgets and strategy. Elisabeth Manipoud, who was assigned to the team by UNICEF together with Christian Voumard (also from UNICEF), later reflected: "One should never forget that this joint and cosponsored programme was imposed on a number of very unwilling Cosponsors who resented more coordination of their respective HIV/AIDS activities. A direct illustration of this is that the six original agencies could never agree on the leader for our transition team. So we started in October 1994 without somebody to give direction, dealing with lots of conflicts and a difficult atmosphere".

This lack of leadership made the speedy appointment of the new Director even more necessary. As with any such appointment, most of the well-known people in the AIDS world were canvassed or made their interest in the job known. Elizabeth Reid from UNDP was one of the most ferocious campaigners for a move away from WHO to a wider-based coordinating body (and also an applicant in the early stages). As she told *Science*[7]: 'It will take a very special person ... someone who can mobilize the world and shake it out of its

---

[7] Balter (1994).

32

denial and reluctance to face up to what is happening'. She might have added that it would also need someone who could contend with the squabbles and conspiracies of some of the cosponsoring agencies, as well as the demands, sometimes conflicting, of the donor countries.

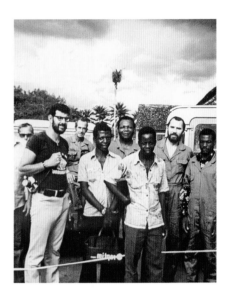

Selection of the Executive Director

The position of Executive Director was not advertised but nominations were requested from Member States and civil society. The Task Force and its Chair, Kastberg, were criticized for this method because it was assumed there would be thousands of names. In fact, there were only 14 nominations. A complicated process followed, overseen by Kastberg and other Task Force members, to ascertain the support behind each proposed candidate and to consider their credentials. A shortlist was produced and sent to the missions in Geneva and to civil society organizations and networks involved through the Task Force but, needless to say, the politics surrounding the process were byzantine and Member States could not agree on one name.

Peter Piot (second from right) in Yambuku, Zaire during the Ebola epidemic of 1976. UNAIDS

Eventually, it became clear that the strongest support, including that of Boutros-Ghali and, notably, civil society, was for Peter Piot, a Belgian scientist who had been Director of the Division of Research and Intervention Development at WHO's Global Programme on AIDS (GPA) since 1992. He had previously worked as Professor of Microbiology and Head of the Department of Infection and Immunity at the Institute of Tropical Medicine in Antwerp. He was one of the first group of scientists to work on AIDS in Africa, had founded Projet Sida with Jonathan Mann and had collaborated with various nongovernmental organizations. Piot was an eminent scientist with the right credentials including direct experience in low-income countries – and, as some colleagues added, he had fewer enemies than the other candidates.

Piot was not a typical UN bureaucrat. On joining GPA in 1992, he was surprised to discover that he enjoyed the international management of public health: "… it was a move from studying the problem to trying to do something about it on a larger scale".

There was no time for Piot to settle in to his new post. After a meeting with Boutros-Ghali in December 1994, when he accepted the post, he returned to the CCO meeting where "they had started discussing pretty openly how they could undermine this new programme and what we would and wouldn't be allowed to do".

Stefano Bertozzi, combining the role of acting Head of GPA after Michael Merson's departure as Director and working with Piot on designing the new Programme, recalls

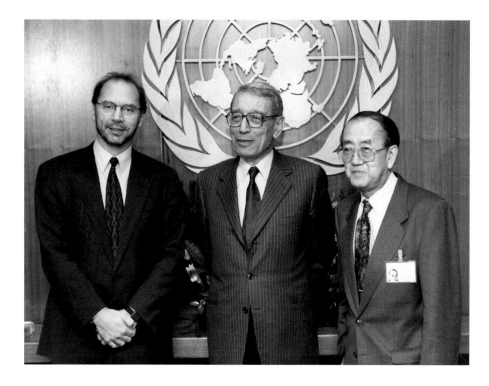

Peter Piot on the day of his appointment as Executive Director of UNAIDS, with United Nations Secretary-General Boutros Boutros-Ghali and Director-General of the World Health Organization Hiroshi Nakajima. New York, 12 December, 1994.
UNAIDS

similar occasions. "Almost from the day the agreement was signed, WHO worked very, very actively to undermine UNAIDS. … I even sat in meetings with [WHO Director-General Hiroshi] Nakajima and the regional directors in which they were talking about UNAIDS' demise so they could resume or reclaim their leadership of HIV/AIDS. Peter should have been receiving support from them at this time but the opposite was true".

1995: establishing governance of the new Joint Programme

The basic principle of how UNAIDS would be governed was strongly contested from the start. In January 1995, the CCO submitted its draft report on the new Joint Programme to ECOSOC and it was discussed at informal consultations on 31 January and again on 10 February. The original 1994 ECOSOC resolution had stated that the Director would report directly to a Programme Coordinating Board (PCB) 'which will serve as the governance structure for the programme. The composition of the Programme Coordinating Board will be determined on the basis of open-ended discussions'. However, the Cosponsors rejected governance and control by Member States. Rather, the agencies wanted to set up a board, selected by themselves, that would make all the decisions about expenditure and hiring people. Piot had to fight against this: "I said, 'our shareholders are the Member States and our accountability can only be to the Member States and not within the [UN] system'. If the CCO had been in control there would have been no accountability, it would have been a matter of [their being] judge and jury".

34

Kastberg recalled that it was easier to achieve coordination on the issue of governance between Member States and civil society than within the UN family. Finally, at the third meeting of the CCO in Vienna, later in February, the Cosponsors agreed to work within the framework proposed by ECOSOC. The PCB, not the CCO, would be the decision-making body.

The composition of the PCB was agreed through ECOSOC among the permanent missions in New York. Piot recalled: "There were people running around with a pocket calculator working out membership according to regions". It was eventually decided that 22 states would be represented on the Board: five each from Africa and Asia, two from Eastern Europe, three from Latin America and the Caribbean, and seven from 'Western Europe and other States'.

Piot's major battle over the PCB was to ensure representation of nongovernmental organizations, but there was strong opposition to this from a few countries. Eventually, it was agreed that five nongovernmental organizations would participate as non-voting members, like the Cosponsors. In early July 1995, ECOSOC adopted a resolution inviting five nongovernmental organizations to take part in the new PCB, three of which were to come from middle- and low-income countries. The selection would be carried out by the nongovernmental organizations themselves. This was an historic decision. UNAIDS was, and still is, the only UN body with nongovernmental organization representatives on its governing body.

It was very clear to Piot that working with Cosponsors would not be easy: "… in essence, no one in the UN system wanted the new programme to happen". He needed allies and friends with whom to discuss strategy and policies. In February 1995, somewhat bruised by the battles over governance, he quietly organized a private 'brainstorming' retreat with some of these friends: "I needed a clandestine place away from the rest of the UN system". A telephone call to Seth Berkley, who was then working for the Rockefeller Foundation and is now President of the International AIDS Vaccine Initiative, brought the offer of the use of their centre at Bellagio, on Lake Como, Italy, at no cost and with funding for the whole weekend meeting. This meeting set a valuable precedent, allowing Piot to retreat from time to time with close allies to discuss strategy and tactics.

The group at the first meeting included Berkley; Jean Baptiste Brunet, responsible for AIDS at the French Ministry of Health at the time; Jim Curran, then Director, Office of HIV/ AIDS at the United States Centers for Disease Control and Prevention; Joseph Decosas, a Canadian scientist; Susan Holck, seconded from WHO's GPA to the Joint Programme; Noerine Kaleeba, founder of The Aids Support Organisation (TASO) in Uganda and a well-known activist; Hans Moerkerk, the Dutch diplomat who was the last Chair of GPA's Management Committee; Rob Moodie, a public health specialist and doctor from Australia who had been a consultant to GPA; Roland Msiska, then Manager of the National AIDS Programme in Zambia; Werasit Sittitrai, a Thai AIDS activist with the Red Cross, and Winston Zulu, a Zambian AIDS activist living with HIV.

UNAIDS was, and still is, the only UN body with nongovernmental organization representatives on its governing body.

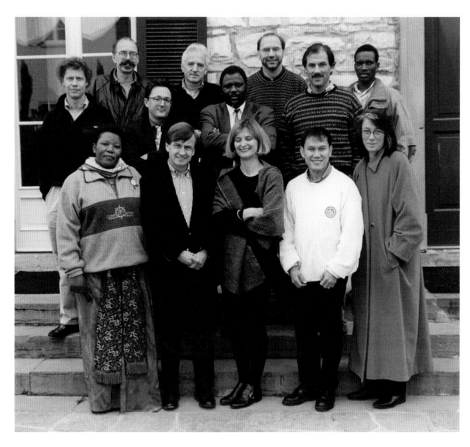

*The group who attended
Peter Piot's first brain-
storming retreat in Bellagio,
Italy, to discuss strategy
and tactics.
UNAIDS*

Kaleeba said it was a unique meeting, one with no formal agenda – "unheard of for the UN"– but with a clear aim, that of strategizing for the new Programme. Kaleeba had decided that she wanted to join this new organization, inspired by Piot's vision of setting up a body that, although within the UN, aimed at balancing the needs and responsibilities of diplomacy with activism. She found this a refreshing change from the bureaucracy she had experienced at other UN meetings.

"I remember one of the statements made at Bellagio which I think has finally been borne out to be true – that we will never be able to prevent AIDS until we restore the health and dignity of people who are being affected. They asked me how do we do that? I said, care for, and support, and involve people with AIDS".

Moodie remembers some of the crucial discussions at Bellagio: "Peter was at that stage struggling with the other UN agencies because he was getting a hell of a lot of fire from WHO, and from UNDP. Even though the whole notion had been developed and born, there was an enormous challenge in actually getting it off the ground and getting the fundamental purpose of coordinating the UN or getting a more integrated response".

In terms of strategy, the consensus of the meeting was that UNAIDS should have a major focus on political advocacy and on working with civil society globally and within countries. The UNAIDS Secretariat planned a series of regional consultations that would bring together all the actors in the AIDS response. As Piot explained, they wanted and needed to 'take the pulse' of the countries they would be working with. It was also an opportunity to market the new Programme and to recruit staff.

It was also at Bellagio, Piot recalls, that he chose the name UNAIDS for the new organization. This was endorsed by the CCO at its meeting in Vienna later in 1995. His 15-year-old daughter Sara designed the first UNAIDS logo.

Strategies and structure

When the initial transition team was disbanded in February 1995, Piot appointed a small preparatory team to work on the strategies and structure of UNAIDS: many came from GPA, others from some of the Cosponsors. Although no team member was guaranteed a job after the end of 1995, it was hard for those from GPA, as so many of their former colleagues were facing unemployment. GPA was not formally disbanded until the end of 1995 but, unusually for the UN, its members were not offered alternative jobs.

Members of the preparatory team have vivid memories of an exciting and exhausting period and of a committed group that spent long hours doing everything from stuffing envelopes to writing budgets. Purnima Mane, originally a social scientist specializing in gender issues in Mumbai, had worked at GPA for a year and joined the UNAIDS' team in 1995 to formulate the strategic plan for the new Programme. She recalled:

"We were a very small team, about ten to twelve. We were really supposed to be Jacks-of-all-trades or Joans-of-all-trades … we did everything. I remember writing job descriptions, sending faxes … there was a spirit of putting together something unique which bound us together; there was no distinction between professional and general staff. It was a very non-hierarchical structure. That's the one good thing people will remember about those days".

Bertozzi recalled a time that was exciting and heady, despite the many problems with the Cosponsors: "We really felt that we were on the cutting edge of UN reform. We felt we had an opportunity of testing new ways of doing business, of being more efficient, being more responsive, of trying to get out of some of the traps that go with any UN bureaucracy".

We really felt that we were on the cutting edge of UN reform. We felt we had an opportunity of testing new ways of doing business, of being more efficient, being more responsive, of trying to get out of some of the traps that go with any UN bureaucracy.

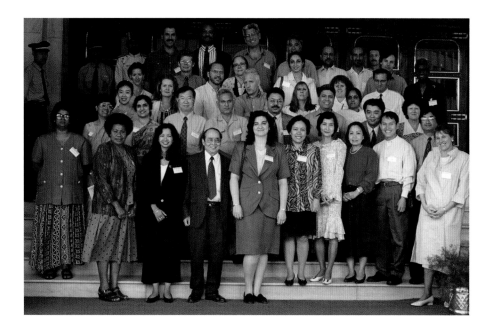

Participants at the UNAIDS regionnal strategic planning meeting in New Delhi, India, 1995.
UNAIDS

Informing countries

During 1995, UNAIDS organized regional strategic planning meetings with different stake-holders around the world – governments, donors, nongovernmental organizations and community-based organizations, networks of people living with HIV, programme imple-menters, policy makers and opinion leaders and members of the academic and research communities. As Mane explained: "We had a basic strategic framework but the interesting thing was Peter asked us to focus a lot on what UNAIDS should not be because the danger was that we would try to be something that we would never be able to fulfil. So, we did those meetings in four months, in five meetings around the world – I attended every single one of them – and put together a strategic plan which was then approved by the Programme Coordinating Board".

Meetings were held in New Delhi, Santiago, Nairobi, Venice and Dakar, and each meeting was organized by the office of a different Cosponsor.

People attending these regional meetings were confused by what they heard about UNAIDS. If UNAIDS was being created because the epidemic was such a major problem, why was it so much smaller than GPA? And what was happening to the funding that GPA used to provide to countries?

Julia Cleves was at the UNAIDS meeting in New Delhi; at the time she was Chief Health and Population Adviser at DFID. "I was predisposed to be positive towards UNAIDS but at the meeting what was said was incomprehensible. Most of the other bilaterals' staff didn't understand either what UNAIDS was or what it intended to be. All the negotiating had taken place at HQs [Headquarters] and the outcomes were not well communicated to country offices. We were also very aware of how badly the UN agencies worked together. It took time for UNAIDS to learn to communicate its own mission".

Clement Chan-Kam joined the preparatory team in mid-1995 from GPA where he had worked for four years after managing the National AIDS Programme in Mauritius. He went on several regional visits: "I remember trying to reassure people, in WHO as well as national programme staff, that far from UNAIDS being a death sentence for WHO's AIDS Programme and far from being a kind of crisis situation for countries in terms of fund flows and technical support, it would actually mean their being able to call upon the collective resources and know-how of six Cosponsors rather than just WHO. Looking back, I feel we must have been very naïve, but we all truly believed in that because that was what UNAIDS was meant to be".

From the beginning, a significant difference between GPA and UNAIDS at country level created difficulties. GPA had funded national AIDS programmes through ministries of health. UNAIDS, however, was intended to coordinate and facilitate funding rather than provide it directly, but such nuancing meant little to those countries that suddenly had no money for AIDS programmes.

In marking out the difference between GPA and UNAIDS, Piot was always concerned with the importance of country 'ownership', that is, whether countries would feel they were making the crucial decisions in planning their response to the epidemic rather than 'outsiders' such as the UN in Geneva. "While working at GPA, I didn't see anywhere the ownership in the developing countries. I had worked enough in Africa to know that if people don't feel 'It's my problem' then they won't really move".

Working with cosponsoring agencies

The UNAIDS preparatory team was housed in a building next to the main WHO headquarters alongside what remained of the GPA staff. As Mane explained, initially there was a lot of anger about UNAIDS and a reluctance to cooperate. "I completely understood – I had lots of colleagues [in GPA] who lost jobs … people felt threatened. At the same time, there were many people who really cared about the response to the disease who … I must admit, went beyond institutional differences and said, 'You know, we've got to make this succeed. This is really too important'".

WHO was responsible for the administrative support of UNAIDS. Bertozzi speculated on whether it might have been better to make a 'clean break' from WHO because: "We spent an enormous amount of our energy fighting with the Nakajima administration to get the kind of support we needed, everything from hiring people, travel policy and suchlike. It was very demoralizing".

Although the relationship with WHO was particularly difficult (for historical and administrative reasons), there was little enthusiasm among the other five agencies for giving UNAIDS the power to coordinate their work. Holck explained: "For way too long the meetings of the cosponsoring organizations were strained and unpleasant. It wasn't all just selfish egotistical stuff. They don't trust each other, they don't trust the other agencies to work collaboratively

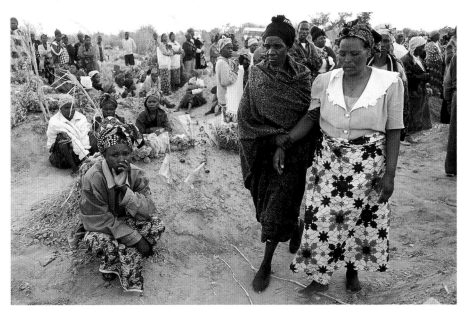

Funerals were becoming a daily occurrence in countries with high rates of HIV infection.
Christian Aid/David Rose

… and the Member States didn't really encourage that either. The Ministers of Health came to the World Health Assembly and would say to WHO, 'don't you dare give up any power or money to UNAIDS' … whereas the Ministers of Education go to UNESCO and say 'don't you dare give up any power'".

Beginning to work together

The World Bank was a very reluctant partner in the UNAIDS project. In memos written in 1995 by their legal adviser, Louis Forget, and by their Human Development Director, Richard Feachem, it was emphasized that the Bank would 'assume no liability' for UNAIDS and wished to have 'as little involvement as possible'[8].

The World Bank was, however, active around AIDS projects in some countries. As Merson explained, in the mid-1990s, the largest amounts of money for AIDS, though not huge, came from the Bank. In 1992, Keith Hansen went to Zimbabwe as a member of the World Bank's health team there. He remembered that the country was rolling out an impressive primary health system, funded by the Bank. A few days after he arrived, he attended a meeting with a university professor who briefed them on the extent of the spread of AIDS in Zimbabwe. "After

---

[8] Quoted in Gellman B (2000). 'Death watch: the global response to AIDS in Africa'. *Washington Post*, 5 July.

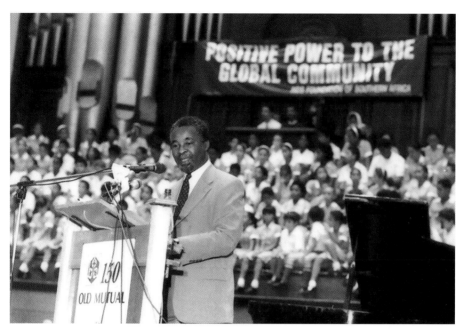

Deputy President of South Africa, Thabo Mbeki, addressing the Seventh International Conference of People living with HIV/AIDS, Cape Town, March 1995. Gideon Mendel/GNP+

20 minutes I realized that everything I had just seen was going to be swept away if this was true … and if it were this powerful in the rest of southern eastern Africa … much of what the Bank was supporting was all in peril". That very morning, he and his colleagues put together a programme of support for HIV and sexually transmitted infections, and he managed that for a couple of years. "But as late as the mid-90s", he said, "the Bank was nowhere near to bringing the full brunt of its resources and influence to bear on the epidemic".

Chan-Kam recalled how determined the preparatory team members were to work with the Cosponsors. "All of us involved in AIDS for several years knew it was all about prevention, about getting through to young people … political leadership. There was a real imperative to get all these different agencies to subscribe in a formal way to the UN effort, to do it jointly". He smiled wryly: "Famous last words".

As the small team worked long hours in Geneva to ensure that UNAIDS would be fully functioning by January 1996, whatever the pressures it might confront, Piot and his colleagues set about building the broad coalition of partners they believed was essential for any effective response. In March 1995, Piot attended his first major meeting as Head of the new Programme, the Seventh International Conference of People living with HIV/AIDS, held that year in Cape Town. It was a great opportunity to meet nongovernmental organizations and discuss their involvement.

Thabo Mbeki, then Deputy President of South Africa, spoke at the Cape Town meeting very powerfully, Piot recalls, thinking he would be a strong ally. South African activist Zackie Achmat also remembers Mbeki's "remarkable" speech. "It was Thabo Mbeki, not Nelson Mandela". The future would tell a different and more complex story.

Throughout 1995, UNAIDS staff met with major nongovernmental organizations working in the AIDS field including the Global Network of People living with HIV/AIDS (GNP+), the International HIV/AIDS Alliance and TASO in Uganda. USAID contributed US$ 500 000 to UNAIDS for the follow-up to the Paris AIDS Summit at which the GIPA principle[9] had been agreed. This funding was mainly used for strengthening and supporting networks of nongovernmental organizations and people living with HIV, such as the International Council of AIDS Service Organizations (ICASO) and the International Community of Women living with HIV/AIDS.

The involvement of people living with HIV was an essential part of the UNAIDS vision, explained Michel Carael, a sociologist who had worked at GPA and joined UNAIDS in its first year. "It was a new way of doing business. Involving people living with HIV was more symbolic than real at GPA. UNAIDS also had a much stronger vision of working across different sectors than GPA where [multisectoralism] was not really taken seriously. Working with civil society was enriching, part of [our] self-development".

The first Programme Coordinating Board meeting

The 'injunction to "just say no" has ... been no more successful in curbing HIV than the earlier epidemics of syphilis, gonorrhoea and heroin use'.

July 1995 witnessed another crucial stage in UNAIDS' development. The PCB met for the first time – in a conference room of the International Labour Organization (ILO), one of WHO's neighbours in Geneva. Piot's report reminded everyone that its business was 'one of the major tragedies of our time ... [the AIDS epidemic is continuing] to grow invisibly at a rate of over 8000 new infections every day ... No country will be able to insulate itself from the shock waves of HIV/AIDS'. Much of the Board's discussions were about the way in which UNAIDS would work, its plans and its objectives, but no member could ever be allowed to forget the epidemic's toll on human life: an estimated 17.9 million people living with HIV in 1995.

Piot's first report as Executive Director spelt out the unique features of the AIDS epidemic. Unlike smallpox, for example, the epidemic is not amenable simply to biomedical control: 'a vaccine and a cure remain elusive', nor is there a simple, non-technical solution. The 'injunction to "just say no" has ... been no more successful in curbing HIV than the earlier epidemics of syphilis, gonorrhoea and heroin use'. However, there had been a number of demonstrably successful HIV prevention programmes, many owing their success to community-based organizations and nongovernmental organizations. They tended to combine several approaches – condom promotion, AIDS information through the media and treatment for sexually transmitted infections – and 'attempted to create a supportive environment in which people are *motivated and enabled* to engage in safe behaviour'.

On the other hand, most prevention programmes were small scale, and in almost every affected country there were the challenges of denial, stigma and the lack of political

---

[9] The principle of the Greater Involvement of People living with or affected by HIV/AIDS was formalized in the declaration signed by 42 countries at the Paris AIDS Summit on 1 December 1994. It was taking the 'Denver principles' (see Chapter 1) a step further and building on them, stressing the importance of involving people living with HIV in policy making and programming around the epidemic.

42

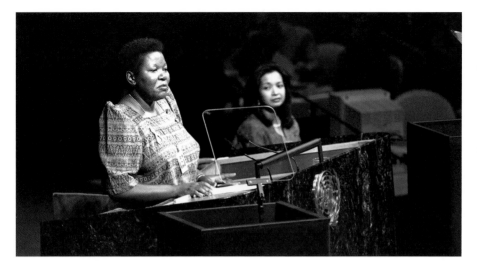

Noerine Kaleeba, founder of The AIDS Support Organisation in Uganda and a member of the original staff of UNAIDS with Marina Mahathir from Malaysia, former nongovernmental organization representative in the UNAIDS Programme Coordinating Board, speaking at the 51st United Nations General Assembly in 1996.
UNAIDS

commitment. Furthermore, there was no easy fix for the socioeconomic and political factors that drove the epidemic in so many countries, such as poverty, inequality of women, conflict and forced migration.

Piot's report spelt out the three mutually reinforcing roles that apply to activities at country, intercountry and global levels. The organization would be a major source of globally relevant policy on AIDS, and would develop, promote and strengthen international best practice and research. It would work on programmes, catalyse and provide technical support to help build and strengthen the capability for an expanded response to AIDS, particularly in middle- and low-income countries.

There were many expectations about what UNAIDS could deliver. Not merely was UNAIDS expected to focus the world's attention on AIDS and to gain political commitment, but it was also meant to ensure an expanded response to AIDS at country level, broad based and multisectoral, incorporating AIDS into all aspects of human development and economic planning. These objectives were based on the assumption that the six cosponsoring agencies would work together at all levels in a harmonious and supportive manner, that UNAIDS would draw on the special strengths and advantages of all six Cosponsors, and that the Cosponsors would integrate work on AIDS into all their relevant programmes. This was not to be the case for at least the first two to three years of the programmes.

Manipoud, External Relations Officer in UNAIDS, explained: "Some order had to be put into the situation. There was so much duplication – UNICEF, UNESCO [and] WHO had a number of similar programmes, creating lots of competition for funding. You're not doing coordination and coherence for the sake of coordination and coherence; you're doing it to benefit and strengthen the national responses which countries are putting together: better support of the UN system to the countries; that was the expectation".

Agreeing the budget

There were major disagreements over the UNAIDS budget at the first PCB meeting. Mane recalled: "They talked about a budget which was one third of what Peter Piot was [asking for], and the Board was up in arms because there were so many different views that they had to … call time-out for people to consult bilaterally because, otherwise, we would never have had consensus. … Peter actually walked up to some of the donors and said, 'Listen, you set this up. If you want it to succeed, you have to fund it right or I'm out'. He didn't have any staff and he was very, very firm. He said, '… this is non-negotiable because you're starting this up … to fail'".

Kastberg supported him, telling the meeting: "Up to now, Sweden has always played a mediating role. I, as of today, cannot play a mediating role because for Sweden it's unacceptable to consider any budget that goes below US\$ 140 million, the first biennium of UNAIDS".

Six agencies signed the Memorandum of Understanding on a Joint and Cosponsored UN Programme on HIV/AIDS.

"So," explained Mane, "they adjourned the Board for an hour so that people could have those conversations and come to some agreement and move forward".

Eventually the PCB compromised and mandated UNAIDS to develop a budget within an indicative range from US\$ 120 to140 million for the biennium 1996-1997 and to proceed with recruitment of staff.

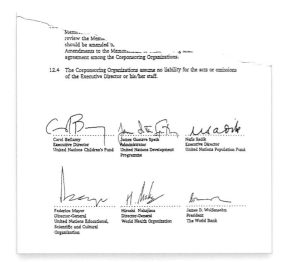

Memorandum of Understanding (1995)

In October 1995, three months before UNAIDS was to open for business and after eight to nine months of discussion and long hours of detailed work, five agencies signed the Memorandum of Understanding on a Joint and Cosponsored UN Programme on HIV/AIDS. The World Bank added its signature in 1996.

By the end of the year, a large number of UNAIDS staff had been recruited from a wide range of backgrounds – academia, journalism, country, activism, research, nongovernmental organizations as well as some from GPA. They brought with them a richness of experience and reflected the broad coalition that UNAIDS planned to work with globally and nationally. Sally Cowal, a former US ambassador, joined as Director of External Relations. She spoke of some "marvellously creative, energetic, intelligent people … [a] really powerhouse team, like nothing else I've seen in the UN. There were also a lot of characters, a lot of people who nobody else would have signed on to the UN system but we did, and I think that was good".

It was decided to launch UNAIDS at the UN in New York on World AIDS Day, 1 December 1995. The event was not a success, despite considerable efforts by UNAIDS staff. Piot was to make a speech in the ECOSOC chamber in the main UN building, with an invited audience of all the delegations and the public in the gallery upstairs. Boutros-Ghali spoke, and a number of celebrities had been invited including Elizabeth Taylor and some opera singers from the Metropolitan Opera House.

Sadly, explained Cowal, it was not the high-profile success hoped for. "The UN never had their act together, they never managed to tell security they were expecting the public so nobody could get in. It always said something to me ... that's how it started, with no visibility on either the organization or the crisis which had caused the organization to come into being".

Anne Winter had joined UNAIDS as Communications Chief a month or so before the launch. "In the beginning, it was quite a struggle to get media attention. It was an unknown organization with an unknown boss. You'd ring journalists and they'd say, 'What?' 'Who?'"

However, that visibility was not the major struggle facing the new organization. UNAIDS was confronting the challenge of perhaps the most serious epidemic known to humankind and it needed all the support that had been committed from within the UN system. But that support was not forthcoming.

"My impression is that UNAIDS was disabled from the start", concluded Merson, "because the donor governments did not insist that all the UN agencies behave responsibly. I sat in the room with Secretary-General Boutros-Ghali and heard every one of them [the heads of agencies] commit themselves fully to the establishment of UNAIDS. But then there are the governing boards of the agencies, the Member States. We can criticize the agencies but where were the governments that had pushed so strongly to have UNAIDS created? Once UNAIDS was established, why didn't they follow on and make of it what it was supposed to be? I'm talking in particular about the rich countries that highly influence the governing boards of each agency. Why didn't they hold the agencies more accountable from the outset? Why did some of them provide fewer resources to UNAIDS than they had to the WHO Global Programme on AIDS?"

The *Five Year Evaluation of UNAIDS* (published in 2002) commented: 'A significant point is that there was no global consensus from which the joint programme emerged. Unlike

UNAIDS was confronting the challenge of perhaps the most serious epidemic known to humankind and it needed all the support that had been committed from within the UN system.

many other global programmes, UNAIDS was not created by a conference or convention. It was driven by a group of OECD bilateral donors, supported by activists seeking a stronger response and designed by ECOSOC. The forces leading to establishment of the joint programme were a mixture of technical and political. They illustrate the range of expectations that built up. Some were dashed at the outset, by the chosen structure. Others have been the focus of the programme's efforts. All have remained to some extent as a challenge to the programme'.

An important part of UNAIDS' history concerns how it dealt with those expectations and challenges over the decade that followed its launch.

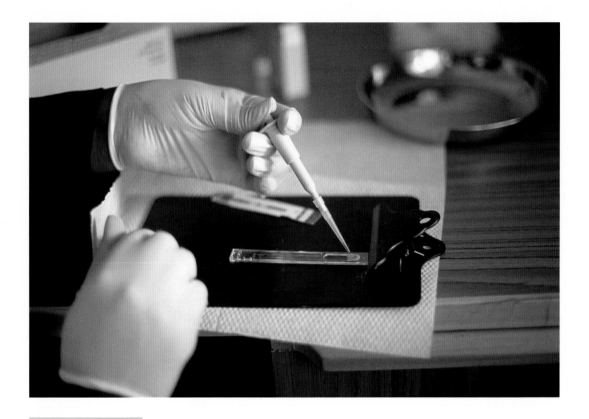

In order to provide antiretroviral
treatment, resources were also needed
to ensure safe testing of blood.
UNAIDS

Chapter 3:
UNAIDS opens for business, 1996–1997

"The biggest challenge was waking up the leaders, it's not just the leaders but their key ministers, then their key bureaucrats".

UNAIDS/World Health Organization (WHO) estimate that in 1995 nearly 17.9 million people were living with HIV globally and nearly 3.6 million had died from AIDS since the beginning of the epidemic[1]. In 1996, the annual resources available for AIDS amounted to US$ 292 million and in 1997, US$ 485 million[2].

On 1 January 1996, after a series of meetings, reports, working groups, whispered conversations and angry confrontations in corridors and telephone calls around the world, UNAIDS became operational. With a staff of 91 in the Geneva-based Secretariat and 10 in various regions – more would be recruited during that year – the fledgling organization would quickly have to learn how to fly. Although, in theory, UNAIDS combined the Secretariat in Geneva and staff in countries plus six United Nations (UN) cosponsoring agencies and could therefore call on a large number of staff, considerable time would be needed before there was any serious consensus or effective collaborative working practices between the Secretariat and the Cosponsors.

Retreat of the UNAIDS Senior Management Team in Talloires, France, September 1996. UNAIDS

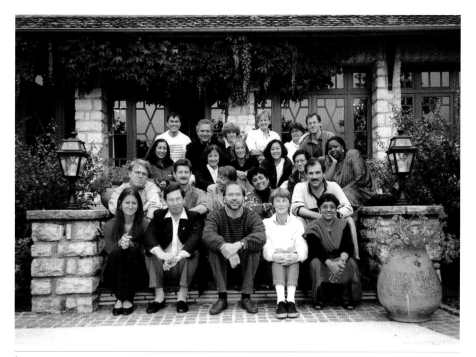

---

[1] UNAIDS/WHO *2007 AIDS epidemic update*, November 2007.
[2] UNAIDS Resource Tracking Consortium, July 2004.

48

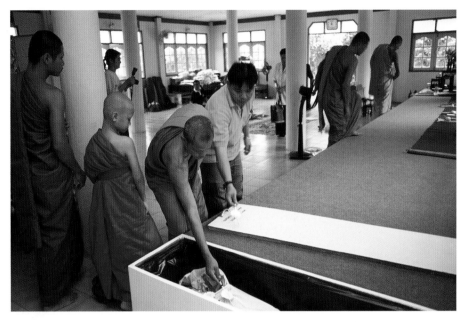

In Thailand as in many countries across the world, religious figures play a key role in the response to AIDS.
UNAIDS/
Shehzad Noorani

As the number of cases of HIV continued to rise, there was a real sense of urgency at UNAIDS. It now had staff, a budget and a strategic plan. The groundwork had been laid in the previous months – including long days in Geneva and meetings in every region of the world. The pace would not slacken.

Political advocacy was high on UNAIDS' list of priorities. By June 1996, UNAIDS staff had met with political, economic and social leaders in more than 50 countries to brief them on UNAIDS' mandate and work. Sally Cowal, Director of External Relations at UNAIDS, was new to the 'AIDS world'. "At first I had doubts [about not having a medical background] but as I came to understand more about the epidemic, it became clear to me that the political motivation around it, the need to overcome denial and complacency, were probably as important as anything we could do".

"The biggest challenge was waking up the leaders," said Rob Moodie, first Director of UNAIDS' Country Support department. "It's not just the leaders but their key ministers, then their key bureaucrats".

It was useful that Peter Piot, UNAIDS Executive Director, and Cowal had quite different sets of contacts and networks. "It was serendipitous at times", she remarked. "Peter had respect in the medical community for his early work. And then he had in his work with the Global Programme, and before, established awfully good connections in a lot of the activists' organizations. I had mostly US political connections through having been an Assistant Secretary of State and an ambassador … so I was able to pull those in. The Secretary of Health and Human Services was Donna Shalala at that time, she was one of my best buddies, we went trekking every summer. That is how we met Madeleine Albright [US Secretary of State] and Richard Holbrooke [UN Ambassador]".

She added that it was, nevertheless, still extremely hard to get anybody's attention. "Governments have difficulties in dealing with these complex issues that go into the making of a crisis, it's all [to do with] public policy about private behaviour". The United States (US) Government was slow to build up a strong response to the epidemic in its own country, let alone internationally, and Cowal recalled the many times she and Piot did the rounds in Washington, DC, and "laid out the facts" – with no result.

Piot undertook several missions with Awa Coll-Seck, Director of the Policy, Strategy and Research department, who joined UNAIDS in mid-1996, after holding positions as Head of the Infectious Diseases department at the University of Dakar, and Coordinator of clinic and counselling for the National AIDS Programme in Senegal. "We had to explain to some Heads of State that … AIDS [was] killing their people, impacting the development of the country … it was really not obvious to everybody that it was a problem".

"We had to explain to some Heads of State that … AIDS [was] killing their people, impacting the development of the country … it was really not obvious to everybody that it was a problem".

Coll-Seck stressed the importance of both sides being prepared for such meetings. A head of state would have been well briefed by his or her technical people, "… and it was sometimes the first time their technicians had access to this level". On such visits, UNAIDS would also present leaders with evidence of change, of good practice, in countries such as Uganda, where prevalence had begun to decline, and Senegal, where prevalence was low. "We would explain … Senegal and Uganda have been very successful because they had [the] very clear commitment of their leaders, and they were not denying this is a real story". She also stresses they were showing leaders that they were not alone in facing this challenge.

Work at country level

By 1996, the epidemic had spread into every region of the world. Sub-Saharan Africa was the most severely affected – almost 15.4 million people there were living with HIV. In Asia, nearly 1.8 million people were living with HIV, and in Latin America and the Caribbean more than one million. The other regions were: Northern America and Western and Central Europe, 1.5 million; North Africa and Middle East, nearly 300 000; Eastern Europe and Central Asia, over 80 000[3].

But as the report of a 1996 symposium around the International AIDS Conference in Vancouver[4] explained: '… the pandemic has become immensely complex. It has become fragmented and is now a mosaic composed of a multitude of epidemics, which can be distinguished on the basis of: predominant modes of transmission; geographic focus; [HIV sub-types]; age, sex, socioeconomic or behavioural characteristics of populations most affected; rapidity of or potential for HIV spread; stage of maturity and, in some communities and countries, declining HIV incidence'.

---

[3] Ibid.
[4] 'The status and trends of the global HIV/AIDS pandemic'. The symposium was jointly organized by the AIDS Control and Prevention Project of Family Health International, the Francois-Xavier Bagnoud Center for Health and Human Rights of the Harvard School of Public Health and UNAIDS, 5–6 July 1996.

Despite the diversity of epidemics, the challenges of the epidemic to individuals, families and societies were very similar. The economic impact on families was often devastating; loss of income because of sickness was aggravated by the cost of drugs and medical care (where available) and ultimately funeral costs.

There was also growing evidence of the impact of the epidemic on countries' economies, as increasing numbers of people of working age fell sick and died. Productivity declined, tax revenues dropped, while pressures on health services increased. In Africa, particularly, the number of children orphaned by AIDS grew. Women's vulnerability to HIV infection was clear in these early years. By mid-1996, UNAIDS estimated that women accounted for over 47% of nearly 21 million adults living with HIV[5]. In Africa, the figures among young women (aged 15–24) were greater; young women with HIV outnumbered their male peers by a ratio of 2:1[6]. Over the following 10 years of UNAIDS' existence, these challenges would increase as the numbers of infected and affected people increased.

Countries desperately needed help. As the external *Five Year Evaluation of UNAIDS*, published in 2002, explained, 'the driving imperative behind the creation of UNAIDS was to reinforce national capacity to respond to the epidemic'.

In theory, a strong national response would be achieved partly through coordinating the work of the UN, especially that of the six cosponsoring agencies. Such coordination would incorporate the normative work on policy, strategy and technical matters undertaken by UNAIDS at global level into their AIDS and related activities at country level, and promote collaborative action among the UN agencies through UN Theme Groups on HIV/AIDS.

United Nations Theme Groups on HIV/AIDS

UN Theme Groups consisted of the Heads of the cosponsoring UN agencies in the country plus the UNAIDS Country Programme Adviser (CPA) or 'Focal Point'. Groups were tasked to plan, manage and monitor the UN system's actions in the country as well as strengthen the interface between the UN system and a country's National Coordination Mechanisms related to AIDS. Theme Groups also linked countries to global policy and research forums. A major role of the Theme Groups was to support national governments in forming a national strategic plan for responding to the epidemic, then attracting the resources to carry out the plan.

As Clement Chan-Kam, who from 1996 was in charge of the Asia Pacific region for UNAIDS, explained, Theme Groups were (and still are) supposed to be the mechanism for, and an expression of, UN collaboration and joint action, aiming to make best use of its collective

---

[5] UNAIDS/WHO *2007 AIDS epidemic update*, November 2007.
[6] UNAIDS (1996). *Point of View: Reducing Women's Vulnerability to HIV Infection*. Geneva, UNAIDS.

resources. "The UN collectively offers a unique platform from which to support countries" because of the mix of technical skills that it can mobilize through the different agencies.

The UN Theme Group was not a new entity, specific to AIDS. In many countries, UN Theme Groups worked on issues such as population, gender, environment and basic education. They had been introduced as part of the UN effort to encourage improved collaboration among agencies. Paul De Lay, who was working for the United States Agency for International Development (USAID) in 1996, described how they "were [often] established to get the

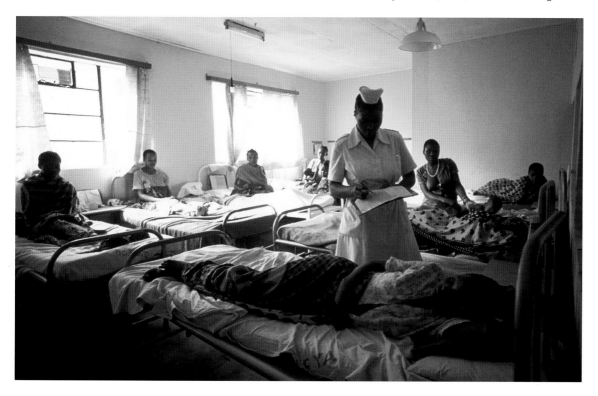

The involvement of civil society was essential to the AIDS response. This included faith-based organizations that provided the majority of care in many countries, such as this mission hospital run by the Catholic Church in the United Republic of Tanzania.
UNAIDS/I.Gubb

UN to work together and especially used for emergencies. For example, when there was a cholera outbreak or a famine, the UN [agencies] would create a Theme Group to deal with this, creating a space where the World Food Programme (WFP) would be motivated to work collaboratively with WHO". But those that were created to deal with the AIDS epidemic represented a unique creation, having both a formal mandate and a cosponsored programme to support them.

The aim was to avoid the duplication of work and competition for funds among agencies that in part led to the demise of the GPA, and to provide one clear UN voice to advise and support governments in combating AIDS. Ensuring the smooth running of the Theme Group on HIV/AIDS was part of the role of the Resident Coordinator, the highest ranking UN official in each country, responsible for coordinating the UN system in the country.

As Director of Country Support, Moodie was responsible for getting the Theme Groups up and running as quickly, and in as many key countries, as possible. "Getting the Theme Groups going, it always struck me as being like a dysfunctional family at Christmas. You go to dinner with everyone but as soon as it's over you want to go. People were dragged reluctantly to the table but it was absolutely the right way to go".

The essential challenge was neatly summarized in the report to the fifth meeting of the PCB in November 1997: 'UN Theme Groups on HIV/AIDS attempt to bring together agencies with 50 years of separate institutional development in a common effort to support the national response. Each of these institutions has a different relationship with government agencies and bilateral donors, with nongovernmental organizations and community groups. With this as a starting point, it was not surprising that the experience of the 132 Theme Groups on HIV/AIDS had so far been mixed'.

At the same meeting, members spoke of their experience of Theme Groups. Teething problems had in several cases been overcome – for example, the initial lack of interest among Heads of cosponsoring agencies or the agencies' determination to protect their own mandates rather than work together on the epidemic. Others had more positive experiences and had managed to strengthen relationships with governments and attract more funding. One commented that the Theme Group had broadened the national response that was "previously almost exclusively biomedical in approach" – exactly the type of result envisaged in creating UNAIDS.

Several members commented that the most successful Theme Groups were those that had formed strong partnerships with nongovernmental organizations and affected communities as well as government.

The advent of the Theme Group on HIV/AIDS was welcomed by civil society groups, particularly in countries where these groups were sidelined by government or did not have a strong role.

The advent of the Theme Group on HIV/AIDS was welcomed by civil society groups, particularly in countries where these groups were sidelined by government or did not have a strong role. In China in the mid-1990s, for example, civil society organizations were only just beginning to emerge and make their voices heard. In India, on the other hand, such groups were already very vocal and active, especially among marginalized groups such as sex workers, drug users and gay men. Like most governments, the Indian government had difficulty managing the relationship with these groups, for whom the establishment of UNAIDS, and specifically UNAIDS Secretariat, represented "a new dawn", said Chan-Kam.

Inevitably, civil society had high expectations of the new Joint Programme. At the third meeting of the PCB in April 1997, for example, Luis Gautier, the nongovernmental organization representative for Latin America/Caribbean on the PCB and Coordinator of *Red de Acción Comunitaria*, Chile, expressed his disappointment at the slow progress of Theme

Groups in moving from the provision of information to implementation of strategic plans of action, and the lack of participation of nongovernmental organizations and people living with HIV.

As far as donors were concerned, Theme Groups were an untested and untried mechanism, explained Julia Cleves, who was working for the United Kingdom Department for International Development (DFID) in India in 1996. They might have been useful for human- itarian emergencies, but governments or civil society did not understand them in any other context. She believes that "in the early days of UNAIDS the huge cost of setting up the processes of Theme Groups in the light of the urgency and magnitude of the epidemic, seemed at the time to far outweigh any benefits we could see being delivered".

Country Programme Advisers

Theme Groups' successful functioning very much depended on the willingness of agency representatives to work with each other, but they also depended on the talent of UNAIDS' CPAs.

By May 1996, 16 CPAs were working in countries and a further 50 would be recruited. The CPA's role was to support the Theme Group in carrying out its tasks as well as providing the government with technical and managerial support, promoting UNAIDS policies and strat- egies, and facilitating identification of technical support and training needs to be provided by UNAIDS and its Cosponsors.

"For some CPAs", said Chan-Kam, "it was a baptism of fire, especially if they were new to the UN. There wasn't much trust from the Cosponsors, [probably] born out of a failure to understand or an unwillingness to try and understand … but looking at the way the epidemic was evolving … there was a real moral imperative to work together".

"I remember clearly what Rob [at our] Friday evening drinks used to say: 'After all, what did we really expect? We are dealing with a bureaucracy that's had 40 years or more of … func- tioning in a certain way and trying to change that. You could not expect that to happen just because of HIV/AIDS'. So, we were – and still are – struggling with that. And, yes, of course, for those of us who were working full-time on HIV/AIDS, we could not understand why people would still lock themselves behind those doors of, you know, 'I've got my mandate' and so on and so forth. You know, I think some of us expected miracles, just because there had been all these pronouncements about a Joint UN Programme but, of course, a bit of logic would have told us that this was going to take a bit of time".

Tony Lisle was one of the first CPAs. He had previously managed Save the Children Fund and Australia's AusAID-funded health and social development programme in the Lao People's Democratic Republic for five years. After an intense, three-week training in Geneva with other new recruits, he was sent to the Lao People's Democratic Republic. "It was still very much the transition period from GPA, this new programme called UNAIDS that no one quite understood". His experience was not unusual. He was provided with a 'shoebox' office on the second floor of the United Nations Development Programme (UNDP) building, a very dilapidated wooden desk and chair, an ancient computer and golf-ball printer – all fairly dysfunctional. He vividly remembers the first time he had to write a memo; as he started to print it the ball of the printer flew off and that was that! CPAs were supposed to receive functioning resources from the Cosponsors.

More troublingly, Lisle had to contend with outright hostility from the Head of one cospon-soring agency. Every other member of the Theme Group welcomed him and worked with him but this one person refused to meet him and discouraged the Ministry of Health officials from doing so. Lisle was unable to work with them for the first three months. So one day he calmly went to the office of this Cosponsor and told the secretary that if necessary he would stay there all night, until her boss met with him. Finally the meeting did happen at 6pm. but it was made clear to Lisle that he was quite the wrong person for the job and that closing GPA was a crime.

George Tembo was UNAIDS' first CPA in Africa, in Kenya, from 1996. Previously he had been Medical Officer in Uganda for WHO's GPA. He saw the involvement of civil society as paramount. "People didn't realize we weren't like GPA, that we were working beyond the Ministry of Health. More importantly, we were mobilizing civil society and working with NGOs and including people living with HIV. I always used to explain – we were giving a voice to the voiceless".

Tembo experienced fewer practical difficulties than Lisle in the Lao People's Democratic Republic. The Resident Coordinator "really understood the concept of UN reform and that UNAIDS was … moving that agenda forward, so I was given quite some prominence". And he had an adequate office. However, it was not an easy country in which to work because at that time there was considerable denial about HIV: "negative talk about condoms" and churches were burning literature on the epidemic.

One of the hardest tasks for the first group of CPAs was defining their role and that of UNAIDS. "It was all so new, we hadn't really focused on our niche, on where we had a comparative advantage", explained Tembo. "At that time people liked to use the term that we were building our boat while … sailing at the same time".

De Lay explained: "And they [CPAs] had to be true renaissance men and women: they were supposed to cover everything and bring everybody together. But there were many instances where Theme Groups would meet and the CPA wouldn't be invited because they were too low in rank. You would have the Resident Representative of UNICEF [and] the Head of WHO [for instance], who didn't want to be coordinated or reached to by some little pipsqueak … who's basically considered just a social advocate. So the situation for CPAs meant that they had almost no budget and little technical credibility, as far as they weren't education specialists, behaviour theorists [or] behaviour change specialists, and these issues became a major challenge for them".

Certainly many CPAs felt challenged or frustrated by the lack of tangible results from their work. But there were clearly rewarding moments. Maria Tallarico, the first CPA in Mozambique in 1996, recalled how the sustained advocacy of the UN Theme Group and the UNAIDS office resulted in AIDS becoming a political priority for the President and his government. This was despite all the other challenges facing a country emerging from a civil war that had lasted for 16 years. Tallarico believed it was an achievement because the role of UNAIDS at country level was clear at the time. She paid credit to the parts played by the Theme Group Chair (the World Bank) and the UN Resident Coordinator, who were both committed to political advocacy at the highest level.

A clear example of such advocacy occurred on World AIDS Day in Mozambique in 1997, when the President, Joaquim Chissano, together with his political and military opponent of many years, Afonso Dhlakama, sat side by side at the World AIDS Day activities in Beira in the Sofala province, which had been at the core of the fighting. In the words of Tallarico: "They came together for the issue of AIDS … They were sitting together with the same level of power in a very controversial region of the country … Together they pledged their commitment to the fight against AIDS. Believe me … that was something really touching. Can you imagine, for the Mozambican people to see these two people fighting each other … then they shake hands, they agree on this issue".

The importance of the event was further marked by the presence of all UN representatives, together with the representatives of the bilateral and international organizations working on AIDS in the country. Most of these representatives had travelled the 1000 kilometres from Maputo to Beira to witness and support the occasion.

Tallarico, who is now UNAIDS Country Coordinator in Honduras, looks back with fondness to her time in Mozambique: "Mozambique was the experience that charged my batteries, my activism … I am still living with this energy and this commitment".

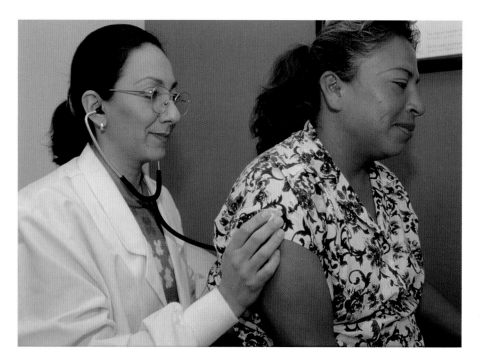

*ASI clinic / doctor with
patient, Guatemala city.
UNAIDS/C. Sattlberger*

As Chan-Kam stressed when asked about the requirements for a successful CPA, it was impossible to provide a blueprint because the country environments differed so much. "You might have a supportive Theme Chair but you might have a Resident Coordinator who's at odds with the Theme Chair. You might have a very strong civil society ... perpetually in combat with authority and you are kind of caught between the two ... So what we found in those early years was that you would go to a country and you would hear from five of your interlocutors, 'Your country programme is fantastic' and you go to another five and they say 'Get rid of that person' (a) because they not did not get from that person what they wanted, and (b) very often they did not really understand what the role of the Country Programme Adviser was".

Need for funding

Unlike GPA, UNAIDS was not a funding body, but it soon became clear that many countries' AIDS work would suffer if the flow of funds was suddenly cut, as many countries had benefited from significant GPA funding. So for the first two years, UNAIDS committed itself to funding some national AIDS programmes – that is, the programmes managed by the Ministry of Health. As Chan-Kam explained, these were "bridging funds to make the pill a little less bitter". Although the funding was an interim measure, from 1996 to 1997, it inevitably created expectations. After two years, there was little new money forthcoming from the Cosponsors. Moodie explained: "If agencies don't want to play ball by increasing their resources, because they don't have ownership of the new model that's been foisted on them from above, then there's considerable resistance". And of course the result was no money for the country.

The UNAIDS PCB decided that 'core financial support to national AIDS programmes should not be provided by UNAIDS and that alternative sources of financial support should be identified'[7]. But the PCB did recommend provision in the next biennium budget (1998-1999) for programme development funds intended for country-level catalytic and innovative activities.

Getting the numbers right

"Being at the hub of the knowledge is the best place to be if you want to coordinate the response. If you do that well, everyone wants to play". And as for advocacy? "If you don't have the data you don't have the discussion point".

Essential to UNAIDS' advocacy work, globally and in countries, was the collection and dissemination of sound epidemiological data that would be used to illustrate and predict (mainly through mathematical modelling) the development and impact of the epidemic. Tracking the epidemic was a key objective of the UNAIDS Secretariat. Nils Kastberg, the Swedish diplomat and Chair of the GPA Taskforce that had patiently and determinedly developed and overseen the birth of UNAIDS, said that one of the important aspects of having one UN voice at global level was to have one set of numbers, one global reference point.

Moodie explained that having credible data – knowing what the epidemic is doing – is central to the work of UNAIDS. "Being at the hub of the knowledge is the best place to be if you want to coordinate the response. If you do that well, everyone wants to play". And as for advocacy? "If you don't have the data you don't have the discussion point".

In 1996, responsibility for managing prevalence statistics was moved from WHO to UNAIDS, and staff started to collaborate with the other major groups working on HIV/AIDS data around the world. Early that year, meetings were held with Jonathan Mann and Daniel Tarantola who had both moved to Harvard, where they had been developing their own sets of estimates. Moodie and Stefano Bertozzi, Deputy Director of the Policy, Strategy and Research department (acting Head until Coll-Seck joined mid-1996) also began working with the US Census Bureau, which had been studying the impact of the epidemic on populations in every country in the world since the early 1980s and collecting all available data on HIV prevalence.

The US Census Bureau had developed the HIV/AIDS Surveillance Data Base on seroprevalence, available to everyone concerned with tracking the epidemic. Karen Stanecki was Chief of the Health Studies branch. "We were working closely within the US Government

---

[7] UNAIDS (1997). *Executive Director's Report to the Fourth Meeting of the UNAIDS PCB,* March. Geneva, UNAIDS.

58

and the various agencies such as the State Department and the US Agency for International Development to develop models [measuring the impact of the epidemic on populations]. The HIV/AIDS Surveillance Database continued to grow and it was a major source of information for evaluating the trends and patterns of the HIV epidemics". UNAIDS certainly did not want to duplicate this work, rather, it wished to build a relationship with the US Census Bureau and others to help them measure the epidemic.

Partnership was always crucial to UNAIDS' epidemiological work, stressed Bernhard Schwartländer, an epidemiologist and Head of the German National AIDS Programme, who joined UNAIDS as Chief Epidemiologist in October 1996. He recalled: "… very enthusiastic, committed, skilled people who were driven by a sense of urgency, by a sense of we need to get things done". He brought together all the key players to agree on the best way of cooperating on tracking the epidemic and making estimates for the future.

"There was a concerted effort to involve everybody who had any modelling experience or knowledge of the dynamics of the HIV epidemic to best estimate at the country level what was happening in terms of HIV prevalence", explained Stanecki.

In November 1996, the UNAIDS/WHO Working Group on Global HIV/AIDS and STI Surveillance was initiated, the main coordination and implementation mechanism for the two organizations to compile the best information available and to improve the quality of data needed for informed decision making and planning at all levels.

Vancouver: breaking the communications barrier

11th International AIDS Conference logo
International AIDS Society

During the first few months of 1996, Anne Winter, then UNAIDS Communications Chief, and her small communications team battled to raise the profile of both the epidemic and the efforts of UNAIDS to respond to it. It was not easy for people to grasp the nature of something as novel as a cosponsored programme. Nor was it a straightforward task, though central to the organization's mandate, to raise public awareness of the AIDS epidemic and its disastrous impact in the developing world.

New ways of thinking were also needed in-house as UNAIDS' staff came mainly from technical backgrounds with little direct experience of communications. Media requests were handled through formal clearance processes and there were few proactive

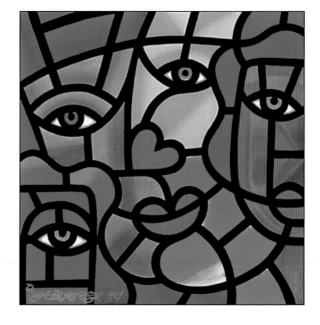

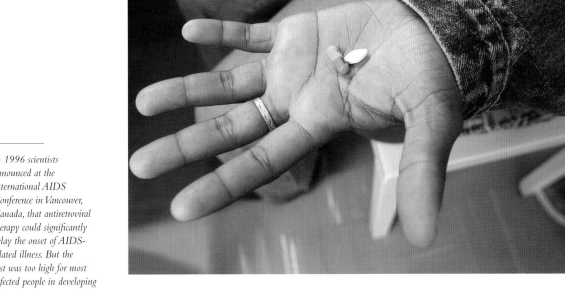

In 1996 scientists announced at the International AIDS Conference in Vancouver, Canada, that antiretroviral therapy could significantly delay the onset of AIDS-related illness. But the cost was too high for most infected people in developing countries.
UNAIDS/E.Miller

efforts to inform and interest journalists. Winter knew this was not good enough; she brought a more sophisticated approach from her United Nations Children's Fund (UNICEF) experience, including media training for many UNAIDS staff. Its success would soon be tested, in July, at the first major event for UNAIDS – the 11th International AIDS Conference, the biennial gathering of the world's leading medical and scientific AIDS experts and grassroots organizations.

The conference was held in Vancouver, on the west coast of Canada. (Unlike the United States, Canada had an open door policy to people with HIV.) "This was key", said Winter, "to seeing whether UNAIDS was actually going to make its mark", because it was a significant opportunity for advocacy and publicizing its work to an audience of around 15 000 delegates and 2000 members of the international media community.

At previous international AIDS conferences, the mood had tended to be pessimistic; Vancouver heralded a new era of hope with the announcement of new scientific advances. The major news at the conference was that highly active antiretroviral therapy (the combination of three or more different antiretroviral drugs, taken simultaneously and regularly) could significantly delay the onset of AIDS in people living with HIV. Typical media headlines were: 'Usual air of desperation gone'; 'Glimmers of hope'; 'At last a treatable disease'.

But it also became clear that the conference slogan 'One World, One Hope' was at best a vision for the future. The theme was intended to emphasize the need for people to work together in combating the epidemic and mitigating its impact. However, the majority of activists attending were from the developed world and, as many would admit, were not yet involved with the developing world's problems.

Many activists and speakers deplored the existence of two starkly different AIDS worlds. In one world, there was wealth and pills (an estimated US$ 20 000 per treatment per year in the USA). In the other, AIDS care and treatment was inaccessible to most people living with HIV. AIDS activist Eric Sawyer (founder of ACT UP) said: "The cure isn't here. We are a long way from a cure, even for the rich. And for the poor, we're no closer than we were 10 years ago. Most people with AIDS can't get aspirin". For many, AIDS was still someone else's problem – the political world had not formed a united front against it.

Jeffrey Sturchio, Vice-president External Affairs of Merck & Co, Inc, illustrated how the activists promoted their cause at the Vancouver conference: "What I remember about the Vancouver meeting was that at one point the congress hall was full of people throwing fake money printed with the names of pharmaceutical companies to dramatise the point that prices needed to come down. So, from then to the Geneva conference, those two years, [there] was that kind of public pressure".

Because UNAIDS was as yet an unknown entity, it had been a struggle to persuade the conference organizers to let Piot speak at the opening ceremony, but they finally agreed. He announced: "It remains unacceptable that people living with AIDS, especially – but not only – in the developing world, should have to live without the essential drugs they need for their HIV-related illnesses … bold action is needed on many fronts. This will take pressure from all of us – including people living with HIV and NGOs in developing countries".

This was the first time any of the UN organizations or any international development official had stated that pursuing treatment access in middle- and low-income countries would be a matter of policy. It was the kind of vision that would require mobilization and movement on a worldwide scale. But this would not happen for several years, and only after major negotiations between senior UN officials, political leaders and Chief Executive Officers of pharmaceutical industries, and activism on a huge and impressively sophisticated scale by individuals and groups in the South and the North.

At the conference, journalists sensed a change from previous gatherings. A piece in the *San Francisco Chronicle* summarized the proceedings:

'The major focus of yesterday's opening ceremony was political. It concentrated on governments that still drag their feet on the AIDS front, and on major pharmaceutical companies whose new drug combinations – however effective in drugs so far – drive expenses for people with AIDS to US$ 10 000–15 000 a year … [Peter] Piot voiced anger … at roadblocks to distribution of the latest medicine to those infected, "most of these drugs could be made accessible … if governments had the right drug policies and if doctors prescribed appropriately"'[8].

This was the first time any of the UN organizations or any international development official had stated that pursuing treatment access in developing countries would be a matter of policy. It was the kind of vision that would require mobilization and movement on a worldwide scale.

[8] Perlman D (1996). 'Worry, hope at AIDS conference: breakthroughs have too high a price for many'. *San Francisco Chronicle*, 8 July.

In collaboration with the Francois-Xavier Bagnoud Center for Health and Human Rights of the Harvard School of Public Health and the AIDS Control and Prevention Project of Family Health International, for the first time UNAIDS presented harmonized epidemiological statistics. In the Johns Hopkins HIV Report[9], Thomas C Quinn wrote that: 'Some of the most sobering statistics at the meeting were from the newly formed UNAIDS … It is now estimated that 33.2 million adults and children worldwide are living with HIV/AIDS, of whom 31.1 million (94%) live in the developing world … In 1995 alone, 3.0 million new adult HIV infections occurred, averaging 8000 new infections each day. Of these about 290 000, an average of nearly 800 new infections per day, occurred in Southeast Asia and 2.4 million infections (close to 6,600 new infections per day) were in sub-Saharan Africa. The industrialized world, in contrast, accounted for 98 000 new HIV infections in 1995, or 3% of the global total'.

This conference was undoubtedly a success for UNAIDS, and helped to position the organization as a key reference point. Vancouver was the first international AIDS conference where the developing world was firmly on the agenda, and UNAIDS contributed to this change in perspective. Weeks of preparation and negotiations had paid off.

Policy making

As well as tracking the epidemic, UNAIDS was to become a major source of globally relevant policy on AIDS[10] and would promote a 'range of multi-sectoral approaches and interventions, which are strategically, ethically and technically sound, aimed at HIV/AIDS-specific prevention, care and support …'[11] The Policy, Strategy and Research department had brought together people from varying backgrounds – nongovernmental organizations, academia, health services, activism – with considerable expertise, but it was a small team to cover a wide range of topics. The aim was also to involve experts from the Cosponsors, for example, through interagency task teams (or working groups), but these were too often talking – or even shouting – shops and did not result in major pieces of policy for some years.

Collaboration with researchers and policy makers around the world was more successful, as was the dissemination of effective policies and strategies through a range of documents from brief fact sheets to lengthy, detailed case studies.

UNAIDS released new data from countries and new research as advocacy and for the use of policy makers, for example, the evidence from Thailand and Uganda that prevalence was falling and the reasons for the decline. These countries, plus Senegal, where low prevalence was maintained, were 'beacons of hope' in a grim landscape. They remained the best examples of successful prevention for several years.

---

[9] 'The status and trends of the global HIV/AIDS pandemic' symposium, 5-6 July 1996.
[10] UNAIDS (1995). *Executive Director's Report to the First Meeting of the UNAIDS PCB*, July. Geneva, UNAIDS.
[11] Ibid.

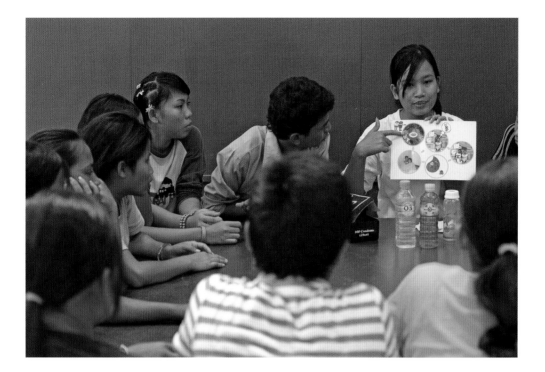

Information was also provided about good examples of innovative support, such as The AIDS Support Organisation's (TASO) 'post-test clubs' in Uganda, bringing together HIV positive and negative people to exchange experience and provide mutual support. 'Particularly effective approaches are a combination of several elements; they enjoy government backing, are protective of human rights, they are adequately resourced and grounded in community action'[12]. Other countries were encouraged to replicate these good practices.

HIV prevention education grounded in community action was an essential task for UNAIDS to promote. UNAIDS/ O.O'Hanlon

In October 1997, UNAIDS put out a press release to highlight the publication of a review of 68 reports on sexual health education from a number of countries. Their key finding was that sexual health education does not lead to increased sexual activity. This work provided an essential counterweight to opponents of early sex education, and is still cited as an important piece of research.

Mahesh Mahalingam was working in Nepal for UNDP at the time; he later joined UNAIDS as adviser on young people. He commented: "UNAIDS used information very tactically. It was happy to disseminate information from other institutions as well as generate it itself, and it anticipated future needs. ... It was path-breaking in terms of profiling the fact that children are being infected, and that it could be prevented. Even now, the fact that sex education does not lead to early sex or risky behaviour comes from [the work] that UNAIDS commissioned, and there's been very little new research on this since".

---

[12] UNAIDS (1996). Press Release for World AIDS Day, 15 March. Geneva, UNAIDS.

Prevention: the crucial issue

The prevention of mother-to-child transmission was an essential intervention for UNAIDS to promote, but achieving this presented real difficulties. First, women in low-income countries could not afford to buy the expensive drugs required. Second, the breastfeeding issue was most controversial. For years, UNICEF and WHO had promoted breastfeeding because it was undoubtedly healthier for newborn babies, but now they were confronted with the fact that HIV could be transmitted through the mother's breast milk. Michael Merson, former Director of GPA, recalled a meeting with Jim Grant, then Director of UNICEF: "I said 'Jim, let me show you the data on breastfeeding [and HIV transmission]' and he almost fell off his chair. It was too painful for him to accept". Merson's arguments with UNICEF in the early 1990s were to be played out again with UNAIDS from 1996 onwards.

UNAIDS was working on prevention in general with experts such as Tarantola, who had moved to Harvard to work with Mann. There was an increasing recognition of the need for a better understanding of people's vulnerability to HIV infections – not simply the interventions necessary to reduce risky behaviour (e.g. information education and communication to maintain or promote 'safer sex behaviours') but also the need to address the 'contextual, socioeconomic factors that determine the vulnerability of people'. A major factor[13] was the 'poverty spiral': the impact of the epidemic on national development and of development on the epidemic. 'This is producing a negative spiral with the epidemic undermining development efforts, and the lack of progress in development, in turn, further increasing the vulnerability of the population to the epidemic'. An example of such effects would be the massive migration of men to work on a road-building project (or the mines in South Africa) where, living in poor conditions apart from partners and families, they have unprotected sex with sex workers attracted to such projects because of the money available.

Bunmi Makinwa from Nigeria joined UNAIDS department of Policy, Strategy and Research in 1997, as a Prevention Adviser, after some years spent working for Family Health International in Washington, DC, and Nairobi. He recalled an era of denial and relativism. In one country he visited, he was told that more people were dying from car accidents than from AIDS. "We had to tell them, 'that may be the case today but if you look at ten years to come, it will be very, very different'".

Makinwa's travels involved identifying the best and most appropriate strategies in the various areas of prevention. "We worked with organizations that were leading in condom programming, condom manufacturing and distribution, condom social marketing; who are looking at sex work and coming up with … the best practices". These strategies were often documented in UNAIDS' series of Best Practice publications on a wide range of issues, and countries found them very useful in providing guidance and direction. Over 10 years later,

---

[13] UNAIDS (1997).

the Best Practice Collection is composed of more than 140 titles (many available in translation) providing case studies of effective programmes and a range of other information useful to policy makers and planners.

UNAIDS was also involved in supporting research and development into technology for prevention – vaccine development, vaginal microbicides and diagnostics for sexually transmitted infections.

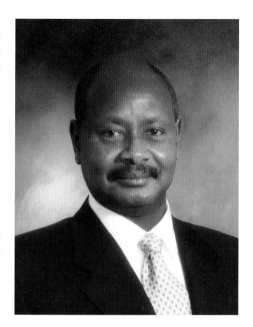

Speaking at the opening ceremony of the 10th International Conference on AIDS and STIs in Africa (ICASA) in Abidjan, in December 1997, Piot said that perhaps the "brightest spot" was Uganda, where HIV rates were continuing to drop. The 1997 data being analysed at the time showed that levels of HIV among pregnant women were one fifth lower than those the year before. Yet "this is a country which a decade ago some privately called the AIDS capital of Africa".

President Yoweri Museveni, Uganda.
UNAIDS

Piot considered the lessons to be learnt. "First, they did it through openness at the very highest level. President [Yoweri] Museveni … spoke out and became a role model for Ugandans, sending them a loud and clear message that AIDS is a reality – [which] they need to come to terms with and confront". Second, Ugandans realized there would be no 'overnight solution' and that a multisectoral response was vital. Third, Ugandans infected and affected had come together in AIDS support organizations such as TASO. "In so doing, they gave AIDS a human face and brought the epidemic into the open". In 2007, it is only too easy to forget how important it was in 1997 to promote Uganda's example – Uganda's response was so unusual.

Piot also spoke of other countries where prevention programmes were "small islands of hope": Zimbabwe's school system had launched model AIDS education programmes with the collaboration of UNICEF and UNAIDS; Swaziland's sugar companies were carrying out excellent workplace programmes; in Burkino Faso, Chad and Mali, HIV prevention was being woven into community programmes in collaboration with the World Bank.

There were also cross-border initiatives, such as those in West Africa on HIV, migration and prostitution, funded by bilateral donor agencies and the World Bank, and the efforts of the International Planned Parenthood Federation to integrate sexually transmitted diseases and AIDS into their sexual and reproductive health programmes in the region.

Establishing the broad coalition

One of UNAIDS' major objectives was to work with a broad coalition of people and organizations involved with HIV/AIDS. During 1995, strong links had been made with nongovernmental organizations, community-based organizations and networks of people living with HIV. Now UNAIDS began to reach out to other players in civil society.

In 1996, Cowal began making contacts with religious bodies, including the Vatican. The approach to the Roman Catholic Church was through the UK-based nongovernmental organization, the Catholic Fund for Overseas Development which laid out the roadmap for Cowal and recommended an approach to Caritas Internationalis, a confederation of more than 160 Catholic development and social service organizations 'working to build a better world, especially for the poor and oppressed in over 200 countries and territories, and an organization that promotes partnership'[14]. Cowal and Piot had at least two meetings with Cardinal Lozano Barragan, President of the Pontifical Commission for Pastoral Care, during these two years. As Cowal explained, they argued that, even if the church continued to say that an artificial means of contraception should not be used, "there's a greater good out there and if the condom can be used as life-saving, that's the greater good. … But we could never quite get there". However, in the following years, UNAIDS worked closely with a range of faith-based organizations. During that time, with the Catholic Church as with others, there has been far greater openness and dialogue.

More down-to-earth debates were held with the business community than with faith-based groups. A small but growing number of major corporations, especially in southern Africa, had begun to recognize the potential seriousness of the epidemic's impact on their work – both on employee productivity and on their markets. A study of African enterprises found that HIV-related absenteeism accounted for 37% of increased labour costs[15].

By the mid-1990s, the Uganda Railway Corporation had an annual employee turnover rate of 15%. There were suggestions that more than 10% of its workforce had died from AIDS-related illnesses[16]. In South Africa, the electricity utility company Eskom had pioneered workplace HIV prevention programmes in the late 1980s. In 1995, the company's Chief Medical officer, Charles Roos, instituted a surveillance study of HIV within Eskom. This indicated that, without any interventions, about 25% of the workforce would be HIV-positive by 2003[17].

---

[14] Caritas website, 2007.

[15] Coutinho A G (2000). *An Assessment of the Economic Impact of HIV/AIDS on the Royal Swaziland Sugar Corporation*. MA research report, Department of Community Health, University of the Witwatersrand, Johannesburg.

[16] Barnett A, Whiteside A (2002). *AIDS in the Twenty-First Century. Disease and Globalization*. New York, Palgrave Macmillan.

[17] Knight L (2005). *Access to Treatment in the Private Sector Workplace*. Best Practice Collection. Geneva, UNAIDS.

The global business sector needed to understand that involvement with the AIDS response wasn't simply a matter of humanitarian concern but would affect their ultimate profitability – the bottom line. In December 1996, UNAIDS held a meeting for businesses and other institutions interested in the business response.

Ben Plumley, then working for GlaxoWellcome, remembered the reaction: "We were very wary of UNAIDS. We felt this was an attempt to fund-raise through the business community and it was absolutely clear to us there was simply no way the business community would raise money for the UN. That tension lasted for some years – was UNAIDS interested in mobilizing the business response or just fund-raising?"

In February 1997, UNAIDS was able to take advantage of an ideal opportunity for meeting business leaders as well as senior politicians – the World Economic Forum annual meeting in the Alpine village of Davos. Cowal had contacts in the World Economic Forum and, through these, had attended the meeting in 1996 and taken part in a healthcare working group. "And that's when I said 'We've got to get [President Nelson] Mandela here'... in the earlier years of that forum, it had put together important people from developing countries and developed countries and the business, government and NGO worlds. So things appeared to happen in this magical little village".

"We will never do better than this. There's Peter on the podium with Mandela, and Mandela is saying to all these people 'if you don't do something about AIDS, you can forget about development'".

Through Cowal's endeavours, both Mandela and Piot were invited to the 1997 meeting. Piot would take part in a panel session on business in the world of AIDS, and Mandela, Piot and Sir Richard Sykes, CEO of GlaxoWellcome, would speak at a plenary session. But as the date of the meeting approached, Mandela's office failed to confirm that he would be there. Cowal flew to South Africa and through the Health Minister, Nkosazana Zuma, who was then Chair of UNAIDS' PCB, apparently won the support of Mandela's office. But there was still no formal confirmation and the Davos Group were saying he had to confirm by 10 January.

Nelson Mandela and Klaus Schwab at the World Economic Forum in Davos, Switzerland. World Economic Forum

As Cowal recalled: "I said, 'to hell he's not coming. I mean, it's like Jesus Christ; if he confirms the night before, they're going to figure out how to accommodate him'. And Mandela did come and everybody attended his session". Cowal said she could remember thinking: "We will never do better than this. There's Peter on the podium with Mandela, and Mandela is saying to all these people 'if you don't do something about AIDS, you can forget about development'".

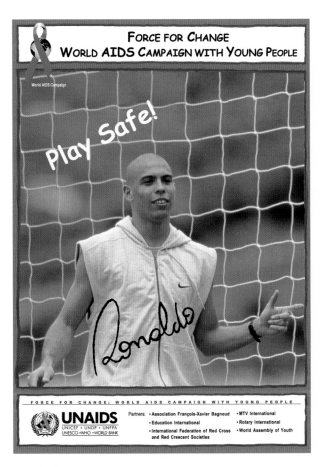

*World AIDS
Campaign 1998
UNAIDS*

The World AIDS Campaign

In 1988, WHO declared 1 December as the first World AIDS Day. It has become one of the world's most successful commemorative days, recognized and celebrated around the globe. In 1997, aware of the need for year-round campaign activity for AIDS, UNAIDS and its Cosponsors launched the World AIDS Campaign with the aim of achieving more tangible results in the advocacy and programmatic areas over a longer period of time. The campaign was intended to make the best use of available resources and increase the reach and impact of the efforts to mobilize societies (one of the objectives always of World AIDS Day) around the world. With a specific theme each year, the campaign could be used as a platform by countries, and materials could be adapted to fit local circumstances.

In 1997, the theme of the first World AIDS Campaign was 'Children living in a world with AIDS'. When the idea was first suggested, UNAIDS was criticized for, as Winter recalled, "trying to do a soft-sell" by concentrating on children rather than the most vulnerable groups, such as gay men. However, this campaign, by using data from around the world, focused public attention on the huge impact that the epidemic was already having on children, as well as its complexity and diversity in different settings.

In following years, themes included 'Men make a difference' (2000–2002), aiming to involve men more fully, 'Stigma and discrimination' (2003) and 'Women, Girls, HIV and AIDS' (2004). The World AIDS Campaign has a formidable penetration worldwide, with events and campaigns taking place throughout the year in most countries.

In 2005, responsibility for running the Campaign was handed over from UNAIDS to an independent organization known as the World AIDS Campaign, based in Amsterdam. A Global Steering Committee sets the strategic direction of the campaign. Their theme, until 2010, is 'Stop AIDS: Keep the promise', an appeal to governments and policy makers to ensure they meet the targets they agreed at the United Nations General Assembly Special Session (UNGASS) in 2001.

68

At the panel session on business and the epidemic, Piot laid out the grim statistics to illustrate how AIDS was affecting business and gave examples of companies that were already taking action. He then called on the leaders present to become involved and to create with UNAIDS a Global Business Council. He certainly convinced Sykes, who instructed Plumley to set up the Council, with the involvement of other interested businesses such as Levis and MTV.

Some eight months later, in October 1997, this council was launched in Edinburgh, Scotland, where the Commonwealth Heads of State and Government meeting was taking place. Mandela was its Honorary President and Sykes was Chair.

"But at the start", recalled Plumley, "the business response was like getting blood out of a stone". Only a few major companies were really involved and until around 2001, it was a "very, very difficult exercise". It took a small number of key leaders, as in other sectors, to start to change thinking in their companies. Also, by 2000, AIDS was becoming more visible, and companies were experiencing more absenteeism caused by HIV.

The Drug Access Initiative: affordable drugs for poorer countries

Following the announcement about antiretroviral therapy at the Vancouver International AIDS Conference in 1996, the pressure was on to provide access to treatment to all who needed it. But the costs of drugs were huge. Even if countries were prepared to consider providing these drugs, they had to weigh the expenditure against their very limited resources for all health problems. Working for DFID in India, Cleves confronted this dilemma: "I was looking at how much money we had for AIDS [and the budget was considerable] but if we had paid for drugs for just a small number of people with AIDS, there would have been no money for anything else".

At the ICASA meeting in Abidjan, on 7 December 1997, President Jacques Chirac of France argued for setting up an international fund to provide drugs – the International Therapeutic Solidarity Fund for People living with HIV/AIDS – but other donors opposed his suggestion. They questioned the sustainability of such a

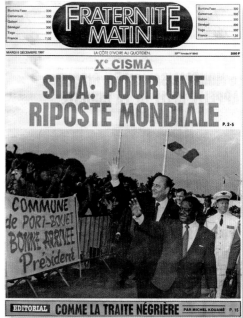

President Jacques Chirac of France at the 10th International Conference on AIDS and STIs in Africa, Abidjan, December 1997. Fraternité Matin

project given the costs and the parlous nature of most developing countries' health services. Treatment activists piled on the pressure and UNAIDS was certainly involved in the debate. At the third PCB meeting in 1996, a request was made for UNAIDS by PCB members to 'enhance its activities in the areas of access to ART [antiretroviral treatment], drugs for associated conditions, and care'.

"UNAIDS did seem to be able to believe beyond the possible, even though it could be a pain in the neck for everyone else", said Cleves. Indeed, UNAIDS was responsible for the first pilot projects on antiretroviral treatment in Africa and in the campaign for reducing drug prices.

The UNAIDS HIV Drug Access Initiative, launched in November 1997, was a collaboration between UNAIDS and brand-name pharmaceutical companies to develop strategies for increasing access to antiretroviral drugs in middle- and low-income countries.

As a pilot project, it involved only four countries: Chile, Côte d'Ivoire, Uganda and Viet Nam. Pharmaceutical companies were invited to supply the drugs at subsidized prices, usually at around 40% below the developed world price of US$ 10 000 to US$ 12 000 per person per year, while UNAIDS tried to adapt the health infrastructure in these countries in order to ensure effective distribution of HIV-related drugs. If the pilot proved to be successful, UNAIDS would expand the Programme to other countries.

At the launch press conference, the initiative's coordinator, Joseph Saba, a Clinical Research Specialist at UNAIDS, explained: "This programme will provide the information we need to determine whether HIV/AIDS-related drugs can be obtained and distributed effectively in developing countries. Armed with this information, countries will then be able to mobilize the necessary resources to treat infected individuals, and to help control the global epidemic".

Although they agreed to sign up to the Drug Access Initiative, the pharmaceutical companies were dubious about the feasibility of treatment in resource-constrained environments. Sturchio from Merck & Co, Inc, recalled: "They came to talk to us in about 1997 about whether we would provide Crixivan at a discount for use in Uganda. We were sceptical. Our argument about the Drug Access Initiative at the time was that, even if we made our medicine available for free, the infrastructure wasn't there, so people wouldn't be able to use the medicines effectively".

In the course of this initiative, UNAIDS conducted elaborate discussions with the countries to make sure that the concerns of the pharmaceutical companies were addressed and that the medicines would reach those who needed them. First, there could not be any diversion of discounted products to developed country markets. Second, the companies wanted guarantees that the drugs would be used in a rational manner, that the treatment programmes would be structured in such a way that their products would be used for maximum benefit and not lead to waste. Third, UNAIDS had to structure the availability of these products so that any intermediaries in the supply chain could not use the price discounts given by the originator companies to enrich themselves. Last but not least, the companies and the UN agencies agreed on the importance of protecting intellectual property interests, to ensure continued investment in research and development for new HIV medicines.

In 1997, antiretroviral treatment cost around US$ 10 000 – US$ 12 000 per person per year. Under the Drug Access Initiative, the prices came down to about US$ 7200 for a year's worth of triple therapy. While this reduction in price was not particularly significant, it did start things moving. Eventually, all companies participating in the initiative offered discounted prices and adhered to the principle of differential pricing for low-income countries.

Struggling with the Cosponsors

In late October 1997, the newly appointed UN Secretary-General, Kofi Annan, addressed the Committee of Cosponsoring Organizations (CCO) of UNAIDS. It was his first meeting with the group. He spoke of some achievements, then explained: "Much remains to be done. The Joint Programme is still young. It is not easy for organizations that work largely alone in programming their resources and budgets to adjust to the requirements of operating a truly joint programme". One might call this an understatement. But he continued: "I expect the UNAIDS experience to show us how to reap the full benefits of a genuinely collective effort which will be greater than the sum of its parts. We cannot afford to fail".

Cowal said working with Cosponsors was "like trying to turn round the Queen Mary ... I didn't know whether the behaviour change to prevent ... an AIDS epidemic ... or the behaviour change in the UN system was more difficult. They didn't like the fact that the creation of UNAIDS had been primarily donor-driven". The meetings of the CCO were generally very tense, with hardly any real dialogue among the agencies and often outright hostility towards the UNAIDS Secretariat. All this would gradually change for the better over the next few years.

Piot said that during those early years he felt as though he was moving around with a large ball and chain around his ankle. The donors were constantly asking, "Where are the results? What are you doing?"

UNAIDS was expected to produce results on a relatively tight budget and spending on AIDS globally was very low at this time. In 1996, the annual resources available for AIDS amounted to US$ 292 million and in 1997, US$ 485 million[18]. In the Executive Director's report to the fourth PCB meeting in March 1997, he wrote that out of a total of US$ 18 million requested to support Cosponsor activities for the biennium 1996-1997, only US$ 4.8 million had been received or pledged.

Eventually, the budget would be fully funded but, as Piot recalled, for some years the PCB set very low budgets for the Secretariat and its country-level staffing.

---

[18] UNAIDS was expected to raise funds from donors for its staffing and the Cosponsors' work at global level, though not at country level, where they could raise money themselves. (This added another tension because donors were not yet convinced that their new creation would work.)

Bertozzi also talks about the challenges of the reduced funding. He recalled a group sitting around Piot's kitchen table and being involved in the initial design. "We certainly had the sense we could be leaner and meaner. There was this sort of cowboy sense in the team that we were going to have a new way of doing things; that we were going to be able to be more effective per person and therefore more cost-effective and therefore in need of fewer resources. Perhaps everyone underestimated the speed at which mainstreaming could occur with fewer resources. In retrospect, it was unrealistic and in some ways cruel for the donors to expect that UNAIDS would suddenly catalyse all this mainstreaming that would magically be squeezed out of the regular budgets of the Cosponsors".

Throughout its short life, UNAIDS has had to deal with the fact that a very diverse group of people and organizations have great expectations of what it can and will do. Inevitably, it disappoints some and pleases others at different times. Not only is there a lack of under-standing about the 'nature of the beast' – the Joint and Cosponsored Programme – there is also a lack of understanding about how the UN works and of its constraints. South African activist Zackie Achmat explained this very well: "I come from a tradition where international solidarity has always played a critical part in work such as the anti-Apartheid movement and the Treatment Action Campaign (TAC). So for me, international organizations are very important". But he, too, is sceptical about the UN system because he believes the "power structure globally prevents the UN from fulfilling its mandate … [for] achieving universal human rights".

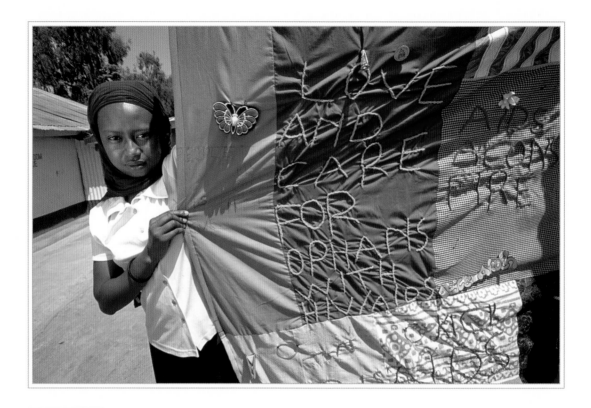

*This quilt has been made by
young people in the Kicosehp
nongovernmental organization,
Kibera Community Centre,
Kenya, Africa's largest slum.
"Love and Care for orphans with
AIDS."
UNAIDS/G.Pirozzi*

CHAPTER 4:

Changing the political landscape, 1998-1999

UNAIDS/World Health Organization (WHO) estimated that in 1997 there were approximately 22 million people living with HIV, and that more than five million people had died since the beginning of the epidemic. Some 80% of cases were in sub-Saharan Africa, which contains 12% of the world's population[1]. The annual global expenditure on AIDS in 1998 was US$ 479 million. In 1999, global expenditure was US$ 893 million[2].

In retrospect, it is clear that together with the work of activists, UNAIDS' activities during 1998 and 1999, especially in the area of political advocacy, contributed to a change in attitude towards the epidemic. These activities would in turn lead to significant events and actions at the start of the twenty-first century that could never have been predicted in 1999.

Looking back to this period, UNAIDS Executive Director Peter Piot stressed the importance of activism: "It is the most potent force to get political leaders to overcome their unwillingness to act promptly on AIDS … As so often in history, top leadership [is made up of] personal vision and responding to pressure from civil society"[3].

By the end of 1999, more senior leaders – presidents and prime ministers as well as leaders in civil society – were beginning to speak out about the epidemic and showing commitment to action. In some countries, this was the result of behind-the-scenes diplomacy and hard negotiations between UNAIDS and political leaders in both the South and North. Considerable patience and persistence were required.

At the beginning of 1998, the statistics on the epidemic were much worse than previously estimated, especially in sub-Saharan Africa, where AIDS deaths were pushing up mortality rates, notably among young adults – a pattern otherwise seen only in wartime[4]. At a demographic impact workshop at the World Bank in January 1998, organized with the UNAIDS Secretariat with the hope of increasing the World Bank's involvement, several reports had suggested that, in some high-prevalence countries, life expectancy at birth had begun to drop back to levels not seen since the 1960s. AIDS was escalating from being a serious health crisis into a full-blown development crisis. The public health models created for diseases such as smallpox and polio would not be sufficient to contain and reverse this epidemic.

Epidemiological surveys and country profiles demonstrated, for example, the need to reduce young women's vulnerability to infection. Gender had been on UNAIDS' agenda from the

---

[1] UNAIDS/WHO *2007 AIDS epidemic update*, November 2007.

[2]   UNAIDS Resource Tracking Consortium, July 2004.

[3] Piot P (2005). Why AIDS is Exceptional. Lecture given at the London School of Economics, London, 8 February.

[4] UNAIDS (1998). *Executive Director's Report to the Sixth Meeting of the UNAIDS PCB*, May. Geneva, UNAIDS.

beginning, as the rates of infection among women were increasing annually, especially in sub-Saharan Africa, but it would take some years before there was full engagement with the issue – partly as a result of lack of resources in the Secretariat and the Cosponsors.

Addressing the challenges of the epidemic

In Western countries, many people believed that the AIDS crisis was over, mainly because of the introduction of antiretroviral therapy (popularly mistaken for a cure) and the consequent reduction in mortality. There was little awareness of the growing disaster in low-income countries, where few people could afford the simplest medication for opportunistic infections such as thrush, let alone expensive new drugs. UNAIDS took on the challenge of combating such complacency in order to leverage a stronger and better-funded response from the developed world.

AIDS was escalating from being a serious health crisis into a full-blown development crisis.

Uganda was one of the first countries to show reduced prevalence rates. Former UNAIDS Community Mobilization Adviser Noerine Kaleeba recalled how President Yoweri Museveni provided leadership in Uganda from the mid-1980s[5]. "He had just delivered us Ugandans from the era of dictatorship … He made a very smart decision to say, 'OK, I have just led you from one evil, but there's another evil waiting'. He said at one meeting: 'Now I'm calling upon you to rise and challenge AIDS'. He made it politically correct for everyone to talk on AIDS, because if the President has sent out a call, if you are seen working on the issue, it is politically correct. There were other countries where if you were seen to be working on AIDS, you were immediately a subject of suspicion – It was a very, very interesting contrast that I saw very early".

Some countries provided encouraging examples of good practice in terms of prevention. But most prevention programmes were small scale – they were dubbed 'boutiques' – and did not provide nationwide coverage. The need to 'scale up' was a constant theme but this was impossible without political action.

How to make people act? UNAIDS staff criss-crossed the globe to press politicians, business leaders, and other members of civil society to step up their response. Such missions were part of a growing politicization of the epidemic. Activists, people who were positive, members of nongovernmental organizations; all joined the growing movement to put the epidemic firmly at the top of global priorities. Some leaders were prepared to make hard political choices, risking their popularity. One such example was President Ernesto Zedillo of Mexico who, in May 1998, stood firm in the face of criticism of the country's outspoken messages on safer sex and condom promotion. He made it clear that the Mexican Government would not give into pressures, particularly from religious authorities, against HIV prevention campaigns.

---

[5] Interview with Noerine Kaleeba for *Frontline: the Age of AIDS*, PBS TV, 2007.

But too many political leaders were still in denial, and resources for HIV prevention and care were risible compared with what was needed. UNAIDS itself was struggling to attract the resources to operate effectively.

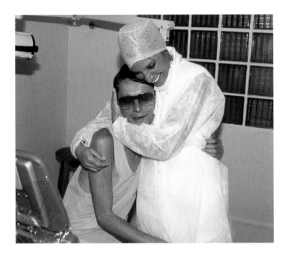

The Western media were beginning to write more seriously and more often about the challenge of the epidemic. UNAIDS contributed to this increasing awareness around the world through regular press releases, campaigns, the World AIDS Campaign and media partnerships. A media analysis of the programme undertaken by CARMA International[6], an independent evaluator of performance in the press, revealed 'that UNAIDS has already obtained substantial results not only when raising awareness about the epidemic, but also when soliciting media coverage of what needs to be done and what UNAIDS is currently doing to respond to the epidemic'.

Access to care remained a central challenge to moving the AIDS response forward.
WHO/A.Waak

However, faced with grim pictures of skeletal men and women, and of young orphans caring for even younger brothers and sisters, there seemed little room for optimism about combating the epidemic in the developing world as a whole.

Access to care remained a central challenge. As the health economist, William McGreevey, told an invitation-only World Bank audience in May 1998: "The brutal fact [is that] 'those who could pay' for Africa's AIDS therapy – the pharmaceutical industry, by way of price cuts, and 'rich country taxpayers' by way of foreign aid – are very unlikely to do so"[7].

Most activists were too preoccupied with their own battles, especially in the United States of America (USA) where drugs were available but unaffordable to many, to tackle the challenges of the South. As Gregg Gonsalves from New York's Gay Men's Health Crisis explained, "when antiretroviral therapy arrived on the scene in the US, cost was still an issue because of the absence of a national healthcare system. … There are 48 to 50 million Americans uninsured, so there was a waiting list for AIDS drugs – the issue of access came up pretty quickly".

UNAIDS' Drug Access Initiative, launched in 1997 (see previous chapter) had shown, admittedly on a small scale, that treatment could be provided in low-income countries. Dr Joseph Perriëns, now Director of AIDS Medicines and Diagnostic Services at WHO, was one of the people who initiated the programme. "This initiative was very important because, between 1997 and early 2000, UNAIDS was able to demonstrate that, with moderate investment in the supply chain and in clinical service delivery, mainly training and some investment in laboratory infrastructure, it was possible to generate positive treatment

[6] UNAIDS (1997). *Progress Report, 1996–1997.* Geneva, UNAIDS.
[7] Gellman B (2000). 'An unequal calculus of life and death'. *Washington Post*, 27 December.

outcomes with antiretrovirals in low-income countries. So the myth that antiretroviral therapy was too difficult [to be provided in poor countries] had been slashed".

Reflecting on the initiative's success, three experts wrote in 2007: 'The Drug Access Initiative was a milestone towards the now well-accepted principle of differential pricing for medicines for developing countries at a time when there were few generic suppliers of antiretroviral drugs'[8].

In 1999, when the generic companies began to enter the market in a more significant way, some nongovernmental organizations and activists criticized UNAIDS for engaging only with the big pharmaceutical companies. Perriëns explained: "The main source of criticism was from the anti-globalization activists who thought that we had made ourselves hostage to the research-based pharmaceutical industry and their intellectual property agenda".

Initially, UNAIDS had concerns about introducing generic drugs into the Drug Access Initiative. The quality of generic drugs was not internationally recognized and there was as yet no legal framework, as the Doha Agreement would provide some years later. 'But then in Uganda, one of the treatment centres involved in the initiative started sourcing generics from the Chemical, Industrial and Pharmaceutical Laboratories (CIPLA) in India, and the Drug Access Initiative in Côte d'Ivoire began sourcing Zidovudine from Combino Pharm in Spain. The experience of the Brazilian AIDS control programme with local production of antiretrovirals at lower cost added to evidence of efficacy of generic drugs[9].

From its earliest days, the UNAIDS Secretariat was criticized by activists and some members of cosponsoring agencies for engaging with brand-name pharmaceutical companies. But broad-ranging partnerships have always been an essential part of UNAIDS' strategy.

Building partnerships

UNAIDS' intensive partnership-building (including with pharmaceutical companies) over the first two years was beginning to reap results, resulting in alliances with nongovernmental organizations, people living with HIV and the private sector. Partnership with experts in epidemiology was perhaps the most productive.

Bernhard Schwartländer, former Chief of the UNAIDS epidemiology unit and now Director for Performance Evaluation and Policy at the Global Fund to Fight AIDS, Tuberculosis and Malaria, spoke about the value of partnerships to UNAIDS' work: "UNAIDS is only as good as the partnerships it can engage in … Partnership pushes our work to the highest possible

---

[8] Schwartländer B, Grubb I, Perriëns J (2007). 'The 10-year struggle to provide antiretroviral treatment to people with HIV in developing countries'. *The Lancet*, 368.
[9] Ibid.

technical standards and encourages a joint goal and joint vision. The role of the Secretariat is to inspire and meld a wide variety of partners together".

Sally Cowal, Director of External Relations at UNAIDS, recalled: "We were beginning to get agreement on what sort of modelling [there] should be and therefore how you could come up with figures. So that was an early and rather significant achievement".

"In UNAIDS there wasn't really any other game in town, we had a clear goal".

Rob Moodie, Director of UNAIDS' Country Support department, agreed: "The epidemiology team rose above turf wars among academic and other groups, working towards a common good. They understood there's a higher and more common good and also [they] had better connections across the agencies".

Statistician Neff Walker joined the UNAIDS epidemiology unit in early 1998: "You could start with a fresh slate. I think UNAIDS is one place where the hope that AIDS would be multidisciplinary, that different organizations would work together and share and agree on common approaches, really worked out [because there wasn't any past history to overcome]". He has noticed a difference in working with estimates for child survival or mortality where there are several competing groups: "In UNAIDS there wasn't really any other game in town, we had a clear goal".

UNAIDS strongly supported and worked with networks of positive people, including the Network of African People living with HIV/AIDS and the Asia-Pacific Network of People living with HIV/AIDS. Kaleeba was at the forefront of this work and, looking back, she said one of the best things UNAIDS has done is to persuade countries "kicking and screaming" to involve people living with HIV. If UNAIDS had not insisted that"… your strategic plan is incomplete without civil society", she said, "many countries would not have involved them".

In collaboration with the United Nations Volunteers (UNV), the United Nations Development Programme (UNDP) and the Network of African People living with HIV, UNAIDS supported pilot projects in Malawi and Zambia where positive people served as United Nations (UN) volunteers. These volunteers were placed in government ministries and nongovernmental organizations. "The primary objective … [was] to increase the effectiveness of national programmes by ensuring that the expertise and knowledge of those most directly affected contribute to national policy development"[10]. It also gave HIV 'a human face' and aimed to reduce stigma. As a result of such a placement in a hospital in Malawi, for example, the number of people seeking an HIV test and returning for the results more than doubled during the year of the project because they had met a healthy, positive person working there.

The Greater Involvement of People living with HIV/AIDS (GIPA) Workplace Project in South Africa was the result of a partnership between UNAIDS, UNDP, UNV and WHO, and some

---

[10] UNAIDS (1997). *Progress Report, 1996–1997*. Geneva, UNAIDS.

would say it has been the most successful work the UN has done in that country. Put simply, the aim of the programme was to place trained fieldworkers, living openly with HIV, in various organizations in the public and private sectors. These men and women would help to set up, or review or enrich existing workplace policies and programmes on HIV. It was promoting the principle of GIPA and supporting government plans in South Africa to combat stigma, increase the involvement of positive people and support all sectors of society to form a Partnership against AIDS[11].

UNDP undertook to help partner organizations where fieldworkers were placed with the workers' salaries for one year, at US$ 500 per person per month. It also undertook to manage the implementation, advocacy, monitoring and evaluation strategies, and to establish support structures for GIPA fieldworkers to avoid burnout. WHO provided accommodation and equipment for the project.

After months of planning among the UNAIDS Inter-Country Team, UNDP/UNV, the Department of Health and the National Association of People living with HIV/AIDS, adverts to recruit fieldworkers were placed in two national newspapers in July 1998. Key requirements were that candidates must be HIV-positive and willing to be open about their status.

The 10 people chosen were taken through a broad training course to prepare them for their placements (by 2002, 24 fieldworkers had been trained and placed in different organizations). Two people were placed on one-year contracts with Eskom, the national electricity utility. They were joining existing workplace programmes and stayed on after the first year, in high-profile positions[12]. By 2000, for example, Musa Njoko – who after her diagnosis 'had been told to go home and wait to die'[13] – had become a regional coordinator for Eskom and a key implementer of their workplace programme. Martin Vosloo's work at Eskom focused on training peer educators and managers on HIV and AIDS-related issues. Eskom now ensures that the GIPA principle is an integral part of the design and implementation of its HIV/AIDS business plan and strategy. People living with HIV serve as mentors and identify new areas of work on which to focus.

The 'star' of the GIPA Workplace Project was Lucky Mazibuko, whose placement was on the newspaper *The Sowetan*. He had always been interested in writing and had edited his school magazine. He now writes a regular column on living with HIV in the daily and Sunday editions of the newspaper, and receives large numbers of letters from readers who are positive or are affected by HIV. In 2002, he and Njoko presented a 13-part TV series, *Positive*, produced and broadcast by the national TV channel SABC2. It focused on stigma, discrimination, care and support.

---

[11] President Mbeki's Declaration of the Partnership against AIDS, 9 October 1998.
[12] UNAIDS (2002). *The Faces, Voices and Skills Behind the GIPA Workplace Model in South Africa*. UNAIDS Case Study. June. Geneva, UNAIDS.
[13] Ibid.

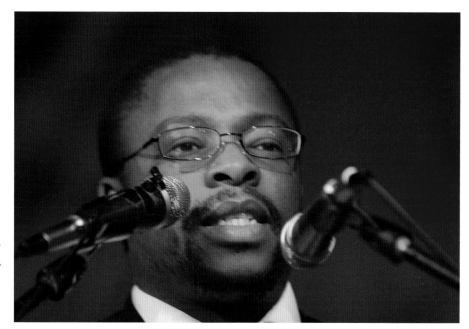

As the UNAIDS Case Study concluded, 'these are eloquent examples of people living with HIV/AIDS standing up for themselves and their rights, educating themselves and making major contributions to their communities. The fact that ... two set up their own companies is a strong indicator of success, reflecting also the fieldworkers' enhanced self-esteem, self-confidence and self-affirmation'.

Working with faith-based organizations

In many countries, especially in Africa, from the start of the epidemic, churches and religious organizations have provided the bulk of the care and support for people living with HIV. Calle Almedal came from the Norwegian Red Cross to UNAIDS in 1997 as Senior Adviser on Partnerships Development, where he assumed responsibility for working with civil society, including faith-based organizations. Almedal explained: "... there are millions of extremely dedicated people out there, doing a good job, not being recognized by anyone ... churches were the first to take care of people with AIDS, they were the first to counsel people with AIDS". At the same time, however, much of the stigma aimed at HIV comes from religious people and bodies.

Piot admitted that he was very critical of the church in the beginning. However, he also observed: "... they were one of the obstacles to be overcome and to turn into allies. I was convinced we needed to develop this broad-based coalition and they are an essential part of that".

UNAIDS has worked consistently over the years to involve and collaborate with organizations from a wide range of faiths, including Buddhism, Christianity, Hinduism and Islam. In 1998, a UNAIDS Case Study produced with the Islamic Medical Association of Uganda, *AIDS education through Imams: a spiritually motivated community effort in Uganda*, described the work of a number of HIV prevention programmes run by or involving Imams, and addressed sensitive cultural issues such as empowering women and promoting condom use. The study also includes a number of illustrated case studies of positive people who are Muslim.

In January 1999, UNAIDS signed a Memorandum Of Understanding with Caritas Internationalis, one of the world's largest nongovernmental organization networks, comprising more than 160 Catholic development and social service organizations, designed to foster cooperation on a response to HIV at local, national and international levels.

Despite inevitable disagreements with the Catholic Church over condom use, UNAIDS has worked with this church at different levels over the past 10 years. The Executive Director has visited the Vatican three times and, as Almedal explained, the Secretariat has a good working relationship with the Papal Nuncio in Geneva. UNAIDS country-based staff also work with faith-based organizations. It was UNAIDS' key role to work across all sectors, and to rise above the inevitable disagreements.

Anne Winter, then Chief of Communications, explained: "An organization which has different constituencies has to act as a broker between them if it wants to achieve results; it has interests which are aligned with part of the agenda of each of those constituencies … in the case of UNAIDS, its bottom line was to defend the interests of developing countries and those most closely affected by the epidemic. So with each group, UNAIDS had to work out the areas of common interest, and how then they could work together to push the agenda forward. But you can't broker the fundamental disputes. What you can do is, in a pragmatic way, broker specific consensus around very specific issues; that's often the most you can do".

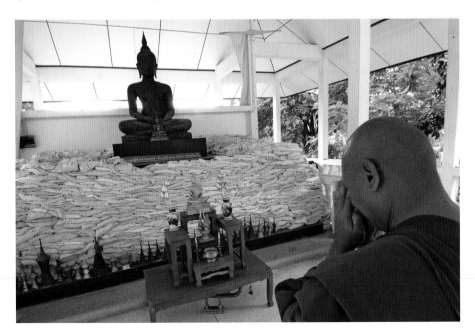

UNAIDS recognized the importance of working with faith-based organizations, who provide so much support to HIV positive people and their families. Wat Pra Baht Nam Phu Temple in Lop Buri, Thailand, has been converted into a hospice for people living with AIDS. A monk prays in front of bags of cremated ashes not yet collected by families.
Corbis / John Van Hasselt

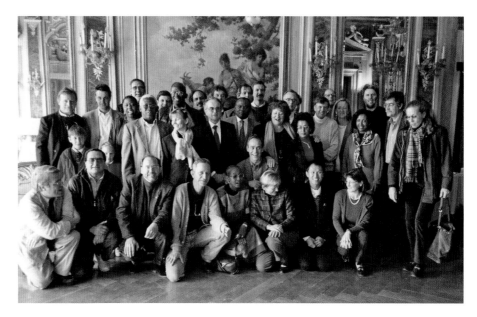

Participants at the Cosponsor Retreat, hosted by UNESCO in Venice, March 1998. UNAIDS

Cosponsors – striving to achieve collaboration

In an article for *Science*[14], Jonathan Mann, former Director of the Global Programme on AIDS (GPA), told the journalist Michael Balter that getting the Cosponsors to work together was one of the trickiest parts of the job for the Executive Director: '… like walking six cats on a leash'.

The Executive Director's presentation to the sixth Programme Coordinating Board (PCB) meeting in Geneva in May 1998 summed up the situation clearly: "We are seeing a major tension at country level between the urgency of action on AIDS and the sometimes slow pace of the UN reform process. In Theme Groups where consensus is hard to reach, UNAIDS faces a tough choice between operating at the pace of consensus – and losing credibility with the host government and the more active Cosponsors – and choosing one Cosponsor's views over another's, which complicates our relationships".

Nevertheless, the 1997 Theme Group assessment showed some progress since the 1996 report. About half the Theme Groups surveyed had put together an integrated work plan in which they charted a course for working together to support host countries in expanding the AIDS response.

Individual Cosponsors contributed in different ways. Mark Malloch Brown, former Deputy Secretary-General of the UN, remembered his first visit to Southern Africa in 1999 as the new Administrator of UNDP. He recalled seeing villages that looked as though they'd been "hit by the slave trade, because adults of an economically active and sexually active phase of their lives were gone, leaving villages of grandparents and kids". This image stayed with Malloch Brown as he reorganized UNDP into a series of 'practice areas', including AIDS, the better to focus its work.

---

[14] Balter M (1998). 'United Nations: global program struggles to stem the flood of new cases'. *Science*, 280.

In Botswana, the UN Country Team was very active on AIDS issues. The UN system, under the leadership of Resident Coordinator Deborah Landey (now Deputy Executive Director, Management and External Relations, UNAIDS), had led the development of a substantial programme of support to the government and other key stakeholders.

Malloch Brown stressed the impact of UNDP's Botswana *Human Development Report*, published in 2000. The report, which was directed by Macharia Kamau, who had succeeded Landey as Resident Coordinator, included a foreword by Botswana's President Festus Mogae. Malloch Brown stated that Mogae would attribute "his own conversion" to the report, "which pointed out that Botswana is like the Singapore of Southern Africa", [in that it] has [higher] per capita income and development rates than any of its neighbours because of its diamonds. Nevertheless, Botswana has the same, if not higher, infection rates as poorer neighbouring countries, which caused the country's development gains to be wiped out. After absorbing the significance of the Human Development Report, Mogae announced that the government would begin providing free antiretroviral treatment to those who needed it. Thus, the Human Development Report changed a country. Malloch Brown commented: "I realized that this sort of powerful advocacy really mattered".

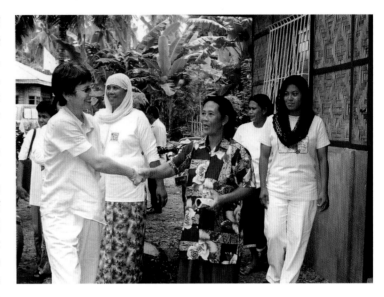

Deborah Landey, United Nations Resident Coordinator visiting beneficiaries of UN multi-donor programme, Mindanao, Philippines
UNAIDS

UNAIDS Cosponsor United Nations Population Fund (UNFPA) was also evolving in its thinking and practice on AIDS. At the first International Conference on Population and Development (ICPD), in 1994, the international community noted that AIDS required an urgent response, but no targets were set. But the 'International Conference on Population and Development plus five' review document published in 1999 had clear targets for HIV prevention, stating, for example, that 'governments, with assistance from UNAIDS and donors should, by 2005, ensure that at least 90%, and by 2010 at least 95%, of young men and women aged 15 to 24 have access to the information, education and services necessary to develop the life skills required to reduce their vulnerability to HIV infection'.

According to Thoraya Obaid, Executive Director of UNFPA, "joining UNAIDS has been instrumental in ensuring that we make the link between sexual and reproductive health and HIV. After the five-year review of the ICPD Programme of Action, HIV took a more prominent position in our work".

The United Nations Office on Drugs and Crime (UNODC) and UNAIDS were also carrying out important work within countries. Kristan Schoultz arrived in Pakistan as Country Programme Adviser (CPA) in 1998, became UN Resident Coordinator in Botswana, and is now Director, Global Coalition on Women and AIDS. In 1998, Pakistan was a country with very low prevalence – less than 1% – but it was thought that a potentially important driver of infection was injecting drug use. The problem was that there were no data to support this theory.

UNODC (which became the seventh UNAIDS Cosponsor in 1999) largely focused on crime and drug supply issues in Pakistan, but it also had a smaller mandate to look at demand reduction; within their demand reduction portfolio, it decided to look at issues related to HIV prevention. A survey carried out with their government partners had indicated that there were approximately 500 000 heroin users in the country, and UNODC was concerned about the possibilities of transmission of HIV in that population. So they approached UNAIDS to discuss a way forward.

UNAIDS agreed to collaborate and to assist in resource mobilization for this effort. Schoultz explained: "The collaboration began with a joint study of behaviours and prevalence among injecting drug users. The study was undertaken by a local nongovernmental organization called Nai Zindagi ('New Life' in Urdu) which was and still is one of the premier drug treatment and rehabilitation organizations in the country. Nai Zindagi conducted the survey of street drug users in one city of Pakistan, Lahore, and tested for both HIV and hepatitis C prevalence, in addition to exploring risk behaviours and attitudes. Though no cases of HIV were found, there was an indication of extremely high hepatitis C". Schoultz recalled that "… almost 90% were hepatitis-C positive and this was a call for action. … It was quite scary when we found this evidence".

Schoultz then focused on process: "On the basis of that study … we, as the UN system, immediately went into action with advocacy efforts. We … engaged the anti-narcotics force in the Expanded Theme Group on AIDS in addition to the Ministry of Health and the Ministry of Local Government, who managed the police, [and] started doing … TV shows, making presentations to the newspapers, holding press conferences". ['We' referred to the Chair of the UN Theme Group on HIV/AIDS and the UNODC representative.] Following the advocacy work, it was agreed to set up a pilot project on harm reduction. This pilot project received only about US$ 70 000, for one year, which was used to develop what Schoultz believed to be "a fairly comprehensive harm-reduction project, which included needle exchange and a full range of harm-reduction interventions such as basic primary health care, counselling, condom provision, and referral for drug treatment – all made possible through extensive street outreach".

The project was considered successful by all partners, including the Government of Pakistan, which actually included the words 'harm reduction' in its national Master Plan for drug control. Schoultz explained: "Largely as a result of what was learned in the Lahore pilot project, there were a couple [of] follow-on projects that were financed by UNODC in other cities of the country. Then, through the continuing advocacy of the UN, civil society partners, and the

Government of Pakistan through the National AIDS Control Programme, the World Bank project designed to support the national response to AIDS included a significant component for a comprehensive approach to HIV infection among drug users".

"And, in what I think is a very good example of a public-private partnership, the Government of Pakistan, using the World Bank project financing, basically outsourced the entire harm reduction effort in the province of Punjab to Nai Zindagi and its partner nongovernmental organizations".

Schoultz considered that this was "... an example of how the UN can take a very small amount of catalytic funding and, working through strategic partnerships, turn that into a very big difference in the way a nation responds to a particular issue – and harm reduction, as we all know, is a very controversial issue globally. But despite this controversy, Pakistan moved forward quickly and pragmatically and with relative success because, I believe, of the way it was handled from the very beginning. One of our primary roles as the UN is to be bringers of knowledge and bringers of innovation and I think that the story of harm reduction in Pakistan is an example of doing exactly that".

"The idea is, nobody's too rich not to need support or too poor not to offer support".

Horizontal collaboration

Compared with the GPA, which sent out hundreds of foreign consultants to advise ministries of health, the UNAIDS Secretariat had limited technical assistance resources to offer to countries. In a radical departure from the consultancy route, the UNAIDS Secretariat promoted a strategy of strengthening and supporting technical resource networks (that is, of consultants and institutions offering technical support) within regions and countries. This was also a way to strengthen institutional capacity within countries and to promote country ownership, as opposed to imposing ideas and experts from the North.

The most successful example of such assistance was the Horizontal Technical Collaboration Group, established by national AIDS Programme Managers in Latin America and the Caribbean to facilitate collaboration on issues such as epidemiology, care, counselling and national strategic planning. "It was based on exchange of ideas and [the principle of] equality", explained Luiz Loures, a physician and public health specialist who had worked for the National AIDS Programme in Brazil and then joined UNAIDS in 1997, and who is now Associate Director for Global Initiatives. "The idea is, nobody's too rich not to need support or too poor not to offer support". UNAIDS supported this initiative from the start, and today more than 25 countries are involved in the Horizontal Technical Collaboration Group.

Prevention of mother-to-child transmission

One of UNAIDS' challenges was to clarify its catalytic role in policy making and program-matic work in order to determine how it could best mobilize the UN system's collective resources – for example, in supporting the scaling up of care, counselling and health

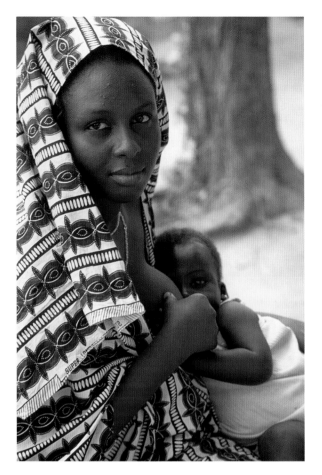

Mother-to-child transmission remained a tough prevention battle for UNAIDS.
UNAIDS/L. Taylor

systems. As the UNAIDS *Progress Report 1996–1997* (published in 1998) stressed: 'We cannot yet describe the global response as one of galvanized support for concerted action on a common set of priorities. We need to constantly remind ourselves that we are not simply observers and analysts of the determinants of this epidemic, but actors capable of fundamentally changing its course. We need to constantly remind ourselves that those most affected by the epidemic are also our potential partners; they are best placed to affect the epidemic's course'.

Information management was clearly at the core of many of UNAIDS' functions. A major objective of the Programme was to identify and promote best practices in responding to the epidemic – whether it be new research on drugs, vaccines, microbicides or on effective prevention programmes such as peer counselling in schools, using the media for messages on condoms or postponing sexual activity. Following that, the aim would be to support countries in turning new research findings and new policies into programmes.

It was harder to reach a consensus with the Cosponsors on some policy issues than others; a prime example was the prevention of mother-to-child transmission of HIV. UNAIDS had initiated research in 1996, and there had been several breakthroughs on drug treatment. In February 1998, the Ministry of Public Health in Thailand and the United States Centers for Disease Control and Prevention had conducted a joint trial, which showed that a short course regimen of Zidovudine was effective in preventing mother-to-child transmission of HIV. In March, UNAIDS hosted a meeting on prevention of mother-to-child transmission of HIV at the request of the United States Agency for International Development (USAID). Paul De Lay, at that time Head of the HIV Programme of USAID, recalled that by then USAID was using the new programme for key issues such as the prevention of mother-to-child transmission. De Lay explained: "We had an effective, cheap, realistic intervention and we felt we should just scale this up massively. We needed an honest broker to pull all this together because of all the controversies surrounding confidentiality, stigma, discrimination and whether breast feeding should be recommended when a mother was infected with HIV".

Cowal was asked to run the meeting: "I had no idea that that amount of emotion over breastfeeding could exist. I was still so naïve. They should have issued me with a bullet-proof vest". It took two days to agree on a statement but, said Cowal, "it was on the lowest common denominator … [it said] something like: all women should know their status, should know about the alternative, but that we would never advise anyone".

Several months later, when visiting WHO headquarters, Cowal saw nutrition manuals for new mothers that stated there was no alternative to breastfeeding. "You would have thought it had been written in 1964, not 1998, because you would not have known something called HIV existed".

Susan Holck, now Director of General Management at WHO, recognizes that the issue is a fraught and complex one but said that the main concern of the United Nations Children's Fund (UNICEF) was to protect the strides it had made in its breastfeeding policy: "They were just not prepared to deal with the challenges of this".

After the meeting, a new task force, the Inter-Agency Task Team on Mother-to-Child Transmission, was established to develop and publish guidelines and recommendations. Its initial members were UNICEF, UNFPA, WHO and the UNAIDS Secretariat. But, as De Lay lamented, "[it was] a pity that the MTCT [mother-to-child transmission] programmes were discontinued". The UNAIDS Secretariat and Cosponsors have been criticized by the external evaluation of the Programme for not handling this issue well over the past few years[15]. Even so, he explained, "this exercise was a good example of how UNAIDS' credibility and convening power and authority were what 'we all wanted to use'. For USAID to hold a meeting like that, half the world wouldn't come".

There would be several more tough battles ahead on prevention of mother-to-child transmission and other policy matters, but there was also growing recognition that UNAIDS was a key forum for bringing together the best in research and evidence-based information.

The 12th International AIDS conference debates the gap between the South and North

In the summer of 1998, the city of Geneva hosted the 12th International AIDS Conference. The conference theme was 'Bridging the Gap' – that is, the growing gap between the North and the South in terms of access to treatment. In the opening ceremony, Piot said the biggest AIDS gap of all is "the gap between what we know we can do today and what we are actually doing".

Journalists[16] such as New York Times journalist Lawrence Altman noted a very different mood from the euphoria in Vancouver two years earlier – in Geneva there was considerable pessimism. Not only were there no recent scientific advances to celebrate such as highly active antiretroviral therapy, but participants also learnt of problems with the new drugs (such as side-effects) and with vaccine tests, and the apparent hopelessness of providing treatment

---

[15] UNAIDS (2002). Five Year Evaluation of UNAIDS. Geneva, UNAIDS.
[16] Altman L K (1998). 'AIDS meeting ends with little hope of breakthrough'. New York Times, 5 July.

"I had no idea that that amount of emotion over breastfeeding could exist. I was still so naïve. They should have issued me with a bullet-proof vest".

to those in the low-income countries. Prevention seemed increasingly the solution, yet as Dr Catherine Hankins, now Chief Scientific Adviser at UNAIDS, said: '… over 100% more money is being spent on therapeutics now than on the development of prevention technologies'[17]. Also, as Werasit Sittitrai, UNAIDS' Associate Director, Department of Policy, Strategy and Research said in the same article (he joined in 1996, having been the Deputy Director of the Thai Red Cross Programme on AIDS), 'we know what prevention works but we don't do enough of it'. Action on prevention had slowed down, and some programmes had ceased altogether.

There were many reasons for this, including cultural taboos about discussing sex and sexuality, advocating the use of condoms and so forth. Such taboos existed worldwide. In April 1998 in the USA, President Bill Clinton had refused to lift a nine-year ban on using federal funds for needle-exchange programmes, despite conclusive evidence that such programmes prevented the spread of HIV. Some years later, at the 16th International AIDS Conference in Toronto, Clinton admitted that this refusal had been a major mistake.

The UNAIDS epidemiology team was constantly refining its working methods in collecting data and making estimates. UNAIDS presented the conference with the first set of authoritative HIV surveillance numbers, backed by Harvard University, WHO, the US Census Bureau and others. The numbers showed that over the previous three years, HIV infection rates had doubled in 27 countries. There were about 4.9 million children made orphans by AIDS in 1998, and 92 000 people were becoming infected each day[18].

The first Global AIDS Report, 1998 UNAIDS

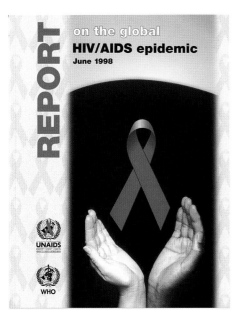

For the first time, also at the Geneva conference, 180 country-specific epidemiological fact sheets were published, reflecting the diversity of the epidemics around the world. Previous estimates had been based on information from regions; because no data were available from some countries, it had been necessary to assume that the pattern of infection in those countries would follow that seen in countries in the same region for which data were available. By 1997, when far more data were available, it had become clear that there were huge differences in the development of the epidemic between countries and communities in the same region.

UNAIDS had been working on methods of improved data analysis since early 1997. A meeting hosted at the Census Bureau in Washington, DC, in 1997, brought together specialists from Latin America, Asia and Africa to look at the data from the Census Bureau from the surveillance studies that had been conducted and to come up with the first country-level estimates. In 1998, this group became the UNAIDS

---

[17] Cate Hankins, quoted in Altman's article, *New York Times*, 5 July 1998.
[18] UNAIDS/WHO *2007 AIDS epidemic update*, November 2007.

Reference Group on Estimates and Modelling. The group continues to meet once or twice a year to guide UNAIDS on the tools and the methodologies for doing country-, regional- and global-level estimates.

After the 1997 meeting at the Census Bureau in Washington, DC, Schwartländer had taken the data away with him. "For the first time, there were serious estimates of the number of new infections and the number of people dying. It was so daunting thinking of the consequences of going public with these numbers. It was a huge responsibility".

He contacted various members of the group to double-check his figures. The data suggested the epidemic was now on a scale he and his colleagues had not believed possible.

In Schwartländer's opinion, the data produced at the Geneva conference were "a real milestone that cannot possibly be overestimated".

The data on HIV and AIDS have always been contentious, a place for 'turf wars'[19]. Some countries protested about their data: UNAIDS explained they had taken the best data they could find. Schwartländer's reply was: "If you have better information, share it with us. We'll then use it. We want to be evidence-based".

The June 1998 figures were criticized as exaggerated by some epidemiologists and health workers. Piot explained: "A lot of the criticism has to do with scientists who believe their disease is more important than someone else's". Such turf wars have continued to the present day.

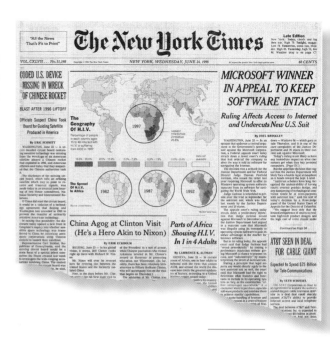

Using data to promote awareness of the spread of the epidemic has always been an essential role for UNAIDS.

Greater engagement and political will

'Peter Piot has a seemingly impossible job', wrote Balter in *Science* magazine[20]. 'With a staff of 130 and a budget of just US$ 60 million a year, Piot is seeking to turn the tide against a disease that has killed more than 11 million people over the past two decades and is relentlessly extending its reach'. Piot was quoted as saying that his 'biggest disappointment is the lack of political commitment in many countries, both rich and poor … Things are happening under people's noses and they don't see it'.

[19] Altman L K (1999). 'In Africa, a deadly silence about AIDS is lifting'. *New York Times*, 13 July.
[20] Balter (1998).

Such feelings led, in July 1998, after the Geneva AIDS conference, to another of Piot's private, informal retreats at Talloires, on the shore of Lake Annecy in France. Piot recalled: "I just felt 'we're not moving, not going anywhere. The AIDS epidemic is getting worse but no results and no support. What do we do?'"

Once again, the advice was to move on the political front, nationally and internationally. The group believed it was no longer possible to make any progress without a quantum leap in political will. Piot said: "That's where we said, 'get into the Security Council, the General Assembly, a Special Session. In countries, go to see Ministers of Finance'".

All agreed that this was a defining moment. Over the next year or so, there would be more room for optimism – not because there was any success in altering the epidemic's upward course, but rather because of some success in making the changes needed in the political landscape to do this. Work behind the scenes would culminate in major events in 2000 and 2001 that testified to the growing involvement of political and other leaders in the developed as well as developing world.

On 1 December 1998, World AIDS Day, an event on an army base in Kwazulu-Natal saw the highest level of engagement in South Africa. Speakers included President Nelson Mandela, Prince Buthelezi and Zulu King Goodwill Zwelithini. It was the first time Mandela had spoken about AIDS in his own country, which was experiencing one of the fastest growing epidemics in the world. He reminded the audience that behind every statistic hid a human being and that political commitment was essential for an effective response to AIDS.

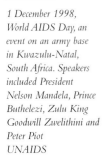

1 December 1998, World AIDS Day, an event on an army base in Kwazulu-Natal, South Africa. Speakers included President Nelson Mandela, Prince Buthelezi, Zulu King Goodwill Zwelithini and Peter Piot
UNAIDS

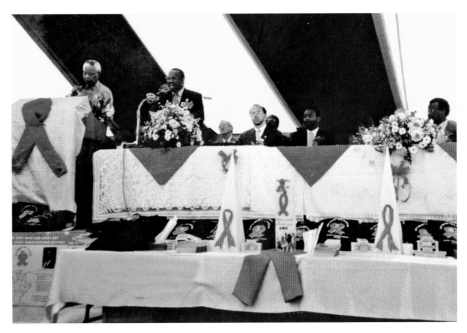

Mandela said: "We are grateful to a province that has the courage to declare that it has a high rate of infection. We admire the brave men, women and children who are with us today to say: 'We are the human face of AIDS – we are breaking the silence!' If we are to succeed then all of us must follow these examples and take responsibility for dealing with this problem. …". Later that month, Piot met with Prime Minister Atal Bihari Vajpayee of India, who expressed concern about the hidden nature of the epidemic. The seventh UNAIDS PCB meeting was being held in New Delhi in December 1998. The Indian Prime Minister had made a national address specifically on AIDS, had personally raised the issue in Parliament and challenged all state ministers to take on HIV/AIDS in their state-level plans.

In February 1999, AIDS was again on the agenda at the World Economic Forum at Davos, Switzerland. Both Piot and MTV President Bill Roedy called on business leaders to focus on young people. Roedy said: "Modern marketing techniques used for selling goods and services to the youth market are most effective in reaching out to youth concerning AIDS. MTV International is using such techniques to design special programming on AIDS issues targeting the young people who make up [our] main audience".

The partnership with MTV – a TV network with a huge global reach especially to the young – started in 1997 when Winter invited Roedy to the launch in Brussels of that year's World AIDS Campaign on children. MTV had already produced some major programming around HIV, weaving story lines and messages about prevention and against stigma into scripts.

The great advantage for UNAIDS is that through MTV it can reach out to a young audience around the world in a credible way – which the UN alone could never do. "We use UNAIDS as the experts for everything [on the epidemic]", explained Roedy. "We fact check everything with them, we're in almost daily contact".

Mandela reminded the audience that behind every statistic hid a human being and that political commitment was essential for an effective response to AIDS.

Tackling the crisis in Africa: the International Partnership against AIDS in Africa

The statistics were worsening in many African countries. In May 1999, the annual World Health Report from WHO had stated that AIDS was the number one overall cause of death in Africa.

'… if political and religious leaders had responded with effective public health programmes much earlier', wrote Altman, 'they might have prevented hundreds of thousands, if not millions, of deaths. Some leaders simply denied the scientific evidence that HIV was being transmitted in their countries. Others mistakenly believed they had more pressing problems to address'[21].

---

[21] Altman (1999).

UNAIDS' partnership with MTV International has been a long and powerful one. Its programmes , with many promoting information about HIV prevention, reach young people all over the world. MTV

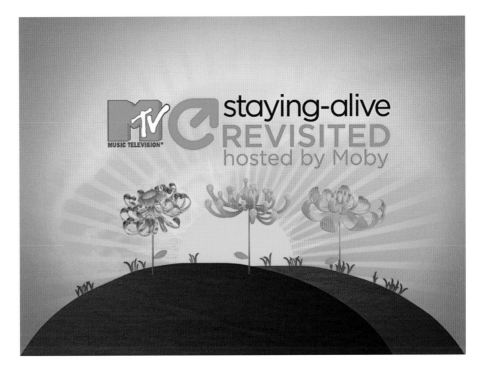

Even those leaders who recognized the dangers of the epidemic did not always act. Mandela told South African activist Zackie Achmat and others at a meeting in March 1999 that he stopped talking about condoms and AIDS "because he was warned [about] white conservative principles and [that] African traditional leaders do not talk about sex, if you want to win the next election. … I think for someone who had been in prison a long time who is really a traditional old man and a royal without being a royalist … having to deal with these things was not easy … but he said [he took] full responsibility for where we are with the infection rate amongst youth".

Fortunately, by 1998, a number of African leaders had begun to address the challenge of AIDS and some governments were increasing their multisectoral efforts against the epidemic. But they needed support, from within countries and outside, if they were to make significant progress.

In June 1998, Piot had addressed the plenary session of the Organization for African Union Summit of Heads of State in Ouagadougou, and a call for action on AIDS in Africa had been included in the final declaration from the heads of state. During 1998, the UNAIDS PCB had called for renewed efforts – by UNAIDS, Cosponsors, national governments and donors – in Africa. At the WHO Regional Committee on Africa meeting in August 1998, participants had begun to accelerate their work on an agreement for a special initiative on AIDS in Africa.

92

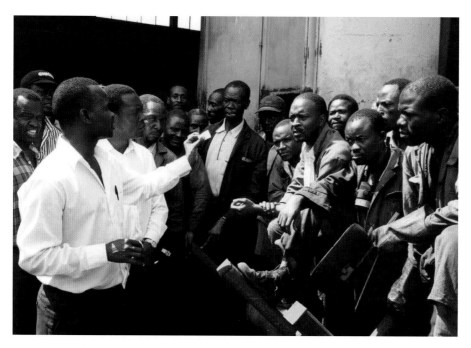

In many countries, business recognized the importance of providing information about preventing HIV infection. UNAIDS/B.Neeleman

At the January 1999 retreat of the Committee of Cosponsoring Organizations (CCO) in Annapolis, Maryland, the Cosponsors and the Secretariat agreed on a concept for intensified action against AIDS in sub-Saharan Africa in the Resolution to Create and Support the Partnership. They resolved to work together on an emergency basis to develop and put into practice an International Partnership against AIDS in Africa (IPAA). The UNAIDS Secretariat was responsible for developing and implementing the partnership.

During 1999, advances were made on many fronts – advocacy with leaders and in the media, technical support to countries and discussions at the highest levels of the UN to gain vital support and work with donors.

In May 1999, at their annual meeting[22] in Addis Ababa, Ethiopia, African finance ministers for the first time put AIDS on the agenda as a separate item and stated that the epidemic was 'a major threat to economic and social development'. Piot addressed the meeting[23]. "After my speech there was dead silence. I thought, 'another of those moments of supreme denial'". "But then", he added, "one after another the Finance Ministers spoke, often making personal references to AIDS in the family or a colleague". That evening, many joined him for a drink: "The problem was how to stop the discussion".

The next day, Ethiopian President Negasso Gidada and His Holiness Abune Paulos, the Patriarch of the Ethiopian Orthodox Church, shook hands with HIV-infected Ethiopians

[22] The meeting is known formally as the Joint Conference of African Ministers of Finance and Economic Development and Planning.
[23] Altman (1999).

A further challenge was to prevent the Partnership from becoming yet another bureaucratic exercise centred on the logistics of coordination and programme delivery

publicly for the first time at the launch of the Dawn of Hope, the first organization of people living with HIV in Ethiopia, a country with 1.1 million people living with HIV in 1999. This action was highly symbolic for an African country at that time.

If the planned initiative on Africa was to have any chance of succeeding, the donors had to be won over. In April 1999, the United Kingdom Department of International Development (DFID) hosted a meeting between a large number of bilateral donors in London and UNAIDS. The aim was to engage them in developing IPAA. Julia Cleves, then Chief Health and Population Adviser at DFID but soon to join UNAIDS as Director of the Executive Director's office, explained: "The donors were critical partners in both financing, political advocacy and technical support, and to further the development of a framework for Africa under which all partners would agree to act". The donors were not yet prepared to make a major commitment but it was an historic meeting – the first time that such a great number of bilateral donors had met specifically to discuss AIDS[24].

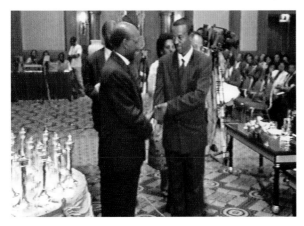

The Partnership was intended to build on existing efforts on AIDS in Africa and to encourage the expansion of Cosponsor, donor and government activities. A major challenge was that the response to the epidemic at all levels was compromised by fragmentation; different actors pursued their agendas in isolation from each other and there were many small-scale projects with their own objectives, management and monitoring and evaluation systems.

Ethiopian President Gidada publicly shakes hands with a person living with HIV for the first time at the launch of the Dawn of Hope, the first organization of people living with HIV in Addis Ababa, Ethiopia, May 1999.
Dawn of Hope

A further challenge was to prevent the Partnership from becoming yet another bureaucratic exercise centred on the logistics of coordination and programme delivery – or just another project that would lose momentum in a year or two. It needed, explained Cleves, a framework within which people could work together, and sign up to. The focus was on collaboration, harmonization, agreeing targets and delivery.

During May and June 1999, some of the Cosponsors expressed active commitment to developing the new Partnership. The World Bank established an AIDS Campaign team in the Bank's Africa vice-presidency (ACT Africa); UNICEF's regional management team for Eastern and Southern Africa endorsed the strategy of its regional task force for HIV/AIDS, which committed substantially higher shares of UNICEF's country programme activities to AIDS, and UNFPA published its review of AIDS-related actions in its reproductive health programmes and embarked on developing an AIDS advocacy project for Africa.

---

[24] UNAIDS (1999). *Executive Director's Report to the Eighth Meeting of the UNAIDS PCB*, June. Geneva, UN-AIDS.

As different partners began to show serious interest, people working on the Partnership knew that the real key to its success would be the involvement of then UN Secretary-General Kofi Annan. Clearly, responding to the epidemic was a priority for him. In June 1999, he had given the first 'Diana, Princess of Wales, Memorial Lecture' on 'The Global Challenge of AIDS'. He spoke of the horrific impact of AIDS worldwide, then focused on Africa where, he said, AIDS is "taking away Africa's future". He stressed the fact that AIDS is everybody's business. It was his first major public speech on AIDS and would be followed by many more during his time as UN Secretary-General.

Step by step, things were coming together. In September, a Memorandum of Understanding was signed between UNAIDS and the Organization of African Unity, in Addis Ababa, to foster collaboration and partnership in the fight against AIDS.

But despite the strong focus on Africa, the main message of UNAIDS' Epidemic Update, 1999, was that there was no room for complacency about AIDS anywhere in the world. In 1999, approximately 26 million people were living with HIV and the number of annual deaths from AIDS reached a new record: 1.4 million people[25].

The beginning of December (6-7) marked a major watershed in the establishment of the Africa Partnership when Annan convened a private meeting of all constituents for IPAA countries – governments, nongovernmental organizations, international organizations, donors and the private sector. It was the first time that all these players had been brought together in the same room to discuss AIDS, as well as the first major involvement of the Secretary-General. UNAIDS had engaged in high-level negotiations to ensure the meeting took place at all. Louise Fréchette, then UN Deputy Secretary-General, was hugely instrumental in preparing Annan's involvement. She explained: "When the Secretary-General [makes] AIDS a personal priority, it does reverberate around the world – most people don't have access to the Head of State, and it makes a huge difference".

Cleves had just moved from being a donor at DFID to work at UNAIDS, as Director of the Executive Director's office. She recalled that the stakes were very high for this meeting about IPAA, because at this point the Secretariat had not yet developed the very good working relationship with the Secretary-General and the Deputy Secretary-General, which was initiated after the event. "We were nervous and worked very hard to get an acceptable text to provide substance to the meeting. It was my first experience of the high adrenalin level of much of the Secretariat's work – knife-edge timing, last minute deadlines, burning the midnight oil".

---

[25] UNAIDS/WHO *2007 AIDS epidemic update*, November 2007.

There was a certain reluctance on the part of donors to attend the meeting, although there were many ministers from Africa, some Chief Executive Officers from the pharmaceutical industry, heads of UN agencies ("several of them very grumbly", recalled Jim Sherry, former Director of the Programme Development and Coordination Group of UNAIDS), and leaders from the nongovernmental organization community. Cleves understood the viewpoint of the donors: "IPAA had been under discussion for a long time at this point, and until this meeting with Annan, UNAIDS had proved incapable of articulating what IPAA actually was. So the donors were losing patience".

The Secretary-General's voice would just have been one voice without the back-up of UNAIDS and equally the reverse.

Sherry explained that upon realizing that no Organisation for Economic Co-operation and Development (OECD) donors would be at the meeting, "in desperation" he called Sandy Thurman, Clinton's AIDS Tsar, and she agreed to change her schedule in order to attend. She "… made her statement … in extraordinarily positive terms about the multilateral effort and the UN and the Secretary-General's leadership", recalled Sherry. Piot brought in Eddy Boutmans, the Belgian Minister of International Development and the only minister from a donor country at the meeting.

Annan charged those present with preparing an unprecedented response commensurate with the scale of AIDS in Africa.

The partners at the meeting committed themselves to working together under a commonly negotiated Framework for Action, focusing on actions in countries. There was some mobilization of money from donors after this, but equally important was their realization that through the Secretary-General's involvement, the response to the epidemic was moving to a higher political level. Annan was showing leadership and, eventually, ownership; his commitment to this work was considerable and constant throughout his mandate.

"So the meeting was a success", recalled Cleves, "and a great relief after so much hard work".

As Malloch Brown said: "There has been a most fortunate synergy in having an African Secretary-General at a time when so much work was needed on AIDS – and [in having] his extraordinary leadership". Both Annan's and UNAIDS' advocacy were important: "The Secretary-General's voice would just have been one voice without the back-up of UNAIDS and equally the reverse. They needed each other. I think it's been a very timely partnership".

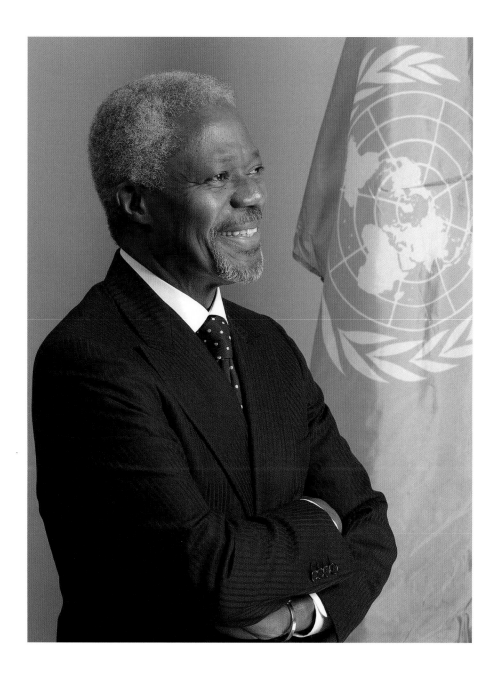

Kofi Annan,
former United Nations
Secretary-General

Annan was aware that the major challenge in engaging leaders in the fight against AIDS was stigma. He commented in an interview for this book: "To break the silence ... to encourage the Heads of State and Government to become involved ... for some Heads of State it was very difficult. I remember trying to encourage [one] to promote the use of condoms. He wouldn't even pronounce the word. He said, 'Mr Secretary-General, you should not be talking about this'. I knew he was a Catholic and told him that I'd even tried to convince the Vatican to change its policy. He said, 'when it comes to condoms, the Pope and I are one and you are not going to change my mind'. That's an African Head of State".

However, increasing numbers of African leaders did not hold such views. For them, the December meeting on IPAA was significant in many ways. It confirmed the involvement of the broad coalition of actors UNAIDS had always aimed for, as well as leadership from the highest levels of the UN and involvement from countries in the South and North. The next two years would see more exciting developments, to some extent based on the work for the Partnership, as well as the beginnings of a major mobilization of resources for tackling AIDS.

Seventh Cosponsor joins UNAIDS

In April 1999, the United Nations International Drug Control Programme (UNDCP) joined UNAIDS as its seventh Cosponsor – an important move as, in so many countries, HIV infection is transmitted through needles shared by injecting drug users.

In December 1999, it was estimated that more than 10% of HIV infections worldwide (nearly 3.5 million people) could be attributed to injecting drug use; injecting drug use was identified as a leading cause of the increase in HIV infections in the Central Asian and Eastern European region.

Kathleen Cravero, then UNAIDS' Deputy Executive Director, said in a speech in March 2002: "When UNDCP joined UNAIDS as our seventh Cosponsor in 1999, it marked a recognition of the close connection between issues of drug use and the HIV epidemic. Not only did it serve to strengthen in a practical way the capacity both of UNDCP and of UNAIDS to tackle the linkage between HIV and drug use, it also sent a signal to the world that this issue was high on the agenda of the United Nations".

For some time, UNDCP – which later became the UN Office on Drugs and Crime (UNODC) – had been active in supporting HIV prevention programmes, particularly targeting young people and other high risk groups, such as injecting drug users.

A significant step was the appearance of a UN position paper in September 2000 on preventing the transmission of HIV among drug users. According to Piot, "this [was] the first United Nations system position paper on this critical issue – where United Nations agencies jointly demonstrate a clear and strong commitment to HIV prevention among drug abusers ... The paper demonstrates that ... we [the UN system] now agree that the drug demand reduction and harm reduction are complementary and mutually supportive approaches, providing a continuum of options"[1].

UNODC's decision to provide support to prison populations in 2004 can be seen as a breakthrough moment for the UN response to AIDS. Prisons and other custodial settings are breeding grounds for infectious diseases. A high proportion of inmates are in prison for drug-related crimes and find ways to continue

---

[1] Interview with Peter Piot in *UN ODCCP Update*, June 2001.

their habit while in prison, often coercing others to follow. Furthermore, unsafe sexual practices, use of unsterile injecting equipment or other crude substitutes, tattooing, violence (including rape) and exposure to blood, all increase prisoners' likelihood of exposure to HIV. [2] HIV prevalence among prisoners iis frequently several times higher than the corresponding national averages in many countries.

UNODC is assisting governments in the implementation of "legislation, policies, and programmes consistent with international human rights norms, and to ensure that prisoners are provided a standard of health care equivalent to that available in the outside community". Antiretroviral treatment and drug substitution therapy are now available in some European prisons, but many countries have yet to implement comprehensive HIV prevention programmes in prisons, or achieve a standard of prison health care equivalent to the standard outside of prison.

Today, the UN system agencies have a strong working relationship around these issues. Christian Kroll, Senior Coordinator of the HIV/AIDS unit at UNODC, recounts: "All our Cosponsors agree that there's a very serious problem among injecting drug-users. This was not always the case before. Now they really support all interventions – HIV/AIDS intervention among injecting drug-users and in prisons. I think that the entire climate in the UNAIDS family has changed dramatically so that we collaborate much better on all these issues".

---

[2] UNODC/UNAIDS/WHO (2007). *HIV/AIDS prevention, care, treatment and support in prison settings – a framework for an effective national response.* New York, United Nations. July.

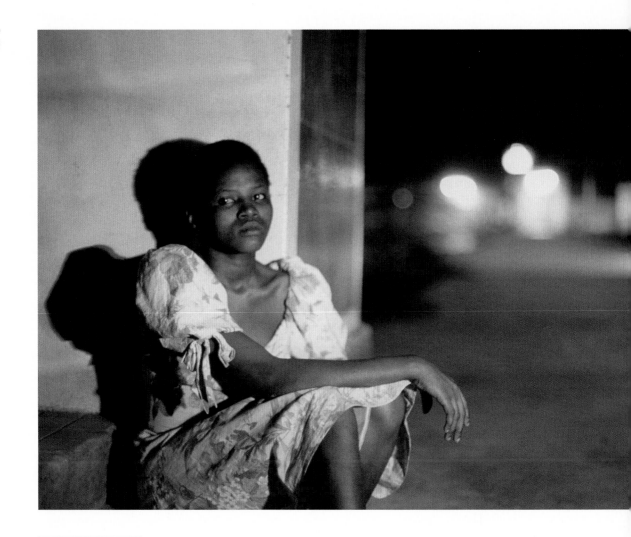

*In West Africa, Côte d'Ivoire has
recorded the highest prevalences of HIV
in the region since the start of sentinel
survailence. UNAIDS/UNICEF/
Giacomo Pirozzi*

Côte d'Ivoire

In West Africa, Cote d'Ivoire has recorded the highest prevalences of HIV in the region since the start of sentinel surveillance. In 1986 prevalence among pregnant women was found to be 3%, increasing to 14% in 1995, while a national survey found estimated prevalence of 9.5%. Among sex workers, the figures emerging from cross-sectional studies have been particularly alarming, ranging from 27% in 1986 to 89% in 1992–1993, decreasing to 28% in 2000. Currently (2007) national adult HIV prevalence is estimated at 7.1%.

The coup d'état in December 1999 and the outbreak of civil conflict in September 2002 resulted in Côte d'Ivoire's mixed success in fighting its epidemic, and these circumstances have also posed challenges to the United Nations system.

One intervention, the Drug Access Initiative, was launched in 1998 by the Ivorian Ministry of Health in collaboration with UNAIDS, the United States Centers for Disease Control and Prevention RETRO-CI project, the Agence Nationale de Recherche sur le SIDA (National Agency for AIDS Research) and the Infectious Disease Clinic of the Hôpital de Treichville. By March 2000, antiretroviral treatment was provided through six medical centres in Abidjan, prescribing treatment to 649 people, while 2144 people in total had passed through the eligibility screening. While these numbers were modest, the programme was the first to provide treatment in Côte d'Ivoire at that time. After the first two years, the programme was absorbed by the Ministry of Health and now represents the main treatment programme in the country. Through the creation of a national solidarity fund of US$ 2.5 million in 1998, the government put in considerable national resources to sustain this treatment programme.

The majority of people who had received treatment by November 2005, a total of 17 600 out of an estimated 111 000 who would need it, accessed it through public sector facilities spread over 33 out of 79 districts in the country. According to the World Health Organization's 2005 *Summary Country Profile for HIV/AIDS Treatment Scale Up – Côte d'Ivoire,* voluntary counselling and testing services are accessible in 95 facilities, again mostly in the public sector.

The National AIDS Programme, RETRO-CI project and the Antwerp Institute of Tropical Medicine are also running a successful HIV prevention and support programme with sex workers – initiated through the Clinique de Confiance launched by Peter Ghys, now Manager of Epidemic and Impact Monitoring at UNAIDS.

As in most countries, the UN Theme Group has provided technical support to the national response through Programme Acceleration Funds (PAF), for example, by strengthening associations of people living with HIV and by initiating prevention activities within the military, situation analysis and strategic planning at the national and decentralized level, and supporting a multisectoral response.

The country has generally displayed signs of political commitment. A national commission for the fight against AIDS was formed in 1987, while the National AIDS Programme in the Ministry of Health was set up in 1992. National strategic planning was undertaken with UNAIDS' assistance in 2001 and again for the period 2007–2010. In 2003, a special ministry to fight AIDS was created to coordinate a multisectoral response. However, the challenge then involved making the various bodies work together in a coordinated and supportive manner. The National Commission does not function well, and the two ministries find it hard to work together, which has a negative effect on implementation.

Overall coordination and implementation of strategic and sectoral plans were thwarted by the conflict that erupted in 2002, causing part of the country to be cut off from government and development support. In response to the conflict, UN interventions changed in focus towards provision of prevention information and condoms to uniformed services (by the United Nations Population Fund [UNFPA]) and increased support to blood safety (by WHO). A situation of conflict may bring an increase in the number of new infections resulting from, for instance, the displacement of people, increased sex work (forced or due to poverty) and (sexual) violence. The efforts of integrating HIV care and prevention efforts into the humanitarian mission may be seen as insufficient.

As a result of the conflict and the isolation of parts of the country, surveillance of the epidemic and prevention, care and treatment interventions have been compromised. While adverse circumstances such as violence and displacement may affect prevalence, the sentinel surveillance survey of 2004 did not confirm this. Instead, it reported a non-significant drop in prevalence between 2002 and 2004, although this survey covered only urban areas. Yet it was noteworthy that more than half of all the pregnant women covered by the survey were between 15 and 24 years old, a substantially larger proportion of young women than at the last survey. Three sites in formerly besieged areas reported that a quarter of all pregnant women were aged 15–19 years. At the same time, there were increased infection rates in this age group, which was also a group with very low education levels. This suggests that the conflict has had a profound impact on young, uneducated women[1].

---

[1] *Ivory Coast National Report, 2007.*

Substantial financial resources are available through the U.S. President's Emergency Plan for AIDS Relief (PEPFAR) and the Global Fund (and potentially the World Bank's Multi-Country HIV/AIDS Programme for Africa [MAP]), greatly assisting the country in its efforts to achieve universal access to prevention, treatment and care. With continued support from the UN system, bilateral donors and its own national resources, the country has, in theory, the means to continue and scale up its efforts. However, beyond the unstable political situation, the most important challenges in fighting the epidemic are related to the lack of harmonization and coordination, causing, for example, shortages of antiretrovirals, in spite of both PEPFAR and Global Fund money. These deficiencies have also postponed the disbursement of money for Phase 2 of the Global Fund proposal. The lack of coordination comes at a cost.

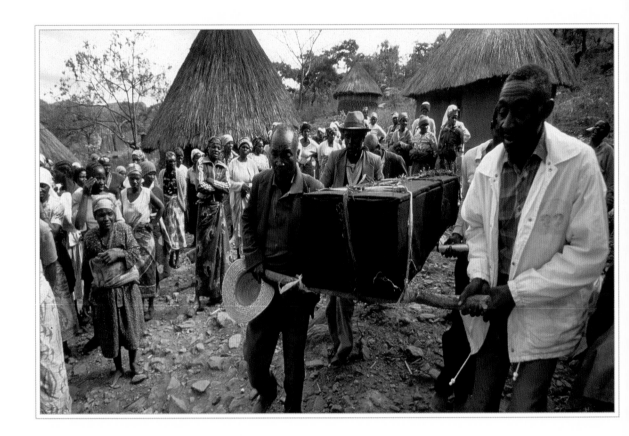

In Nyakomba village, Zambia, villagers offer their respect at the funeral of a man dead from AIDS. By 2000 a major change in attitude to AIDS would lead to much greater political commitment to action. But already several millions had died from AIDS-related illnesses.
UNAIDS/ M.Szulc-Kryzanowski

Chapter 5:
The end of the beginning:
a clear global mandate, 2000-2001

By the end of 1999, about 26 million adults and children – two thirds of whom were in Africa – were living with HIV. More than 9,000 new infections occurred every day, or over six every minute. More than 20% of these were among young people aged 15–24. Already, there were in excess of 5.9 million orphans in Africa because of AIDS[1]. Global expenditure on AIDS in 2000 was US$ 1359 million. In 2001, it was US$ 1623 million[2].

The new millennium brought a major change in attitudes to AIDS and, over the next two years, the epidemic and its impact became a key item on the agenda of global leaders and organizations. On 10 January 2000, the United Nations Security Council discussed AIDS in Africa as a major human security concern as well as an obstacle to development – it was also the first time the Security Council had considered a health issue as a relevant subject for debate. The Vice-President of the United States of America, Al Gore, chaired the debate while the speakers included the UNAIDS Executive Director, the UN Secretary-General and the President of the World Bank, James Wolfensohn.

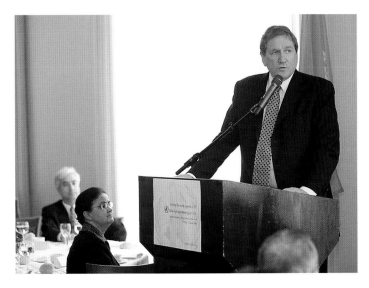

*Former United States Ambassador to the UN, Richard Holbrooke
UNAIDS/J. Rae*

The session had been engineered by Richard Holbrooke, United States Ambassador to the UN since August 1999, in close consultation with UNAIDS Executive Director Peter Piot, and in part as a result of visiting Africa the previous November in his capacity as a Security Council member. Holbrooke returned from this trip convinced that AIDS was a major global problem and should be deliberated at the Security Council. Even before that visit, Piot had discussed the idea of a Security Council session with Holbrooke (it had been part of the strategic road map planned at the Talloires, France, retreat in 1998), but he had not anticipated the speed with which Holbrooke could work. Although Holbrooke met with some resistance, he was determined that the matter should be on the Security Council's agenda because, as he explained to his aide, R P Eddy, 'RP, one of the only UN entities that ever gets anything

---

[1] UNAIDS/WHO, November 2007
[2] UNAIDS Resource Tracking Consortium, July 2004.

done is the Security Council. That's where decisions are made, that's where attention is focused'[3]. So he, his staff and UNAIDS Secretariat staff worked very hard between Christmas and New Year – writing background documents for the meeting, Piot recalls, "...but we took everybody by surprise". Holbrooke did all the political work, including involving Gore, and UNAIDS provided the background, arguments and evidence.

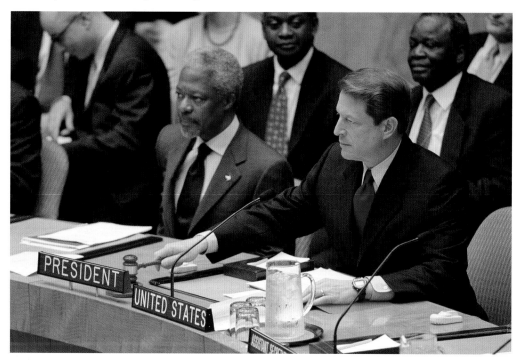

AIDS debated at the United Nations Security Council

Former UN Secretary-General Kofi Annan told the Security Council that the impact of AIDS in Africa was no less destructive than that of warfare itself. By overwhelming the continent's health services, by creating millions of orphans, and by decimating the numbers of health workers and teachers, AIDS was causing socioeconomic crises which in turn threatened political stability. Later that year, another session of the Security Council would lead to work on preventing HIV among peacekeepers and uniformed services.

The Security Council debate brought AIDS to the forefront of the global political agenda. According to Piot[4]: "It opened so many doors, top leaders told me, it was debated in the Security Council, it must be a serious problem. Ridiculous, but I got that sort of response". The momentum would now build. As Jim Sherry, then Director of the Programme Development and Coordination Group, said, "the fuse was lit".

Here with UN Secretary-General Kofi Annan, Al Gore, Vice President of the USA, chaired the first debate on AIDS as a major security issue at the UN Security Council in January 2000.
UN Photo

---

[3] Behrman G (2004). *The Invisible People.* New York, Free Press.
[4] Interview with Peter Piot for *Frontline: the Age of AIDS*, PBS TV, 2007.

Piot recalled: "There had been a massive failure of leadership in all sectors in tackling AIDS, but this started to change around 2000. UNAIDS was a key catalyst in this change, and maybe that is all we've contributed". The greatest change took place among African leaders; it happened more slowly among those in Asia, in the donor countries and in Eastern Europe.

Mbeki's involvement with AIDS "denialists" causes consternation

"There had been a massive failure of leadership in all sectors in tackling AIDS, but this started to change around 2000. UNAIDS was a key catalyst in this change, and maybe that is all we've contributed".

One African leader took a very independent and controversial stance on the epidemic. There was consternation when news broke in March that President Thabo Mbeki of South Africa was conferring with AIDS dissident researchers who did not believe HIV to be the cause of AIDS. By 2000, an estimated 4.3 million South Africans were living with HIV – the highest number in any country in the world.

Mbeki had written a letter on 3 April 2000 to the Secretary-General, copied to United Kingdom Prime Minister Tony Blair and US President Bill Clinton, strongly questioning the efficacy of drugs such as AZT, and asking why the pharmaceutical companies were prepared to pour millions into drugs while failing to address such contextual factors as poverty and lack of education. Many interpreted his stance as reinforcing the views of those who questioned the link between HIV and AIDS.

Apart from his unwillingness to publicly acknowledge the scientifically proven link between HIV and AIDS, Mbeki's comments were fair. Perhaps at the heart of his belief was his assertion in the letter that: 'It is obvious that whatever lessons we have to and may draw from the West about the grave issue of HIV/AIDS, a simple superimposition of Western experience on African reality would be absurd and illogical. Such proceeding would constitute a criminal betrayal of our responsibility to our own people'.

Elhadj As Sy, then team leader of the UNAIDS Eastern and Southern Africa Inter-Country Team based in Pretoria, consulted with Piot. A private meeting between Mbeki and Piot was quietly arranged at the President's home in Pretoria one Saturday evening in early April. As Sy stressed that it was essential, if the situation was to be 'salvaged', to ensure the media was not involved. Piot flew to Johannesburg and was met by As Sy who drove him straight to Mbeki's house in Pretoria. Piot recalled: "I thought, let's talk. That's my preferred approach when there's a problem. We had a very long meeting that went on well into the night. I tried to make a case that HIV causes AIDS, that AIDS is a big issue for development in Southern Africa, and I obviously failed".

In early May, the South African Government organized a two-day meeting of a Presidential AIDS Panel of scientists to debate the cause of HIV. Awa Coll-Seck, UNAIDS Director of Policy, Strategy and Research, and previously an academic, was invited to join.

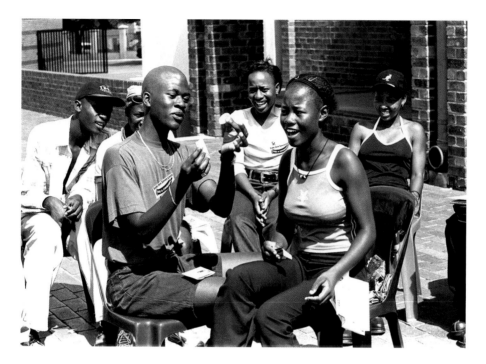

There have been many projects to educate young people about prevention. Here, in a Soweto Youth Centre, young men and women are shown how to use condoms.
UNAIDS/G.Pirozzi

The panel was divided into two camps; those like Coll-Seck who argued that HIV caused AIDS and the others, the so-called AIDS dissidents, arguing against the HIV case. It was, she explained, impossible to reconcile the two.

Mbeki's stance has had profound repercussions on the response in South Africa where, despite high prevalence, the government has been very slow in providing antiretroviral treatment. At the same time, there are some impressive HIV prevention programmes in South Africa – especially for young people – that are replicated as best practice in other countries, and some excellent workplace programmes providing prevention and treatment in major corporations.

In the USA, Clinton had been slow to mobilize a response to AIDS in the developing world. It was not until April 2000 that his administration formally designated the disease a threat to US national security, a threat 'that could topple foreign governments, touch off ethnic wars and undo decades of work in building free-market democracies abroad'[5]. The National Security Council had been instructed to make a rapid reassessment of the government's efforts – the first time it had been involved in combating an infectious disease. Earlier that year, in February, a White House interagency working group had been formed. In May 2000, Clinton signed an Executive Order which aimed to help make AIDS-related drugs and medical technologies more accessible and affordable in sub-Saharan Africa.

---

[5] Gellman B (2000). 'AIDS is declared threat to US national security'. *Washington Post*, 30 April.

Fighting for AIDS treatment in South Africa

The story of South Africa's response to AIDS is complex. Before Mbeki's discovery of, and involvement with, the AIDS denialists' viewpoint, the South African Government passed its Medicines and Related Substances Control Act in the autumn of 1997, allowing it to override patents and produce and import generic drugs such as antiretrovirals. But by February 1998, 39 drug companies had filed suit in Pretoria's High Court to stop South Africa from manufacturing generic drugs including antiretrovirals. For four years, the legislation was held up and South Africa was placed on a US list that threatened trade penalties. Bart Gellman wrote in the *Washington Post*: 'What for South Africa was an exploding health emergency … the United States treated mainly as a problem of trade'.

UNAIDS and the UN worked behind the scenes to try to persuade the drug companies to withdraw their lawsuit which, apart from anything else, was giving these companies terrible media coverage.

A particularly influential voice in this debate belonged to the activist group, the Treatment Action Campaign (TAC). Founded on 10 December 1998 (Human Rights Day) by South African activist Zackie Achmat, it campaigned for equitable access to affordable treatment for all people with HIV and to reduce new HIV infections. TAC supported the government's Medicines Act against the pharmaceutical companies, but soon there was growing hostility between the government and TAC. The government refused to provide the drug nevirapine for preventing mother-to-child transmission of HIV. This drug reduces the risk of transmission by 50%. The government was taken to court by TAC and, eventually, in July 2002, a landmark ruling by the Constitutional Court ordered the government to remove restrictions, to permit and facilitate the provision of nevirapine, and to extend testing and counselling services at hospitals and clinics in the public health sector.

Achmat explained the need for TAC: "AIDS service organizations play an important role … but we need to recognize that … the epidemic is going to be far broader, it needs a far broader response, and [it] needs to become the job of the ANC [African National Congress], the Communist party, the head of Anglo American, the head of the corner shop to understand what the issues are".

TAC's next move was to demand antiretroviral treatment for all those in need. Public demonstrations and a civil disobedience campaign followed but the government pleaded lack of funding. Eventually, permission was granted to international generic manufacturers Chemical, Industrial and Pharmaceutical Laboratories (CIPLA) and Ranbaxy to import generics and, finally, in November 2003, the Cabinet announced a national treatment roll-out plan to provide comprehensive care and treatment for people living with HIV and to help strengthen the country's national health system.

Planning for the United Nations General Assembly Special Session on AIDS – an historic first

In January 2000, at the UN Security Council debate on AIDS, the Ukrainian ambassador to the UN had called for a Special Session on AIDS. A UN General Assembly Special Session (UNGASS), in which the entire UN focuses on one issue, is called to address matters of the greatest global significance. This would be the first time a Special Session addressed a health issue, reflecting a growing consensus in the UN (and beyond) that AIDS was much more than just a health issue, rather a major threat to global human and economic development.

UNGASS was really a high point for everyone, a small team working so hard.

Preparation meetings started in May 2000. As Sy moved to New York to head the UNAIDS office there: he was immediately thrown into preparing for UNGASS the following June. He explained: "Normally, if you prepare for a Special Session, you have three to four years, regional consultations – a whole infrastructure. Here you had a year where everything needed to happen and [so we had to] communicate a sense of urgency to move the whole agenda".

In the spring of 2000, Kathleen Cravero joined UNAIDS as Deputy Executive Director. Her first impression was of a brilliant, talented but rather anarchic group of people. Unlike most of the UNAIDS staff, Cravero was a UN person through and through, having worked at the United Nations Children's Fund (UNICEF), the World Health Organization (WHO) and the United Nations Development Programme (UNDP) for many years, often at country level. Part of her role was working with Cosponsors. Cravero's first major task was to organize UNGASS – this was all-consuming from September 2000 until the actual event in June 2001. "UNGASS was really a high point for everyone, a small team working so hard".

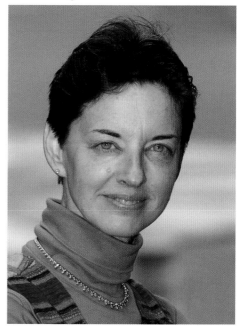

In the spring of 2000, Kathleen Cravero joined UNAIDS as Deputy Executive Director
UNAIDS

Political drama at the Durban International AIDS Conference

Another high point at the start of the new millennium came in July 2000; the 13th International AIDS Conference was held in Durban, South Africa. For the first time, this major AIDS gathering was being held in a low-income country and, specifically, the country with the largest number of people infected with HIV. Significantly, given Mbeki's views on the cause of AIDS, a week before the conference, on 6 July, the highly respected journal *Science* published a statement later known as the Durban Declaration. It was signed by 5000 scientists around the world, affirming that empirical evidence for the link between HIV and AIDS was 'clear-cut, exhaustive and unambiguous'. The theme of the conference was 'Break the silence', emphasizing how much stigma, denial and discrimination were hindering attempts at prevention, care and treatment. The conference confirmed the growing politicization of the response. At the first session, held in a cricket stadium, participants eagerly awaited Mbeki's opening speech, but any hopes for a change in his views on HIV were dashed. In his opening speech, Mbeki used the occasion to reiterate his belief that extreme poverty is the leading killer across Africa.

Reading extensively from a World Health report, Mbeki said: "The world's biggest killer and the greatest cause of ill health and suffering across the globe, including South Africa, is extreme poverty". He added: "As I listened and heard the whole story told about our own country, it seemed to me that we could not blame everything on a single virus".

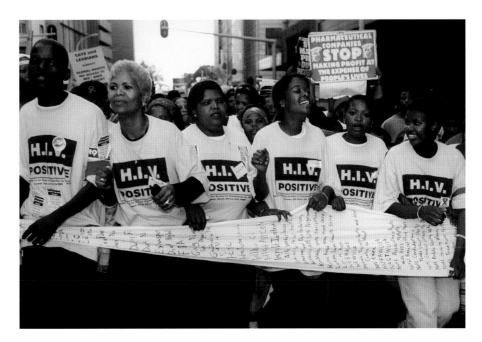

At the 13th International AIDS Conference in Durban, South Africa, delegates including members of the Treatment Action Campaign demonstrated for better access to HIV treatment.
Panos / Gisele Wulfsohn

Piot spoke immediately after Mbeki, which was difficult, as he had to hide his disappointment. He was also making an historic plea. For the first time, he was calling for billions rather than millions – US$ 3 billion a year to be precise – to take basic measures in Africa to deal with the disease. And US$ 10 billion more each year to provide Africa with the standard drugs used in the developed world. US$ 3 billion is 10 times what was then being spent on AIDS in Africa.

"We need billions, not millions, to fight AIDS in this world. We can't fight an epidemic of this magnitude with peanuts". He recalled that his move from the m[illions] word to the b[illions] word speech was very badly received by donor nations. All they said was, "forget it; you're dreaming; you're irresponsible, it's never going to happen". He also called on some of the wealthiest nations to cancel the debt of many of the hardest hit African countries so that some of the US$ 15 billion spent on servicing debt every year could instead be dedicated to health care and HIV prevention.

Commenting on the Durban event, a UNAIDS report later summarized: 'No one who attended the conference, and particularly the closing ceremony, had any doubts that a line had been crossed in the global response to the epidemic. The alliance of science, people living with AIDS, community groups, the UN, governments and civil society demonstrated just how potent a united stand against HIV/AIDS can be. The conference … recognized that AIDS is a crisis of governance. It also recognized that failure to apply the tools and resources available is a political issue. Leadership saves lives … The Durban conference was critical in mapping out the need for an immensely increased resource flow'[6].

Durban was also the conference that put AIDS treatment for all on the global agenda. "It was the turning-point for the social movement for HIV treatment access for all", said Julian Fleet, then Senior Adviser for care and public policy at UNAIDS. Before Durban, many govern-ments and basically all international development agencies and donors had focused only, or mainly, on prevention. South Africa's TAC had started the conference with a fierce rally and a march, demanding access to drugs. It ended the conference by announcing a 'defiance campaign' to smuggle in Fluconazole [a drug to treat severe fungal opportunistic infections] from India, where a company manufactured a generic version costing about one seventh of what Pfizer charged for its patented version in South Africa.

Edwin Cameron, a South African High Court judge, openly gay and openly HIV-positive, gave a moving keynote address at the conference. "I exist as a living embodiment of the iniquity of drug availability and access in Africa. This is not because, in an epidemic in which the heaviest burden of infection and disease are borne by women, I am a male; nor because, on a continent in which the vectors of infection have overwhelmingly been heterosexual, I am proudly gay; nor even because, in a history fraught with racial injustice, I was born white".

He continued: "My presence here embodies the injustices of AIDS in Africa because, on a continent in which 290 million Africans survive on less than one dollar a day, I can afford monthly medication costs of about US$ 400 per month … I am here because I can afford to pay for life itself".

Gregg Gonsalves of Gay Men's Health Crisis in New York looks back: "Durban was a paradigm shift [for] … thinking about global access issues. People came back transformed by that experience and by the calls from the Treatment Action Campaign and Edwin Cameron and others for treatment. It changed the landscape. Northern activists became more involved in the issues facing our colleagues in the South".

Paulo Teixeira, Director of Brazil's National AIDS Programme, came to Durban bearing a message from his government. "We are not able to be the drug supplier for Africa", he said, "but Brazil has offered to share everything it has learned …".

"We need billions, not millions, to fight AIDS in this world. We can't fight an epidemic of this magnitude with peanuts".

---

[6] UNAIDS (2001). *Executive Director's Report to the 11th Meeting of the UNAIDS PCB*, May/June. Geneva, UNAIDS.

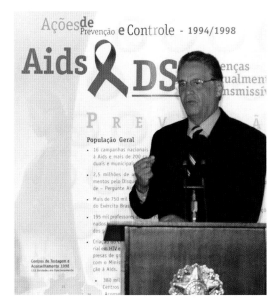

*Former President
Fernando Henrique
Cardoso of Brazil.
UNAIDS*

"We're keen on this partnership", said Ayanda Ntsaluba, the South African Director General of Health, adding that a team from his country would be heading to Brazil "very soon"[7].

Prompted by a strong activist movement, Brazil had pioneered access to antiretroviral treatment to all in need of it. Even though Brazil is a medium-income country, the cost of branded drugs was too high so it started making generic versions of HIV drugs in its own laboratories. For these drugs, the prices tumbled by more than 70% in four years. By 2000, Brazil's AIDS death rate had been halved, and HIV-related hospital admissions had fallen by 80%.

Working with uniformed services and peacekeepers to prevent HIV transmission

Following Durban, the political momentum gathered pace. On 17 July, at another UN Security Council session, AIDS was debated again and Resolution 1308 was passed, requesting the UN to develop further AIDS prevention and education for all peacekeepers as part of pre-deployment orientation and ongoing training. This resolution would lead to developing UNAIDS' work on prevention among peacekeepers, military personnel and other uniformed services worldwide, under the leadership of Ulf Kristofferson (who had previously worked with UNICEF and the Office of the United Nations High Commissioner for Refugees) as Director of its office on AIDS, Security and Humanitarian Response.

It had been clear for some years that armed forces, including UN peacekeepers, were at risk of contracting and spreading HIV. These young people often spend long periods of time away from their families; they are more likely to have multiple partners and unprotected sex, condom use is often incorrect, inconsistent – or entirely lacking[8]. Sex industries often grow around military bases in response to demand.

As a major UNAIDS publication on AIDS and the military described[9], during peacetime, rates of sexually transmitted infections among armed forces are generally two to five times higher than in comparable civilian populations; in times of conflict, they can be more than 50 times higher. But there are exceptions; in Senegal, for example, rates are lower among soldiers than among civilians.

[7] Schoofs M (2000). 'Turning point. The International AIDS Conference makes a commitment to saving third world lives'. *Village Voice*, 19 July.

[8] UNAIDS (Third Revised Reprint, 2005). *On the Front Line: A Review of Policies and Programmes to Address AIDS among Peacekeepers and Uniformed Services.* Geneva, UNAIDS.

[9] Ibid.

114

Young military personnel are especially vulnerable. Half of all new sexually transmitted infections occur among 15 to 24-year-olds, which is the most sexually active age group. Yet education of this age group (especially uniformed services) promises to slow the spread of sexually transmitted infections, including HIV.

UNAIDS' work with the uniformed services recognizes the importance of establishing strong, sustainable partnerships with security forces as well as with other relevant partners. It is also vital to obtain political commitment at the highest level, from ministries of defence and of the interior.

Kristofferson initially found this task challenging, as countries were understandably reluctant to provide prevalence figures among the uniformed services. "It's very strategic information. If I were Minister of Defence would I give that to you? It was very hard to get senior leadership in the military to admit that they had a problem".

However, he and his colleagues persisted and obtained results. A successful pilot programme in Ukraine led to the development and institutionalization of a formal HIV and drug use prevention education programme for the military. UNAIDS has now helped to implement similar programmes in 106 countries, reaching around 7.5 million young men and women in uniform, estimated Kristofferson.

It was very hard to get senior leadership in the military to admit that they had a problem.

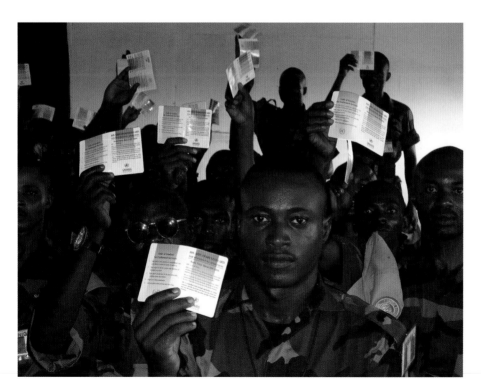

In every country soldiers and peacekeepers are at risk of HIV infection. Soldiers like these in Nigeria have been given cards with basic information on AIDS.
UNAIDS

UNAIDS has developed an additional range of tools to support national programmes, including a comprehensive programming guide and peer education kit. An AIDS Awareness Card strategy includes three distinct cards targeting peacekeepers, uniformed personnel and UN employees with basic information on HIV prevention, and a pocket to carry a condom. Kristofferson explained that he had the idea for the card during the first session of the Security Council meeting in 2000, when Holbrooke took the floor and expressed his frustration. He explained that Holbrooke "held up a 46-page manual on HIV and said, 'I don't understand this, do you?' and I said 'No'". He said: "You can't bring a 46-page manual to a peace-keeper who comes from the Chittagong hill tracts or the outskirts of Nairobi with a very rudimentary educational background".

An HIV/AIDS awareness card in Spanish. They have been produced in 18 languages.

The peacekeeping and uniformed services cards are now available in 18 languages, covering approximately 90% of the nationalities serving in peacekeeping operations worldwide. Kristofferson estimates that even though 1.2 million have been produced, they cannot meet the demand.

Kristofferson explained the importance of seeking political partnerships at the highest level: "We started seeking partnership agreements with political parties – Ministers of Defence, Justice and so on – and today we have signed partnership agreements with 48 governments around the world where they have committed to take part or the whole of our peer education guide as part of the curricula for training police, soldiers and peace-keepers".

In addition to the growing engagement of Member States, leading regional bodies are increasingly acknowledging the need to integrate information on HIV prevention into the operations of uniformed services, including the African Union, the Caribbean Community (CARICOM), the Commonwealth of Independent States and the North Atlantic Treaty Organization.

116

Raising money as well as awareness

For about two years, the heads of both UNAIDS and WHO had been discussing and planning with a range of partners how to raise the enormous sums needed to provide adequate care, support and treatment for people living with HIV in low-income countries (as well as for other serious infectious diseases). Some donors were clearly open to a major initiative, but serious planning and hard negotiations were needed.

In July 2000, the communiqué of the meeting of the Group of Eight (G8) nations in Okinawa, Japan, announced an ambitious plan of action on infectious diseases, acknowledging that health is central to economic development. It recognized that of all the communicable diseases linked to poverty, AIDS has the largest impact on individuals and societies. The seeds were sown for what would eventually become the Global Fund to Fight AIDS, Tuberculosis and Malaria.

At a follow-up G8 meeting in December 2000, several donors, including Canada, the European Commission and the UK, said it was time to move forward. Until this point, the European Union had not shown much political leadership in responding to AIDS, although it had been a

Eastern Europe has seen a steep rise in HIV infections over the past few years. In Kiev, Ukraine, a worker with a mobile needles exchange project hands out clean needles and information in the street as part of an HIV prevention programme for injecting drug users.
Gideon Mendel for the International HIV/ AIDS Alliance/Corbis

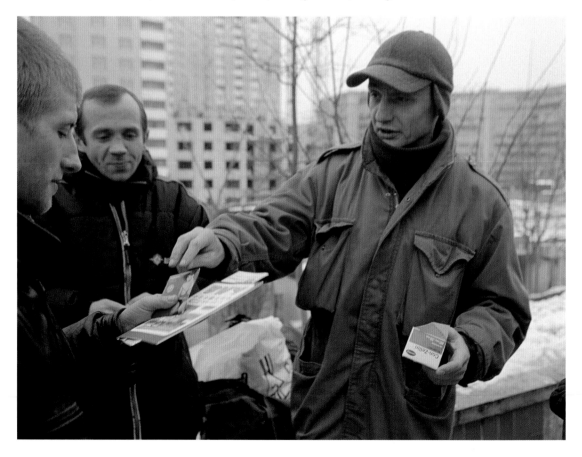

major donor in the early years of the epidemic. But, in September, the European Commission had convened a high-level Round Table meeting on communicable diseases and poverty reduction, chaired by Romano Prodi, President of the Commission, and cosponsored by the UNAIDS Secretariat and WHO. At the Round Table it was decided to focus on AIDS, tuberculosis and malaria. A first step was to design a new plan of action to tackle these diseases.

"The World Bank talking about it helped make AIDS a mainstream development topic".

On 8 September, at the UN Millennium Summit that led to the UN Millennium Declaration, 158 heads of state and government from countries heavily affected and others less so, referred to the fight against AIDS. Several used their precious five minutes to speak exclusively about AIDS. Many referred to AIDS as one of the greatest challenges in the twenty-first century. The UN Secretary-General's report had a major section on promotion of health and combating AIDS.

The World Bank takes action: the Multi–Country HIV/AIDS Programme for Africa

Action was needed, not just words – as well as significant funding. Although certain World Bank staff had been very involved with, and supportive of, UNAIDS right from the outset, the Bank's response in terms of funding had been disappointing to many of its staff as well as those outside. This was partly because of the lack of firm leadership on the issue but also, in fairness, because countries were not themselves proposing projects on HIV/AIDS for loans – a further sign of leaders' denial.

Not everyone at the Bank's head office was convinced of the pandemic's importance[10]. Although the Bank's World Development Report in 1993 acknowledged that by 2000, AIDS might be killing 1.6 million people every year, it also noted that tobacco might kill two million annually (which, of course, was true).

As Keith Hansen, now Sector Manager of Health, Nutrition & Population for Latin America and the Caribbean at the World Bank, explained: "As late as the mid-1990s, the Bank was nowhere near to bringing the full brunt of its resources and influence to bear on the epidemic … It was really only in the late 1990s that … the Bank became engaged at an institutional level". As the Bank's lending for HIV/AIDS fell (from US$ 67 million in 1994) to US$ 41.7 million in 1997, Debrework Zewdie cautioned in 1998 that the progress of the last 20 to 30 years 'on the development front in Africa is now in jeopardy'[11].

The year 1999 brought change at the Bank, partly because of the advocacy of two Bank officials, Zewdie and Hans Binswanger (the latter made it known at a meeting that he himself was positive), mainly because of the increasingly disturbing data coming from UNAIDS and its

---

[10] Mallaby S (2004). *The World's Banker*. New York, Penguin Books.
[11] Behrman (2004).

partners. The most important step, said Hansen, was that the Bank should wake up to the fact that AIDS was a development threat and a development issue. "We began to force it on the agenda with conversations with countries that were not raising it with us … and [to realize] that we had a unique role to play in making AIDS legitimate to discuss as a development issue, not just as a public health concern or a humanitarian problem".

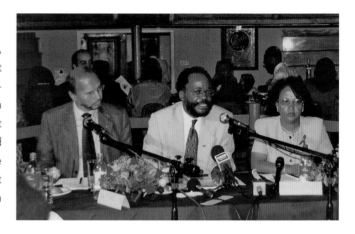

Launch of the World Bank HIV/AIDS Strategic Plan. (left to right) UNAIDS Executive Director Peter Piot; World Bank Vice President, Africa Region, Callisto Madavo; World Bank Director, Global HIV/AIDS Programme Debrework Zewdie. Lusaka, Zambia, September 1999. UNAIDS

In March 1999, Zewdie's group produced its own manifesto for action, and in May she won her campaign to create a new department for AIDS in the African region. The President of the Bank, James Wolfensohn, 'woke up to the scale of the pandemic'[12], and in September 2000 the Bank's board approved a Multi-Country HIV/AIDS Programme for Africa (MAP). The initial sum authorized was US$ 500 million, and another half billion was promised as soon as necessary.

Hansen explained: "The emergence of MAP changed the scale and tone of how we dealt with AIDS … in Africa, at least, it was clearly the Bank's top priority". The Bank expected that it would take about three years for the US$ 500 million to be committed and to get countries interested. It took less than 18 months. Hansen explained: "Both our own reviews and independent evaluations have concluded that the sheer weight, the prominence, the novelty of the MAP, helped break down the barriers and the denial that had existed. And countries that previously wouldn't even discuss it in public were suddenly lining up to get support from this. The World Bank talking about it helped make AIDS a mainstream development topic".

Launch of International Partnership against AIDS in Africa

In early December 2000, the Second Africa Development Forum took place in Addis Ababa. Organized by the UN Economic Commission for Africa together with a number of UN agencies, it brought together more than 1500 African leaders, policy makers, activist organizations and academics. The focus was on 'Leadership at all levels to overcome HIV/AIDS'. Speaking at the Forum, Piot coined the phrase 'social immune system'. Reflecting on a recent visit to Uganda, he said: "… I met with women who are preparing their children to be orphans, organizing everything from memory books to sustainable arrangements for micro-credit. These women are truly leaders … There is no escaping the reality that AIDS can only be curbed through a sustained social mobilization that systematically reduces vulnerability … Reducing vulnerability to AIDS and its impact is about creating a social vaccine or, better still, a social immune system that continually learns, builds and rebuilds itself in protecting against the impact of AIDS".

---

[12] Ibid.

"I let people see that I'm not an HIV statistic but a dynamic young woman full of life and with dignity who happens to have HIV infection".

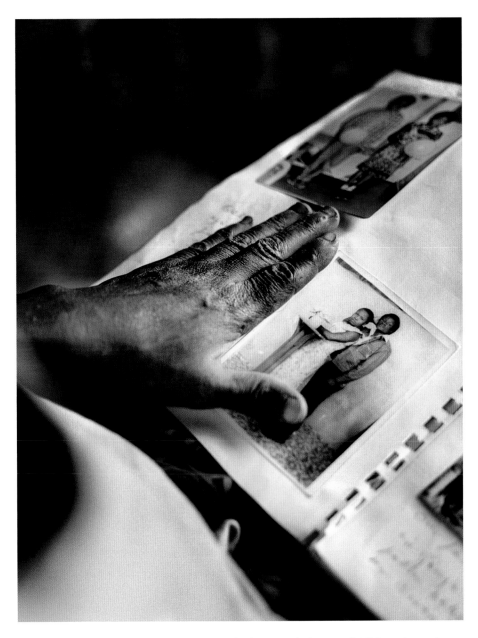

In Uganda and many other countries, mothers dying from AIDS-related illnesses create memory books for their children
Panos/Alfredo Caliz

A cornerstone of the Forum was the principle that people living with HIV are themselves a vital asset for creating any such 'social immune system'[13]. A young, positive woman, Charlotte Mjele, said: 'If you treat yourself as a shameful HIV *victim*, others will be happy to treat you that way as well. But if you treat yourself as a positive *role model*, they'll accept you and respect you. I let people see that I'm not an HIV statistic but a dynamic young woman full of life and with dignity who happens to have HIV infection'[14].

[13] Ibid.
[14] Ibid.

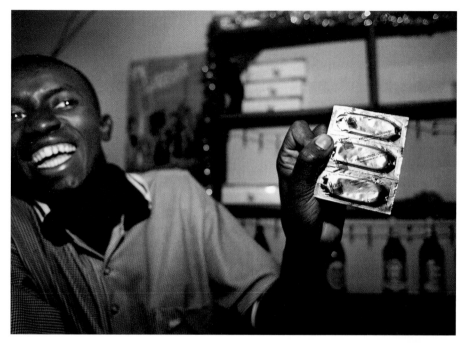

A major task of the newly established International Partnership against AIDS in Africa was to tackle the stigma of AIDS and promote prevention, including condoms – here being sold in Kampala, Uganda.
Panos / Sven Torfinn

Annan formally launched the International Partnership against AIDS in Africa (IPAA) at the Forum, saying that "… the IPAA is the concrete expression of the continent's resolve to act in new ways and with renewed vigour against AIDS".

The formal outcome was the *African Consensus and Plan of Action: Leadership to Overcome HIV/AIDS*. As with all these meetings, the event itself was only the culmination of an extensive preparation process. It was preceded by 23 consultations across Africa, involving governments, the UN, the private sector and civil society, as well as national workshops. UNAIDS had collaborated closely with the UN Economic Commission for Africa.

The regional strategy produced for the Africa Partnership helped to lay the foundations for the global strategies debated and, to a considerable extent agreed, at UNGASS in 2001.

Since 1999, there had been significant progress in increasing African ownership of the Partnership and mobilizing high-ranking political support. The King of Swaziland opened Parliament by describing AIDS as a 'national disaster' and a National HIV/AIDS Crisis Management Committee was established. The Presidents of Ghana, Malawi, Mozambique, Nigeria and Zimbabwe established high-powered AIDS Commissions. The President of Burkina Faso created a National Solidarity Fund and the government was developing AIDS-related initiatives to be funded through debt relief initiative mechanisms.

Policy making: increasing access to treatment

The Drug Access Initiative had, in a limited way, proved that antiretroviral treatment could be provided in places where health services were poorly resourced, and at much lower prices from generic companies. Now there was a need to scale up.

In 1998, WHO's new Director-General, Gro Harlem Brundtland, had joined Piot in a serious dialogue with the pharmaceutical companies to discuss the challenges of providing treatment in the developing world: 'Between 1998 and 2000, Brundtland and Piot partly pressured, partly enticed the company leaders towards a much wider use of differential pricing for antiretrovirals'[15].

In January 2000, the Director-General of WHO had given her speech to the policy-making Executive Board. She stated, "… squarely put, the drugs are in the North and the disease is in the South. This kind of inequity cannot continue … I wish to invite the pharmaceutical industry to join us now in taking a fresh and constructive look at how we can considerably increase access to relevant drugs".

It is worth noting that there was divergence of opinion among the different pharmaceutical companies on the issue of lowering drug prices. At an internal meeting, the Chief Executive Officer of Roche had said: "We have got to get off the subject of prices – they are not the issue"[16]. But Jeffrey Sturchio of Merck & Co, Inc, and Ben Plumley of GlaxoSmithKline felt that the only way to turn perceptions around was to make something affirmative happen by slashing the prices of HIV medicines[17].

In February 2000, the Executive Director of UNAIDS and the Director-General of WHO had a meeting with Ray Gilmartin, CEO of Merck & Co, Inc, during the World Economic Forum at Davos.

Gilmartin was not very positive. Piot recalls: "We said, 'well this was a waste of our time; nothing happened … we'll try again'". But a few weeks later, Ken Weg from Bristol-Myers Squibb and then a representative from Merck & Co, Inc contacted them; now they did want to talk about the price of drugs.

After many months of meetings, the drug companies offered to cut prices and work on a new initiative. As Julia Cleves, Director of UNAIDS Executive Director's office, explained, this offer was initially regarded with some scepticism by the UN. A period of intensive activity ensued which came down to negotiating a joint statement of intent between the UN and the pharmaceutical companies.

---

[15] Schwartländer B, Grubb I, Perriëns J (2007). 'The 10-year struggle to provide antiretroviral treatment to people with HIV in the developing world'. *The Lancet*, 368.

[16] Gellman B (2000). 'A turning point that left millions behind'. *Washington Post*, 28 December.

[17] Ibid.

122

An agreement was finally reached in April 2000. 'Gilmartin said that the five major pharmaceutical companies had committed in principle to substantial discounts on their AIDS medicines in poor countries. The conditions of their offer, broadly drafted, included burden-sharing by governments and reinforced protection of the industry's patents'[18].

In May, the Accelerating Access Initiative (AAI) was announced. A UNAIDS press release summarized the purpose of the effort: 'A new dialogue has begun between five pharmaceutical companies (Boehringer Ingelheim, Bristol-Myers Squibb, GlaxoWellcome, Merck & Co, Inc and F. Hoffman-La Roche) and UN organizations to explore ways to accelerate and improve the provision of HIV/AIDS-related care and treatment in developing countries'[19].

However, at the World Health Assembly, it became clear that many ministers of health from African states did not view the new initiative as the exciting development it appeared to be to UNAIDS staff. Cleves explained that an emergency session had to be called, where several ministers attacked UNAIDS for "going behind their backs" and negotiating with the pharmaceutical companies; in fact, for attacking their sovereignty. Several meetings and papers followed in order to deal with the surprising negativity of these ministers.

As Joseph Perriëns, now Director of AIDS Medicines and Diagnostic Services at WHO, explained, unlike the Drug Access Initiative, AAI offered, fairly openly, discounted or differentially priced drugs to a named series of developing countries; that is, to almost all of the least developed countries plus, in some cases, all of sub-Saharan Africa.

Some months after the AAI was launched, the prices of the first-line drugs offered within the discussions between countries and the pharmaceutical companies dropped very significantly to about US$ 1200 per treatment year. Sturchio remembered that: "We lowered our prices by two-thirds in May of 2000 and began to see a sharp increase in the number of people, even at those prices, who were being treated in Africa". The new initiative was not easy to administer. Roll-out was slow, and was hindered by the fact that each of the 39 countries had to negotiate prices and conditions with the pharmaceutical industry[20].

In a separate effort, Lieve Fransen, HIV/AIDS Coordinator at the European Commission, called for representatives from the AIDS Coalition to Unleash Power (ACT UP) and Médecins

"To be sure, they were only first steps but they were steps and ultimately they made a difference. What I hated was that if you didn't succeed 100%, the NGOs rubbished it".

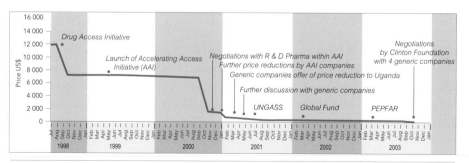

Prices (US$/year) of first-line antiretroviral regimen in Uganda: 1998-2003.
UNAIDS

---

[18] Ibid.
[19] UNAIDS (2000). Press Release, 11 May. Geneva, UNAIDS.
[20] Schwartländer, Grubb, Perriëns (2007).

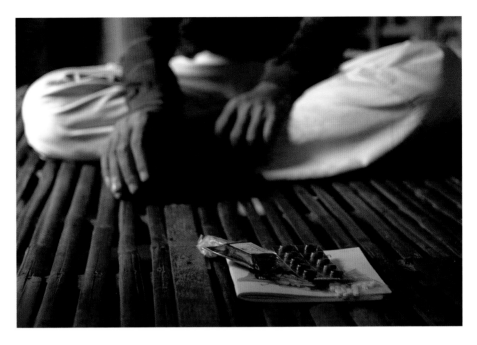

*Still far too many
positive people
in 2000 were
unable to afford
antiretroviral
treatment.
UNAIDS and its
partners worked
closely with some
of the major drug
companies to bring
down drug prices.
UNAIDS/
O.O'Hanlon*

Sans Frontières, generic manufacturers such as CIPLA and Chief Executive Officers from the seven largest pharmaceutical companies to sit down together with the leaders of WHO and UNAIDS and agree on a tiered price structure for the treatment of HIV, tuberculosis and malaria[21]. In September 2000, the Chief Executive Officers expressed their willingness to launch such a scheme and CIPLA announced the availability of generic, first-line antiretrovirals at US$ 350 per patient per year.

There is considerable disagreement between the activists and others over the effectiveness of the AAI in reducing drug prices. Médecins Sans Frontières claims nothing really changed until generic manufacturers began to reduce prices. After the AAI agreement was announced, Bernard Pécoul from Médecins Sans Frontières commented: "The elephant has laboured mightily and brought forth a mouse".

As Cleves later commented, any efforts made by the UN were likely to be denounced as in some way inadequate.

It was easy to underestimate the steps taken by the drug companies, given their culture and track record. According to Sturchio, the AAI helped to highlight the feasibility and urgency of treatment delivery to key decision-makers within the pharmaceutical industry. "While everybody on the outside was jeering that this was too little, too late and the prices were still too high, the reality of the AAI was different. It wasn't until some of the senior people at our companies could see that it was possible to work with UNAIDS and WHO and other agencies, that the pharmaceutical industry could make progress on actually implementing

---

[21] Ibid.

programmes that would help people who needed the medicines. From the inside, AAI was much more significant than it was represented to be in the media".

In April 2001, Annan met with the leaders of six research-based pharmaceutical companies (Abbott Laboratories, Boehringer Ingelheim, Bristol-Myers Squibb, GlaxoSmithKline, Hoffman-La Roche and Pfizer) in Amsterdam, together with the Director-General of WHO and the Executive Director of UNAIDS, to discuss "what further steps can be taken by these companies to make care and treatment more accessible for people living with HIV/AIDS in developing countries".

Annan explained he had called for the meeting because encouraging the active participation of all partners in the fight "has become my personal priority … The pharmaceutical industry is playing a crucial role". He also applauded the contributions from nongovernmental organizations "who are our vital partners in this fight".

At the Amsterdam meeting, the drug companies agreed to continue to accelerate reducing prices substantially, with a special emphasis on the least developed countries[22], particularly those in Africa; to continue to offer affordable medicines to other developing countries, on a country by country basis, and to recognize the need to consider increased access to HIV/AIDS medicines to qualified nongovernmental organizations and appropriate private companies offering health care to employees and local communities in these nations.

Marta Mauras, then Director of the Office of the Deputy Secretary-General of the UN, was involved in arranging the Amsterdam meeting and a subsequent one in New York. She believes these meetings with Annan were probably very instrumental in putting pressure, "very important political pressure", on the drug companies to start lowering prices. It was also clear that despite the research and development companies' objections to generics, their existence and value was at least acknowledged as a political and economic fact.

Looking back at that period, Schwartländer, former Chief of the UNAIDS epidemiology unit and now Director for Performance Evaluation and Policy at the Global Fund, commented: 'A unique combination of generic competition and strong political, activist and media pressure were crucial factors leading to the rapid reduction in prices. The question remains, however, whether reductions could have been achieved earlier'[23].

Whatever the answer to that question, the two UNAIDS drug initiatives were important because they would, in the not too distant future, lead to far more ambitious schemes.

The work on drug pricing was also an example of effective collaboration between the UNAIDS Secretariat and WHO, one of the Cosponsors. Both were essential to this work, and this partnership would continue later as access to treatment became a major focus of their work from 2002 onwards.

---

[22] A category used by the UN to describe poor, commodity-exporting developing countries with little industry where the gross national income per capita is less than US$ 750.

[23] Schwartländer, Grubb, Perriëns (2007).

The Agreement on Trade-Related Aspects of Intellectual Property Rights also paves the way for cheaper drugs

Although 40% of HIV infection was attributed to homosexual transmission in Latin America, less than 20% of public health expenditure on AIDS prevention, not including expenses on blood banks, went to work with this group in 2001.

In May 2001, the World Health Assembly adopted two resolutions that had a particularly important bearing on the debate over the Agreement on Trade-Related Aspects of Intellectual Property Rights (TRIPS), a World Trade Organization (WTO) agreement that protects patent rights including those for drugs. The first resolution addressed the need to strengthen policies to increase the availability of generic drugs, and the second addressed the need to evaluate the impact of TRIPS on access to drugs, local manufacturing capacity and the development of new drugs.

Ellen T'Hoen, Director for Policy and Advocacy at Médecins Sans Frontières' Campaign for Access to Essential Medicines, commented: 'Unable to turn a deaf ear to the growing chorus of critics of TRIPS and its effects on access to medicines, the WTO changed course … The voices had been heard: public health would now feature as a key subject at the Doha conference and the round of trade negotiations that followed'[24].

An important outcome of the Fourth WTO Ministerial Conference in Doha, Qatar, in November 2001, was the Doha Declaration on TRIPS and Public Health, 'a declaration that is considered a key victory for developing and least developed countries, principally because it recognizes the countries' autonomy to implement the TRIPS Agreement in the best possible way for public health'[25].

The Doha Declaration stresses that TRIPS 'can and should be interpreted and implemented in a manner supportive of WTO members' right to protect public health and, in particular, to promote access to medicines for all'. The Declaration states explicitly that 'public health crises, including those relating to HIV/AIDS, TB [tuberculosis], malaria and other epidemics, can represent a national emergency' for which governments can issue a compulsory license authorizing, under certain conditions, the use of patented products'[26].

T'Hoen cited numerous factors leading up to the Doha Declaration, including: the mobilization of developing countries, which acted together in a block; the strong pressure from international nongovernmental organizations and public opinion expressed in the media; the work of WHO and the UNAIDS Secretariat, and the fact that Canada and the USA had threatened to issue a compulsory license against the German company, Bayer, the producer of ciprofloxacin, during the anthrax scare and its use in biological terrorism[27].

[24] T'Hoen E (2003). 'TRIPS, pharmaceutical patents and access to essential medicines: Seattle, Doha and beyond', in J-P Moatti et al. (eds) *Economics of AIDS and Access to HIV/AIDS Care in Developing Countries: Issues and Challenges*. Paris, National Agency for AIDS Research.
[25] Ibid.
[26] UNAIDS (2004). *UNAIDS Global Report 2004*. Geneva, UNAIDS.
[27] T'Hoen (2003).

From 2000 to 2001: increasing efforts and advocacy for prevention

Starting with the UN Security Council and ending with the powerful voices at the Africa Development Forum in Addis Ababa, the year 2000 had been one of enormous activity and of a huge step forward in the visible commitment from leaders across the globe. An increasing number of countries, including Botswana, Ethiopia, Ghana, Kenya, Swaziland and Uganda, had heads of state chairing their HIV/AIDS national body. By the end of 2000, both domestic and international resource flows started to increase for Africa.

The ongoing focus of policy makers and the media on antiretroviral treatment had, according to some, been a detriment to HIV prevention. Arguing that drugs were not the *only* solution, Alan Whiteside[28] wrote that 'there is a real danger that we may lose sight of … other goals. First, treating the symptoms does not get to the cause. Prevention must remain a priority, ensuring new generations do not need treatment'. UNAIDS takes the view that treatment and prevention should go in tandem but many would agree that for several years, the spotlight was more intensely on treatment. Purnima Mane, former Director of UNAIDS' Policy, Evidence and Partnerships Department, and now Deputy Executive Director (Programme) at the United Nations Population Fund (UNFPA), commented: "With the arrival of the Global Fund, prevention fell through the cracks".

While collaboration was improving with some Cosponsors, vital work on AIDS prevention among young people was constrained by interagency disagreements. Too many prevention programmes, even if apparently successful, were small projects.

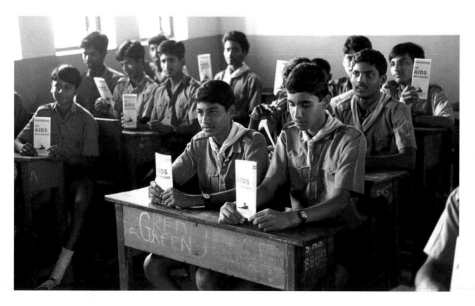

Young Indian school boys are learning about HIV in an AIDS awareness class. In a nearby school, girls received similar lessons. There was an urgent need to scale up prevention projects in many countries. UNAIDS/S.Mathey

---

[28] Whiteside A (2001). 'Drugs: the solution?' *AIDS Analysis Africa*, 11 (6), April/May.

Crucially, condom supplies could not be guaranteed everywhere. A number of African countries had run out of stocks of male condoms and progress was slow on making female condoms widely available. Research published in July 2001 found the overall provision of condoms was just 4.6 per man, per year 'which seems low'. A key report on condom availability asserted that:' Another 1.9 billion condoms need to be provided a year for all countries to equal the level of provision of the six highest providing countries'[29]. The authors of the report estimated that it would cost US$ 47.5 million to close the 1.9 billion condom gap.

The authors added: 'Finding ways to promote condom use and other prevention among high transmitting people is particularly important. Experience in Thailand shows such an approach can greatly reduce sexually transmitted infections and HIV'[30].

The prevention needs of marginalized groups were among the issues discussed at the 10th meeting of the UNAIDS Programme Coordinating Board (PCB) in Rio de Janeiro in December 2000, where concern was expressed about the specific need in that region for scaled-up programmes targeting men who have sex with men. Although 40% of HIV infection was attributed to sex between men in Latin America, less than 20% of public health expenditure on AIDS prevention, not including expenses on blood banks, went to work with this group in 2001. Notable exceptions included Mexico and Peru, which contributed more than 30% of their prevention expenditure towards men who have sex with men. In his report, Piot also spoke of the unfinished prevention agenda; the need to direct resources rapidly to local responses to make young people a priority, to ensure a guaranteed condom supply everywhere, to expand prevention of mother-to-child transmission services and programmes for injecting drug users.

The PCB endorsed the Strategic Framework for Global Leadership on HIV/AIDS, which highlights universally applicable commitments for an expanded AIDS response. The PCB encouraged Member States to translate these commitments into action rapidly at country level, and to make use of the framework to elaborate common goals and formulate specific commitments at the highest levels.

By December 2000, the General Assembly of the United Nations had passed a resolution confirming their decision to hold the Special Session on AIDS, and the two facilitators, Ambassador Penny Wensley from Australia and Ambassador Ibra Deguene Ka from Senegal, had been appointed by the president of the General Assembly.

Sea change in 2001

UNGASS would be a remarkable event for the AIDS community but, already, political commitment was gaining strength in many regions and countries. Increasing numbers of National AIDS Councils had been created, especially in Africa, and there was a new level of donor support for tackling AIDS and other communicable diseases.

[29] Shelton J D, Johnston B (2001). 'Condom gap in Africa: evidence from donor agencies and key informants'. *British Medical Journal*, 323, 21 July.
[30] Ibid.

128

"The year 2001 stands out for me", said Plumley, who had recently joined UNAIDS as Communications Adviser from GlaxoWellcome. "[It's] a year of great sea change, because suddenly we're playing in the big league. In 1996, Peter [Piot] could not have got the Heads of Government and all the countries together in the way [that happened] in 2001. Things came together at UNGASS [including] the movement on drug pricing which I think was a huge achievement for UNAIDS, much under-rated, and then the scaling up of funding".

"The year 2001 stands out for me. [It's] a year of great sea change, because suddenly we're playing in the big league. In 1996, Peter could not have got the Heads of Government and all the countries together in the way [that happened] in 2001".

The Organization for African Unity Summit in Abuja: Annan's call to action and beginnings of a new Global Fund

While the most public event on AIDS in 2001 was UNGASS, key people from UN organizations, donors and countries were also meeting that year to plan what would eventually become the new Global Fund. Political commitment and financial commitment were gaining momentum in parallel.

In early 2001, various donor countries and UN organizations (UNAIDS Secretariat, UNICEF, WHO and the World Bank) took the discussions further, now focusing on the question of whether to push for separate funds for AIDS, for tuberculosis, for malaria or for a more general health fund.

When donors and UN organizations met again in London in April 2001, they agreed on a single Global Fund to Fight AIDS and other deadly diseases.

On 26 April 2001, the final day of the Organization for African Unity Summit on HIV/AIDS, Tuberculosis and Other Infectious Diseases in Abuja, Nigeria, hosted by President Olusegun Obasanjo, the UN Secretary-General issued his now famous global call for action. At the same summit, African leaders pledged 15% of their national budgets to improve health care and recognized HIV/AIDS as the greatest threat to health in Africa.

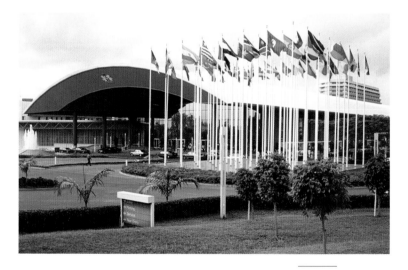

Organization for African Unity Summit on HIV/AIDS, Tuberculosis and Other Infectious Diseases in 2001 in Abuja, Nigeria Engida Wassie, African Union Commission

Annan told the audience that AIDS was Africa's "biggest development challenge" and "that is why I have made the battle against it my personal priority". He gave unequivocal support

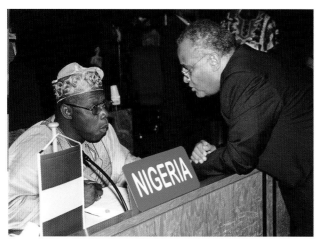

Nigerian President Olusegun Obasanjo and Salim Ahmed Salim, Secretary-General of the Organization for African Unity at Abuja Summit Engida Wassie, African Union Commission

to treatment as well as prevention, and announced: "I propose the creation of a Global Fund, dedicated to the battle against HIV/AIDS and other infectious diseases". Annan called for commitments, a 'war chest' of roughly US$ 7 to US$ 10 billion a year from developing countries and donor countries, over an extended period of time. The sum would cover all work on AIDS, not just the planned Global Fund.

These figures were based on a paper on resource needs for HIV/AIDS that was published in *Science*[31] by a key group of epidemiologists and other experts from UNAIDS and the other organizations and institutes with whom they collaborated. This 'policy forum' estimated that by 2005, the response to AIDS would require about US$ 9 billion annually, with half the resources needed in sub-Saharan Africa. Importantly, the authors wrote that one third to one half of these resources could come from domestic sources, both public and private, with the remainder from international sources. The provision of actual costings for AIDS globally was a major breakthrough.

Louise Fréchette, former UN Deputy Secretary-General, commented: "The Abuja speech … was part of a strategy … and had been preceded by consultations with the heads of the UN agencies. Suddenly, we were … cranking up the machine … it was a precursor in what became a much, much more aggressive public campaign".

On 30 April 2001, Annan addressed the Council on Foundations in Philadelphia (with representatives from some 1800 US philanthropic foundations), reiterating his proposal to create a Global Fund to channel funds for HIV/AIDS and other infectious diseases.

In May 2001, the Secretary-General addressed the World Health Assembly, informing them that plans for the Fund were progressing, and stressed that the Fund must be additional to existing funds and mechanisms, not just a new way of channelling money already earmarked for development. He also made it clear to UNAIDS that he believed the Fund had to be broader than AIDS, and asked the UNAIDS Secretariat and WHO to organize a wider consultation in the first week of June.

On 11 May, US President George W Bush addressed reporters and senior government officials gathered for the visit of Obasanjo and pledged US$ 200 million to what was still an idea – the Global Fund. France and the UK also made pledges of US$ 300 million. Annan personally pledged US$ 100 000 from a prize he had received, which was matched by the International Olympic Committee. In June, pledges of US$ 100 million arrived for the planned Fund from the Bill & Melinda Gates Foundation and US$ 1 million from the Winterthur Insurance/Credit Suisse group.

[31] Schwartländer B, Stover J, Walker N, Bollinger L, Gutierrez J P, McGreevey W, Opuni M, Forsythe S, Kumaranaake L, Watts C, Bertozzi S (2001). 'Resource needs for HIV/AIDS'. *Sciencexpress*, June.

130

In June 2001, a small group of people led by Cleves from the UNAIDS Secretariat and Andrew Cassels, now Director of Health Policy, Development and Services at WHO, had organized the meeting at the President Wilson Hotel overlooking Lake Geneva. Representatives from more than 50 countries from the developed and developing world, multilateral organizations and nongovernmental organizations, private foundations and other stakeholders attended the meeting. It was agreed that 'the Fund should take an integrated approach to fighting HIV/AIDS, TB [tuberculosis] and malaria and build on existing efforts to strengthen local capacity and health systems'[32]. But there were strong tensions between some of the donor countries and the multilateral organizations, which were suspected of wanting to run the fund on their own. The UN was not deemed capable of doing anything in a businesslike way by certain donor representatives. These tensions would at times dominate the planning meetings for the Fund.

Establishing the Pan Caribbean Partnership against HIV/AIDS

Across the Atlantic, the Pan Caribbean Partnership against HIV/AIDS (PANCAP) was established in February 2001. The Partnership was launched in a region that had the second highest prevalence of HIV after Africa (an estimated 390 000 adults and children living with HIV at the end of 2000). The Caribbean Partnership Commitment had six original signatories: Owen Arthur, Prime Minister of Barbados and Chair of CARICOM; Denzil Douglas, Prime Minister of Saint Kitts and Nevis; Edwin Carrington, Secretary-General of CARICOM; Peter Piot, Executive Director of UNAIDS; Sir George Alleyne, Director of Pan American Health Organization/WHO, and Yolanda Simon, Founder and Regional Coordinator of the Caribbean Regional Network of People living with HIV/AIDS (CRN+). Simon commented: "Having a place at the table [for CRN+] from the very beginning helped keep the needs of persons living with HIV, their families, their loved ones and their communities at the forefront of the regional response".

With an overarching goal to 'curtail the spread of HIV/AIDS and to reduce sharply the impact of AIDS on human suffering and on the development of the human, social and economic capital of the region', PANCAP brought together governments of all countries and territories in the region, regional and international organizations in the fields of health, education, development, culture and other sectors, networks of people living with HIV, bilateral and multilateral organizations, the private sector, religious bodies and others. It functions as a network that encourages each partner to work within its own mandate and areas of comparative advantage, while fostering an environment for partners to pursue their respective programmes in a coordinated fashion.

"... it's too easy to dismiss these conferences as 'Oh, well, just diplomatic society, what comes out of it?' Well, what comes out of it is much needed clarity on what ... needs to be done. It is the common song-sheet of the international community".

Posters like this one in Trinidad capture people's attention. Such awareness-raising was essential in a region that had the second highest prevalence rate of HIV in the world. UNAIDS/B.Press

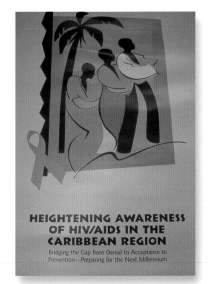

---

[32] Global Fund website, 2007. *History of the Global Fund.*

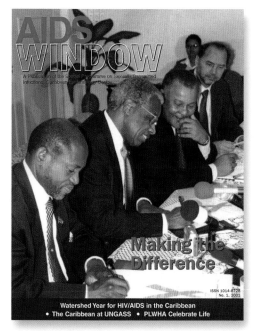

Watershed Year for HIV/AIDS in the Caribbean
• The Caribbean at UNGASS • PLWHA Celebrate Life

Nina Ferencic, UNAIDS Regional Coordinator for Latin America and the Caribbean, explained: "UNAIDS was not [itself] creating a partnership but [was] the force backing up the Caribbean Community Secretariat [i.e. CARICOM] that had the authority to convene". Ferencic continued: "So, we said 'okay, what [UNAIDS] can bring is the technical expertise and the know-how, but what CARICOM can bring is the political influence, the contacts and the buy-in at the highest levels of government in Caribbean countries'".

A regional response suited the Caribbean because 'a common market economy with free movement of professionals and workers with other skills made the political and natural boundaries irrelevant for the fight against AIDS … If some countries did not mount an effective response, it was inevitable that the consequences would be felt in other countries'[33].

The signing of the Pan Caribbean Partnership against HIV/AIDS, February 2001. AIDS Window

A collaborative, coordinated response can help to overcome the very limited human resource (and financial in some cases) capacity of some of the smaller islands, as well as gaining economies of scale and enhancing quality of programmes. A significant result of the partnership is 'strength in numbers' or being able to pull more weight through a united stand[34].

The Caribbean Partnership Committment, 2001 UNAIDS

Although it took at least two years of advocacy to involve prime ministers and presidents, the number of actors involved in the AIDS response in the Caribbean eventually grew to 60. Today, all countries in the Caribbean are engaged in PANCAP.

As a result of consistent advocacy by PANCAP leaders, resources from multilateral and bilateral donors as well as other international sources for the response to AIDS in the Caribbean (including funding from the Global Fund and the World Bank) more than quadrupled in the first three years of the Partnership.

In relation to the Global Fund, PANCAP became the Regional Coordination Mechanism, thus avoiding the need to create a separate structure and an example of how a partnership structure can reduce duplication of efforts.

By 2007, more than 220 projects were operational in the PANCAP constituency, representing a total value of more than US$ 880 million.

Five years into its existence, PANCAP has established itself as a highly active and highly visible partnership – a champion for change.

[33] UNAIDS (2001). *A Study of the Pan Caribbean Partnership against HIV/AIDS (PANCAP). Common Goals, Shared Responses*. Best Practice Collection. Geneva, UNAIDS.
[34] Ibid.

United Nations General Assembly Special Session 2001

For a few months before UNGASS, many UNAIDS staff were focused nearly exclusively on the preparation for the Special Session. UNAIDS staff were managing meeting logistics as well as support for the negotiations over the draft Declaration of Commitment (the actual negotiations were run by the two facilitators, Wensley from Australia and Ka from Senegal), and negotiating with the large numbers of civil society representatives that applied to attend. Several staff practically decamped to New York from Geneva. Cravero recalled: "None of us really knew what we were doing when we began to prepare for UNGASS. I think we would have all been overwhelmed had we really realized what were in for".

The first round of substantive negotiations towards a UN resolution on HIV followed the publication towards the end of February of the Secretary-General's report on the global epidemic.

Although much of the political action was focused on New York, work continued elsewhere. Also in February, the European Commission approved a new Programme of Action to combat HIV/AIDS, malaria and tuberculosis. This included an increase in the money allocated to health, AIDS and population programmes.

The hard work of UNAIDS and its many partners on advocacy bore fruit at UNGASS in 2001. This event was historic for a number of reasons. For three days, AIDS was being discussed at the highest level globally, in the world's most high-profile forum, by many heads of state and senior leaders from other sectors. Every night, the AIDS red ribbon glowed on the UN building, an image symbolic of the new level of political commitment that would circulate around the globe, on television screens and in newspapers.

Fréchette reflected on the event's importance: "It's one thing for the Secretary-General to [make a] key message [as at Abuja] but it's something else for the entire international community to actually explicitly agree on a more detailed plan of action ... it's too easy to dismiss these conferences as 'Oh, well, just diplomatic society, what comes out of it?' Well, what

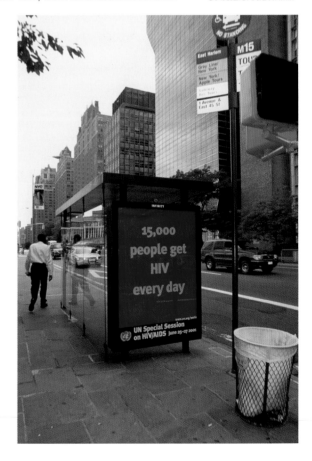

During the UN General Assembly Special Session on HIV/AIDS, posters on New York City bus stops were used to heighten awareness.
UNAIDS/R. Bowman

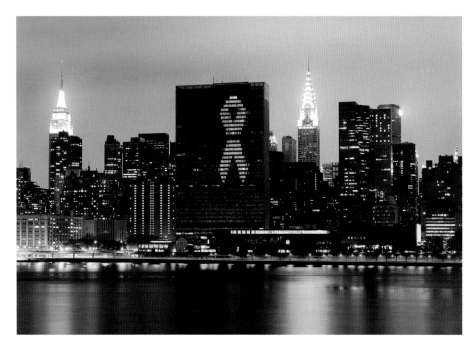

The AIDS red ribbon glowing in neon on the UN headquarters during the UNGASS symbolized the new level of political commitment to combating the epidemic.
UNAIDS/R.Bowman

comes out of it is much needed clarity on what … needs to be done. It is the common song-sheet of the international community".

Fréchette continued: "I am a strong believer in the importance of targets, quantifiable targets . . . they are a way of keeping your feet to the fire, of giving you a way to measure whether what you're doing is making a difference. I think UNGASS was very important in that respect . . . UNGASS is a good illustration of what the UN's role is . . . it can help with technical capacity, it can help in a very practical way at country level, but this more strategic mobilization of the international community is a vital role of the UN . . . it should never be underestimated".

The aim of UNGASS was to come up with a Declaration that all heads of state would commit to, producing a powerful and unique global and national response to the epidemic. Inevitably, there were major disagreements between states (and civil society), in particular about the more sensitive issues such as prevention for sex workers and gay men. Cravero recalls the all-night sessions spent debating the finer but essential points of the Declaration. She said that some activists were very critical of the Declaration without an adequate understanding of the process and the barriers, such as cultural and religious sensitivities, that needed to be carefully negotiated.

Although prevention continued to be seen and identified as the mainstay of the global AIDS response at UNGASS, many heated debates erupted on the topic of AIDS drugs and their strategic place in the fight against the pandemic. The Rio Group, a unified negotiating block at UNGASS comprised of Argentina, Bolivia, Brazil, Chile, Colombia, Ecuador, Mexico, Panama, Paraguay, Peru, Uruguay and Venezuela, provided a strong voice advocating for greater access to affordable drugs. The donors, except for France and Luxemburg, opposed this position.

Eamonn Murphy, who represented a government delegation at UNGASS, explained that some donors felt that the Rio Group was pushing so strongly on the issue of treatment that this could only be achieved at the cost of shifting the focus from prevention programmes.

The Rio Group's official statement, however, suggests that they were fully aware of the importance of prevention. 'We note that the [Declaration of Commitment] makes no specific reference to the question of treatment, even when referring to care and support for persons living with HIV. For the Rio Group, treatment is just as important as prevention'.

According to Murphy, the feasibility of providing wide-scale access to antiretroviral treatment was still a largely unresolved issue in 2001. "From a donor's perspective, quality, capacity for delivery, patient adherence and cost issues were essentially questions without answers. How were these drugs going to be delivered and to whom were they going to be accessible? Are they just going to go to the wealthy in the cities? Plus, for a donor, the question always is, how to make commitments that are sustainable?"

Although the Rio Group succeeded in elevating the importance of providing accessible AIDS treatment in the Declaration of Commitment, no concrete numerical targets were set for this.

Achieving the right balance between prevention and treatment would continue to be a topic of hot debate for years to come.

UNGASS was an example of UNAIDS at its best – serving its core function well by bringing disparate agencies together to achieve more than any one of them could achieve on its own, explained Cravero.

An UNGASS side-event, on 26 June, attracted a large audience and distinguished guests. Organized by the International Federation of Red Cross and Red Crescent Societies, the event was initially planned as an intimate dialogue between UNGASS delegates and people living with HIV. In fact, attendance was by invitation only, but as news of it spread, demand for invitations grew, including one from the Secretary-General's office.

This meeting was another step on the way to an important alliance, brokered by Calle Almedal, UNAIDS' Senior Adviser on Partnerships Development, between the International Federation of the Red Cross and the Red Crescent and the Global Network of People living with HIV/AIDS (GNP+). Annan gathered the GNP+ members and the Federation's positive staff around him for a photo opportunity and welcomed the alliance as sending a "powerful message in breaking the silence around social stigma".

No country and no leader could any longer say they did not know about the exceptional magnitude of the AIDS crisis or about exactly what needed to be done.

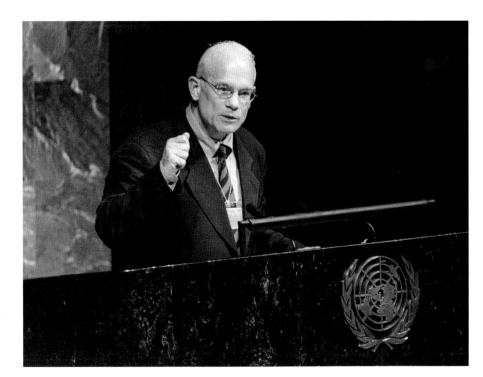

UNGASS helped to put the business response to AIDS on the map. Bill Roedy from MTV and then Chairman of the Global Business Coalition on HIV/AIDS, addressed the plenary of the General Assembly.
MTV

Piot sees UNGASS as a defining moment in the global response to AIDS. "We've had so many useless meetings and conferences, but this one made a real difference … many Presidents and Prime Ministers went back to their country and established a National AIDS Commission under their authority. It provided the road map now for what to do about AIDS … and the funding went up in a big way, despite September 11".

The Declaration of Commitment became a benchmark for global action; it produced a clear global mandate that could be used to hold international leaders to account. Extensive media coverage on a scale unprecedented for a UN event contributed to raising awareness globally of the epidemic and its impact.

No country and no leader could any longer say they did not know about the exceptional magnitude of the AIDS crisis or about exactly what needed to be done. And for the first time ever, there were time-bound targets on HIV prevention, resource mobilization and other aspects of the global AIDS response, serving to make governments clearly accountable[35].

As thousands of weary but generally elated people returned home from New York, work increased on the Global Fund. At UNGASS, several governments of developing countries had pledged millions of dollars of their own resources as a sign of their support for the fund.

---

[35] *Declaration of Commitment on HIV/AIDS* (2001). UN General Assembly 26th Special Session, No. A/RES/S-26.2.

136

In July 2001, at the G8 meeting in Genoa, heads of state of Canada, France, Germany, Italy, Japan, the Russian Federation, the UK and the USA, as well as the European Commission, unanimously affirmed their support for the Global Fund and expressed their determination to make it operational as soon as possible.

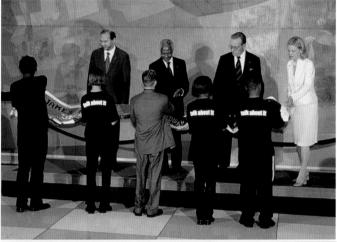

In 2001, the Executive Director of UNAIDS told the PCB that "this year will be remembered as one of the most significant in the history of the epidemic. For the first time, the global perspective joins care for those infected to the task of ensuring those not infected remain so. It is a year when resources are coming, and when political leadership is at unprecedented levels …". While not solely responsible for any of these events or policy developments, the Joint Programme played a critical – often catalytic – role in bringing them about.

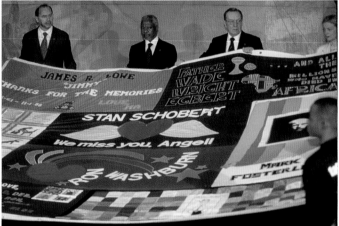

Over the next two years, UNAIDS would build on the successes, to which it had contributed, of 2000-2001. The birth of the Global Fund would eventually ensure more resources for developing countries. The *Five Year Evaluation of UNAIDS* cited many achievements but called for major, and necessary, improvements in country-level work. So 2002 would see a significant change in focus for the organization.

AIDS Quilt presentation at the UNGASS in New York (from left to right) UNAIDS Executive Director Peter Piot; former United Nations Secretary-General Kofi Annan; UNGASS President Harri Holkeri of Finland; and Mrs Nan Annan.
UNAIDS/R. Bowman

The International Labour Organization becomes UNAIDS eighth Cosponsor

In October 2001, the International Labour Organization (ILO) became the eighth Cosponsor of UNAIDS. ILO brought its considerable expertise in the world of work, and, since 2000, with its establishment of a programme on HIV/AIDS and the World of Work, had carried out several country-level activities in Africa, Asia, Eastern Europe and Latin America and the Caribbean.

At UNGASS, ILO published its pioneering *Code of Practice on HIV/AIDS and the World of Work*. It was the result of intensive efforts by the organization's tripartite partners – workers, employers and governments.

The Code establishes key principles for policy development and practical guidelines for programming in the key areas of prevention, care and the protection of human rights.

A key principle of the code is: 'HIV/AIDS is a workplace issue and should be treated like any other serious illness/condition in the workplace. This is necessary not only because it affects the workforce but also because the workplace, being part of the local community, has a role to play in the wider struggle to limit the spread and effects of the epidemic'.

Having promoted an enabling environment, ILO began in earnest to roll out an ambitious campaign promoting policy and programmes that address HIV in the workplace. With critical financial and political support from the US Department of Labor, the International HIV/AIDS Workplace Education Programme was conceived and began modestly in India in 2000.

From an initial grant of US$ 400 000, the pilot project launched in selected Indian States has now expanded to become an interregional initiative with a cumulative allocation of US$ 24.5 million, covering 23 countries and reaching about 300 000 workers in some 300 enterprises worldwide. To date, about 250 national counterparts are involved in guiding the implementation of project work. "At the present level of funding, the programme which operates across sectors from banking to construction, to informal street vendors, expects to directly assist a further 120 000 workers as new country projects come on stream", says Sophia Kisting, Director and Global Coordinator of the ILO Programme on AIDS and the World of Work.

The India experience confirms the critical contributions made by collaborating institutions representing people living with HIV. "Involving persons living with HIV/AIDS is very important. Many top executives and other decision-makers have never met them before. When they notice that they are fit to do their jobs and co-workers are not at risk, the decision-makers cooperate with our goals", says India's National Programme Coordinator Syed Mohamed Afsar.

According to Manoj Pardesi, living with HIV himself and carrying out advocacy work with the India SHARE Project, the involvement of people living with HIV in the project is making a difference. "Enterprises and trade unions are buying the idea of keeping people living with HIV/AIDS in employment and creating a non-discriminatory environment for us", he says.

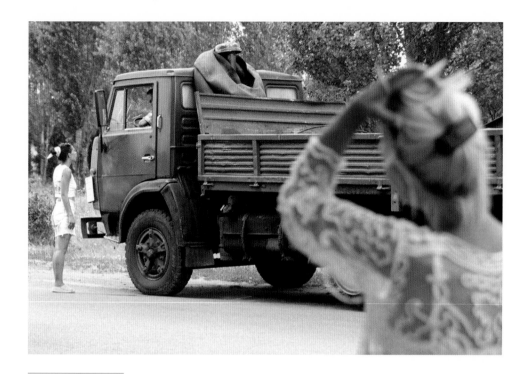

*Sex workers, here flagging down drivers
in Ukraine, are one of the groups most
vulnerable to HIV infection. These
women need money to buy the drugs
they inject.*
WHO/UNAIDS/V.Sukorov

Ukraine

Ukraine has the highest HIV prevalence in all of Eastern Europe and Central Asia: it is estimated at 1.5%, about 410 000 people living with HIV by the end of 2007[1]. Annual HIV diagnoses have more than doubled between 2000 and 2005. The epidemic is predominantly concentrated among groups of people who are most at risk – injecting drug users, sex workers and men who have sex with men – but infection rates among women are also increasing rapidly. More than 45% of new HIV infections reported in the first half of 2007 were among injecting drug users[2].

The sudden increase in HIV infection in Ukraine in the late 1990s was not predicted but there is clearly a link to the process of economic transition following the demise of communism.

The former Director of the Regional Support Team for Eastern Europe and Central Asia, Henning Mikkelsen, explained: "… the rise in infections was very much a reflection of what people went through in that process of economic transition there because, if you look at these places, all of them are characterised by the fact that there was one monopoly industry then suddenly all these new countries [were] established and all the trade links, and so on, brought together, then these industries, they went down; there was nothing left there. There was really no future, and so, what did you do? Well, you went out to the poppy fields and got some poppy … and you could cook your heroin with your friends and you shoot up. But that was not something that we had foreseen at that point in time, the global intelligence didn't see that this was going to happen there, so we were – I was really taken by surprise there".

In seeking to explain the Ukrainian and other epidemics in the region, Mikkelsen tries to look at underlying reasons: "We don't really understand the whole dynamics of why this occurs – I mean, some people say that it's because now so many people are very poor and there's a lot of unemployment and so on, but I don't think that's the whole explanation. There are other societies where people are poor and unemployed but they don't start to shoot up drugs, so you cannot explain everything with this kind of terminology there. I think it reflects a lot that, after the Soviet Union broke down, of course, there was a very difficult economic situation that altered the whole universe of social, moral values, which existed under communism … so many people were completely disoriented in terms of how should they define themselves and their life there. And, in particular, young people, they cannot look back on their parents and [say], 'Well, this was how they were living; I will do it the same way'. That has no value

---

[1] UNAIDS (2007). *Global Report 2007*. Geneva, UNAIDS.

[2] UNAIDS/WHO (2007). *Fact Sheet Eastern Europe and Central Asia, 2007*. Geneva, UNAIDS; UNAIDS/WHO AIDS (2007). *Epidemic Update, 2007*. Geneva, UNAIDS/WHO.

any longer. So, suddenly they are the outcasts and they used to be the superpower. [All these] psychological factors [lie] behind it, also".

As a newly independent state, the concept of development cooperation was novel to Ukraine but, by the late 1990s, there was a small United Nations presence in Ukraine. By 2007, there were three professional staff supported by administrative staff, as well as two people assisting with the implementation of the "Three Ones" and two UN volunteers.

In the early to mid-1990s, civil society was also a relatively new concept in Ukraine, as throughout the whole of Eastern Europe, and community-based responses were just emerging. There was no tradition of working across sectors, so a multisectoral approach had to be encouraged.

Mikkelsen explained: "Even within the health sector, there are very vertical structures. So the people working on sexually transmitted infections don't talk to those working on drug control who don't speak to the AIDS people, and each is running their little empire. But from the beginning, UNAIDS established some pilot projects, such as working with injecting drug users and sex workers. At the same time they worked at a high level with senior government officials including President Kuchma. He was outspoken on AIDS very early on".

Jantine Jacobi, UNAIDS Country Coordinator in Ukraine in 2002 and 2003, recalled that after seven consecutive years in Africa, she enjoyed working in this completely different setting and context and appreciated the working relationship with government counterparts.

The epidemic she encountered was a very different one as, for example, young, well educated people from an affluent background were the most affected. But there were also similarities, such as the stigma and discrimination against injecting drug users with HIV, including from health workers. Sadly this is not untypical of health worker attitudes towards people with HIV in many other countries.

As the UN system was still in its infancy in Ukraine, and global development discussions were not yet centred on harmonization and alignment, Jacobi observed that the UN was initially more inward looking rather than making its own expertise available for supporting national priorities. She therefore facilitated regular meetings and closer links between Theme Groups and Technical Working Groups (as the latter included the membership of civil society), other development partners and government. She also aimed to rally the agencies around the UNAIDS Programme Acceleration Funds (PAF), ensuring their focus was on providing support to national priorities such as young people using drugs. One such PAF-funded undertaking was led by the United Nations Children's Fund with participation from the United Nations

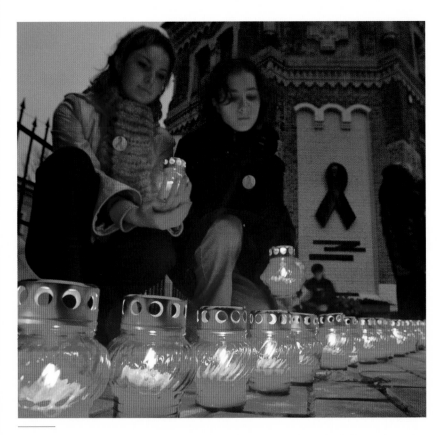

*Girls light candles
during an AIDS
Awareness rally in Kiev,
Ukraine, in 2005.
Reuters/Corbis*

Development Programme, the United Nations Office on Drugs and Crime, the Russian Federation and the World Health Organization . It assessed the practices of drug use among young people. Another joint venture was the setting up of a joint Monitoring and Evaluation Programme, funded predominantly by the U.S. Centers for Disease Control and Prevention but coordinated by UNAIDS, and bringing together the various players in the response, in particular, civil society.

The overall focus initially was on advocacy, ensuring that AIDS would feature on the political agenda at the same time as all the other urgent and emerging issues in a country in transition. The UNDP-supported Race for Life became a major annual advocacy event, as did the World AIDS Day Commemoration, gaining increasing support from civil society. The success in accessing a Round One grant from the Global Fund was of great importance, signifying both political commitment and good collaboration at country level between partners in the response.

In January 2004, the Global Fund announced that it had temporarily suspended its grant in Ukraine, citing the slow progress of Fund-backed HIV programmes. After being among the first countries to have received a first round grant for US$ 92 million, the Fund worked closely with the International HIV/AIDS Alliance, as the new grant recipient, to reinstate the grant within weeks. The grant supports HIV treatment, HIV prevention (including prevention of mother-to-child transmission), care and support services and is now recognized as one of best performing AIDS grants in the Global Fund portfolio.

Though Ukraine in general may not have a strong civil society history and background, the All Ukrainian Network of People Living with HIV has become a strong player and has given a face and voice to the epidemic. Jacobi recalled that the network and the UN organizations were not always able to bridge the communication gap. In setting up regular meetings with the network and including the network as co-chair of the technical working group on treatment and care, UNAIDS tried to strengthen the collaboration. The network played a significant role in the development of the Global Fund proposal and became increasingly engaged in policy discussions. As they gained prominence, their role as key partner in the response was recognized and they became an example to other organizations in the region and exchanges with other networks were supported.

For instance, the network was one of the initiators and key partners of UNAIDS in establishing the Eastern European and Central Asian Union of Organizations of People Living with HIV. They currently serve as the Secretariat to the Union and are globally recognized as one of the strongest national networks of people living with HIV.

The current UNAIDS Country Coordinator, Anna Shakarishvili, praised the members of the network for their work on reducing stigma and discrimination. As a testimony to their role and contribution in this area, they were awarded the first Red Ribbon Award, 'Celebrating Community Leadership and Action on AIDS', at the International AIDS Conference in Toronto in August 2007.

When Shakarishvili joined as UNAIDS Country Coordinator in Ukraine in 2005, there was a small but active Theme Group, chaired by UNICEF, that continues to play an important role in the implementation of the "Three Ones" and in strengthening coordination within and beyond the UN system in Ukraine. The Joint Team on AIDS, established in April 2007, became an entry point for various partners seeking technical assistance from the UN system in Ukraine.

One of the first tasks accomplished by the Joint Team was to assist the National Coordination Council in the development of the country proposal in response to the Global Fund's sixth Call for Proposals for grant funding for HIV – with a total budget of US$ 151 million. In the context of the development of this proposal, a number of important initiatives were undertaken under the auspices of the National Coordinating Council. They included donor harmonization and alignment, developing national targets and a roadmap towards universal access by 2010, a National AIDS Spending Assessment and a gap analysis and costing exercise of the National AIDS Strategy. The Global Fund approved the country proposal, and aims to provide wide-scale prevention, care and support services to most at risk populations in Ukraine. It is in line with the national targets and goals towards achieving universal access by 2010.

Following UNAIDS' and other partners' successful advocacy work, the Ukraine Government substantially increased the amount and scope of funding for HIV services, with an increase of 260% to the national AIDS budget, from US$ 7.3 million in 2007 to US$ 19.6 million in 2007. For the first time in the history of Ukraine, state funds are allocated for the provision of substitution therapy, after a successful registration of methadone in tablet format. This serves as a prerequisite for the substantial scale-up of substitution therapy for injecting drug users, for the effective prevention of HIV and improving adherence to antiretroviral therapy among HIV-infected injecting drug users across Ukraine.

Overall, Ukraine appears on the preferred track of HIV response, with all the elements of the "Three Ones" in place and support from the UK's Department for International Development in line to support its full implementation. Though continuity and coordination at national level may be a challenge, due to leadership issues and change in government, progress is well under way with regard to monitoring and evaluation, revision of the National AIDS Strategy and Programme, the increasing involvement of civil society, including people living with HIV, and good collaboration among stakeholders at all levels.

Ukraine is currently significantly intensifying efforts in the areas of prevention of HIV, treatment, care and support for people living with HIV, and other affected communities, with the support from the US$ 92 million Global Fund grant currently being implemented, a US$ 26 million loan from the World Bank, and additional support from the bilateral donors and the UN.

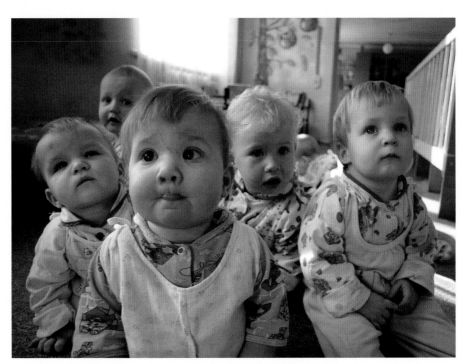

As the rates of HIV soar in Eastern Europe, so do the numbers of orphaned children. These babies live in an orphanage in Makeeva, Ukraine
AFP/Getty Images/
Alexander Khudoteply

144

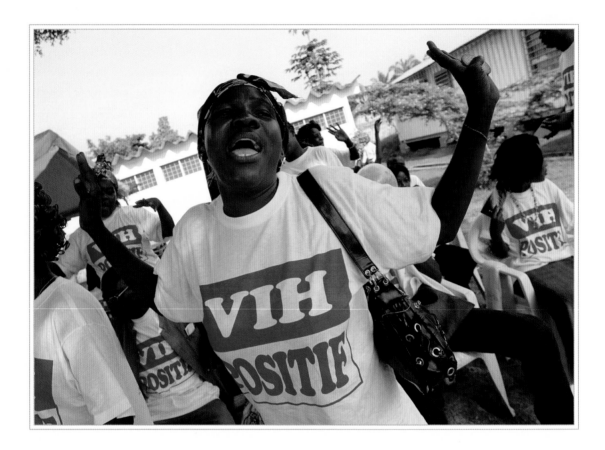

People living with HIV celebrate
World Aids Day in Kinshasa, Congo.
Corbis/Reuter/Jiro Ose

Chapter 6:

Changing the United Nations landscape in countries, 2002–2003

At the end of 2001, nearly 29 million people were living with HIV (about one fifth were aged 15–24), and 3.2 million had been newly infected. In 2002[1], global expenditure on AIDS was US$ 3164 million; in 2003, it was US$ 4730 million[2].

The momentum of the previous years continued, in part spurred on by the 2001 United Nations General Assembly Special Session (UNGASS) on HIV/AIDS. Early in 2002, the Executive Director's testimony to the Committee on Foreign Relations of the United States Senate set the scene for the challenge and expectation of the biennium: "We are now in a position to make a leap forward – a leap that will for the first time put us ahead of HIV".

However, the grand words and Declarations of 2000 and 2001 had yet to be turned into action and concrete resources. The epidemic was not levelling off and, while there were some real results on the ground (for example, declines in HIV prevalence in Addis Ababa, Kigali and Kampala), the performance of national programmes in many countries was still wholly inadequate. Only 1% of pregnant women in heavily affected countries had access to services for the prevention of mother-to-child transmission, despite clear evidence of its effectiveness. In France and the United States of America, fewer than 5% of babies born to HIV-positive mothers were themselves infected; in developing countries, the average remained between 25% and 35%[3]. Most newborn babies infected with HIV die before the age of five years[4].

UNAIDS warned that it would take several more years for current efforts to result in declining HIV prevalence trends, particularly in Southern Africa, a region with 2% of the world's population but almost 30% of the world population living with HIV[5]. A major challenge in countries was the inadequacy of health systems and severe lack of human resources (the result of AIDS deaths and migration to richer countries and better paid jobs in the private sector or nongovernmental organizations) that would hamper the effective spending of extra resources.

---

[1] *2007 AIDS epidemic update*, November 2007.

[2] UNAIDS Resource Tracking Consortium, July 2004.

[3] Dabis F, Ekpini E R (2002). 'HIV/AIDS and maternal and child health in Africa'. *The Lancet*, 359 (9323).

[4] UNAIDS (2004). *Global Report 2004*. Geneva, UNAIDS.

[4] UNAIDS (2004). *AIDS Epidemic Update*. Geneva, UNAIDS.

Women and growing vulnerability to HIV

Another alarming development was the increasing 'feminization' of the epidemic. Since 1985, the percentage of women living with HIV had been rising and, by 2002, almost half the number of adults living with HIV were women; in sub-Saharan Africa, women were at least 1.4 times more likely to be infected with HIV than men[6].

'The face of HIV/AIDS has become that of a young African woman', reported the *Los Angeles Times* in November 2003[7].

'The face of HIV/AIDS has become that of a young African woman'.

Noerine Kaleeba, who started as UNAIDS' Community Mobilization Adviser, had been speaking about this trend from the inception of the Joint Programme. In 1997, she had warned: "If we do not take concrete action on raising the status of women, forget about doing anything about AIDS. ... We were not planning specifically for women and [I knew] if we didn't do that, we would get to a stage where the numbers of women infected would overshoot that of men". Protecting women is crucial to development, she explained, because in many countries they grow the food, bring up families and care for the sick and dying.

In many cultures, gender inequality is at the root of women's increased vulnerability to HIV infection. Women are less likely to have control over their lives or their sexuality; they often marry at an early age, when they are physiologically more vulnerable to HIV and their (usually) older husbands may already be infected. Wives and girlfriends, even when older, have little, if any, influence over their male partners' sexual behaviour; abstinence, being faithful and using condoms may not be an option for them.

Education is seen as a key defence against HIV infection. In many low-income countries, girls receive less education than boys; if families lack money to pay school fees, or sick parents need to be cared for, it is the girls who stay at home. A recent, comprehensive

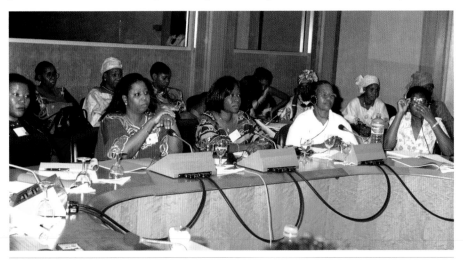

UNAIDS Director of Policy, Strategy and Research, Awa Coll-Seck, participating in the 7th Annual Conference of the Society for Women and AIDS in Africa, in December 1998, in Dakar, Senegal. UNAIDS/Niang

[6] UNAIDS (2003). *AIDS Epidemic Update*. Geneva, UNAIDS.
[7] Farley M (2002). 'Female AIDS cases on the rise'. *Los Angeles Times*, 27 November.

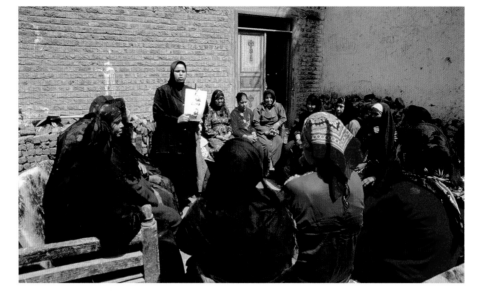

The vulnerability of girls and women to HIV infection goes to the very heart of social and cultural norms about gender, as well as underlining the need for addressing the impact of poverty.

review[8] of the research on girls' education and vulnerability to HIV between 1990 and 2007 in Eastern, Southern and Central Africa confirmed this: 'Put simply, education is key to building "girl power!"' However, the report revealed that early in the epidemic, before 1995, women with a higher level of education were more vulnerable to HIV than those who were less educated. The most likely reason, the researchers concluded, is that more highly educated people have better economic prospects, which influenced their lifestyle choices, making them more mobile. They are also more likely to live in urban areas where HIV prevalence is high, and more likely to have more sexual partners. But as the epidemic has evolved, and there is far more information available about AIDS, more highly educated girls and women are better able to negotiate safer sex and reduce their risk of exposure to HIV. Thus those with less education have been at greater risk.

Women are also among the poorest people in the world. An estimated 70% of the 1.2 billion people living on less than one US dollar a day are women[9], and economic vulnerability increases vulnerability to HIV. Numerous studies show that women often become sex workers or barter sex for economic gain or sheer survival. If their husbands die or leave, sex work may be the only option for women without any education or women who lack any rights to their husband's property. Surveys of sex workers in some urban areas between 1998 and 2002 detected extraordinarily high levels of HIV infection: 74% in Ethiopia; 50% in South Africa; 45% in Guyana and 36% in Nepal[10].

The vulnerability of girls and women to HIV infection underlines the complex challenge of preventing HIV infection. It goes far beyond the provision of information and education about HIV and the provision of condoms – let alone the admonitions about abstinence and fidelity. It goes to the very heart of social and cultural norms about gender, as well as

[8] Hargreaves J, Boler T (2007). *Girl Power. The Impact of Girls' Education on HIV and Sexual Behaviour*. Johannesburg, ActionAid International.

[9] UNDP (2001/2002). *Human Development Reports*. UNDP, New York.

[10] UNAIDS (2002). *Global Report 2002*. Geneva, UNAIDS.

underlining the need for addressing the impact of poverty and inequality on all the populations of the developing world.

Empowerment of women is essential but at the same time boys and men must be involved in prevention programmes too, otherwise there is a risk of alienating them.

In 2003, the United Nations (UN) Secretary-General convened a Task Force on Women, Girls and HIV/AIDS in Southern Africa that identified key actions to reduce girls' and women's prevalence levels. This Task Force would lead to the setting up, in 2004, of the Global Coalition on Women and AIDS (GCWA).

The Five Year Evaluation of UNAIDS

The Five Year Evaluation of UNAIDS inevitably led to a period of reflection and reassessment, changes in policy and use of resources, especially in countries.

The *Evaluation* described the challenges with the Cosponsors, and the fact that financial arrangements brought Cosponsors neither benefits in the form of extra funds, nor their support through commitments to fund; 'in that sense, the word Cosponsor is a complete misnomer'[11]. But the report welcomed the Secretariat's efforts that have 'ultimately born fruit, with a global strategy that is owned jointly by the Cosponsors'. The Programme's successes included reaching a global consensus on policy and programme approaches to fight AIDS, and acceptance by development agencies and civil society organizations of common programming approaches – although 'it is too early to say that public political commitments have been translated into effective action'. A major success had been in securing more finance from the Organisation for Economic Co-operation and Development (OECD) donors; by November 2002, a nearly sevenfold increase in international resources targeted at AIDS in Africa amounted to approximately US$ 1 billion[12]. The scale of response had started to reverse the decline in funding of the 1990s.

Much of UNAIDS' work was praised by the Evaluation Team. It wrote of 'a talented and committed team of people' who have created a unique UN Joint Programme 'that has established itself as a leader in tackling HIV/AIDS, and a centre of knowledge about the disease'. It has been successful in its role of leadership; the advocacy work has been 'innovative, flexible and adaptive'; new types of partnership have been formed, horizontal learning has been developed into a powerful tool and diverse groups such as people living with HIV, nongovernmental organizations and business people have been brought into the process. 'Success at consolidating and presenting the epidemiology of the disease underpinned a strong narrative about the scale and threat to development'.

The major criticism focused on UNAIDS' work in countries. Although the team found that coordination at global levels had been effective, it had been much less so at country level.

'Success at consolidating and presenting the epidemiology of the disease underpinned a strong narrative about the scale and threat to development'.

---

[11] UNAIDS (2002). *Executive Summary of the Five Year Evaluation of UNAIDS*. Geneva, UNAIDS.
[12] UNAIDS (2002). *Executive Director's Report to the 13th Meeting of the UNAIDS PCB*, December. Geneva, UNAIDS.

Major reasons for this were that Theme Groups were relatively new and untested, and their accountability was not clear; the Programme Coordinating Board had limited influence over country-level activities, and there was a lack of incentive for Cosponsors to develop a genuinely integrated approach. For example, promoting coherent, system-wide action on AIDS was still not included in the performance appraisal of UNAIDS Cosponsor staff. The key expectation that UNAIDS would reduce duplication of effort and ensure consistency among UN organizations had not yet been met, according to the Evaluation Team.

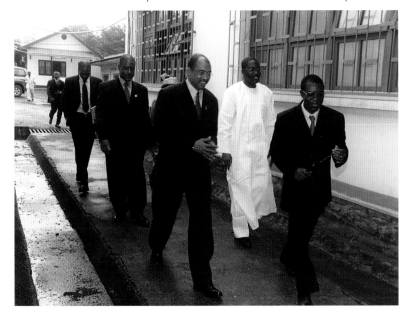

The team recommended high prominence for work on gender, admitting that UNAIDS could be criticized for not making this a higher priority, despite some consistent work over the years.

The primary message of the *Evaluation* was for UNAIDS to shift its focus on efforts to the country level, where there was still a great need for advocacy, resource mobilization and coordination.

Following recommendations from the Evaluation, major efforts were made to focus on country-level work. They were planned and overseen by Michel Sidibe (third from right, here in Cameroon), who had joined UNAIDS as Director of the Country and Regional Support Department in 2001. UNAIDS

Involving a wide range of partners in the fight against AIDS is a key step in building an 'ideal' expanded, country-level response. According to the *Evaluation*, an 'ideal expanded country-level response' is one in which actions would be broadly spread through both health and non-health departments, sector agencies, nongovernmental organizations and communities; basic services and condoms would be widely available; prevention efforts would focus on populations at high risk as well as the general population and young people; voluntary and confidential testing services would be available and lead to treatment for sexually transmitted infections, opportunistic infections, action to prevent mother-to-child transmission and treatment with antiretroviral therapy; legislation and work practice would alleviate stigma and discrimination; and the system would be supported by statistical services enabling monitoring of the epidemic's trends.

Changing the United Nations landscape in countries

In December 2002, the recommendations of the *Evaluation* were accepted by UNAIDS' governing body; consequently, major efforts were made to focus on country-level work. They were planned and overseen by Michel Sidibe, who had joined UNAIDS as Director of the Country and Regional Support Department in 2001, after many years working for the United Nations Children's Fund in Africa and New York.

Sidibe explained that the *Evaluation* was a wonderful foundation for him. It enabled UNAIDS to move forward, to give "a face to UNAIDS actors in country". He saw his role as a bridge between the policy- and decision-makers and the implementers at country level. The original mandate of UNAIDS, he believed, had not sufficiently stressed the importance of country ownership and had not focused on priorities at country level. The "call" from the *Evaluation* was to improve the functioning of the UN system to help to support the national response.

Soon after his arrival at UNAIDS, Sidibe organized the evaluation of the National Strategic Plans on AIDS in 113 countries. This review provided the basis for redesigning UNAIDS' country-level work; it revealed that most of these plans had not been made operational – for example, government officials' fervently expressed resolve to fight the disease had not been translated into specific, time-bound goals and targets, let alone into clear directives for achieving these; furthermore, the few existing operational plans had not been costed. "It was now time to move from conceptualizing, to hard planning, to implementation".

The original mandate had not sufficiently stressed the importance of country ownership and had not focused on priorities at country level.

UNAIDS needed to change its profile at country level; there was a "big gap between Peter Piot's [UNAIDS Executive Director] role at global levels and what the Country Programme Adviser was supposed to do", explained Sidibe. He stressed the importance of understanding the difference between political advocacy and advocacy for implementation, which is an important role for UNAIDS, as is disseminating country-specific information, not only global reports, as had been the case until then.

Programme Advisers to Country Coordinators

One of the key decisions of UNAIDS' governing body in 2002 was to strengthen capacity in the following three areas: monitoring and evaluation, resource mobilization and tracking, and social mobilization and partnership-building. As a consequence, there was a roll-out of more staff to countries, and the Country Programme Advisers (CPAs) were renamed UNAIDS Country Coordinators.

This signified an important upgrading of the role, providing the Country Coordinators with more authority and making them full members of the UN Country Team in each country. There was considerable Cosponsor resistance to this change, in particular from old-style UN Resident Coordinators, despite strong support from Mark Malloch Brown, the United Nations Development Programme Administrator. The UNAIDS Country Coordinators now became central to the coordination of the response in countries, rather than performing a passive, supportive role. This was a major change, explained Sidibe. Under the new arrangement, the UNAIDS Country Coordinator became the prime source of information and intelligence needed to confront the epidemic, and was accountable for the UN's performance.

Roger Salla Ntounga, now UNAIDS Country Coordinator in Ethiopia, who had worked with the Programme in various capacities since the early years, noted a significant change in attitudes towards the UNAIDS Country Coordinators. In 2000, he went with the new CPA to a country where they met middle management in the government. About five years later he went back to introduce the new UNAIDS Country Coordinator and "we met the Ambassadors themselves, the Ministers". So the new UNAIDS Country Coordinators immediately started work at a very different level from their predecessors. "This is a reflection of the credibility we have now".

Bunmi Makinwa became UNAIDS Country Coordinator in Ethiopia in 2003, having been Head of the Inter-Country Team for East and Southern Africa, based in South Africa, for three years. He explained that Addis Ababa is the political hub of Africa, the seat of the African Union and home of the Economic Commission for Africa "where the political horse-trading in Africa takes place".

Makinwa aimed to get AIDS integrated into that political hub in a way that would be permanent "and we succeeded. AIDS is part of the agenda permanently of the African leaders now". There is now an office in the African Union dedicated to work on the epidemic, and UNAIDS also put in place an annual review of the performance of African countries on AIDS. This review (based on the leaders' declaration at Abuja in 2001 and therefore giving some clear indicators) is carried out by the African Union with UNAIDS' support.

In several countries, social mobilization officers were appointed as well as new monitoring and evaluation staff. The latter are essential to ensure that governments receive better strategic information in order to make decisions and to monitor progress and track the epidemic. There are now 41 monitoring and evaluation advisers operating in UNAIDS country offices and Regional Support Teams, the largest force on monitoring and evaluation around AIDS in the world and a major monitoring and evaluation resource for development in general.

Improving United Nations functioning in countries

Other changes were made to improve the coordination and accountability of the UN system at country level. Regional Directors of the Cosponsoring agencies now meet regularly to review the performance of their country representatives. Sidibe stressed the importance of this 'bridge' between headquarters, region and country for the various agencies. The other important change was to move from UNAIDS Inter-Country Teams, which had focused mainly on advocacy according to the original mandate, to Regional Support Teams. This shift signified the progressive decentralization of UNAIDS operations at regional and country levels.

152

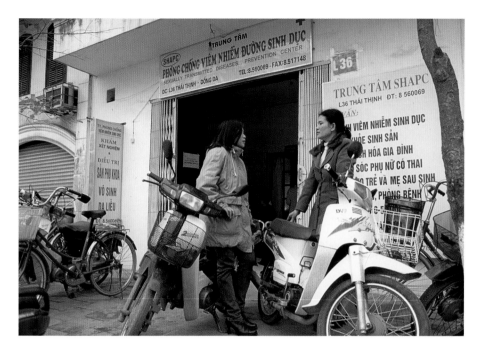

In order to improve UN functioning, it was felt that, first, the UN's own house should be in order, and activities related to HIV in the UN System Workplace were initiated. For instance, UNAIDS prepared a staff survey on HIV awareness among staff, and in-country workshops for UN staff were organized to ensure that staff themselves were better informed, e.g. on their rights and on the UN HIV/AIDS personnel policy.

Another important change occurred in 2003, as the process of gathering surveillance estimates became increasingly country owned and country based. Karen Stanecki, Senior Adviser at UNAIDS' Epidemic and Impact Monitoring Department, explained: "In the past two rounds of the *Global Report*, we actually made a concerted effort to train country people responsible for HIV surveillance on how to do national HIV estimates, so that they would feel ownership of the estimates. In 2003 and in 2005, we conducted over a dozen regional workshops where we trained epidemiologists from over 150 countries on how to use the UNAIDS tools and methodologies recommended by our Reference Group. Our hope was that this would lead to country ownership of the estimates and that it would not be viewed as a Geneva-based process".

Stanecki and her colleagues also believe this process has improved their estimates because these are now based on data available in countries and more in-depth country knowledge. "As countries expand their own surveillance systems, they have more information to use in this process and they have a better knowledge of the limitations of their data".

Continuing advocacy

"As countries expand their own surveillance systems, they have more information to use in this process and they have a better knowledge of the limitations of their data".

UNAIDS also continued to work with a wide range of leaders in the developing world to strengthen the response to the epidemic. Legislators, who have such influence and responsibility, were increasingly focusing their attention on AIDS. UNAIDS and the Inter-Parliamentary Union produced *The Handbook for Legislators on Law, Human Rights and HIV/AIDS*, helping legislators to become more active in the response. South Africa, for example, has passed an Employment and Equity Act that forbids discrimination based on HIV status.

The UN and China work together to fight stigma and discrimination

As in all affected countries, stigma and discrimination are major barriers to combating the epidemic in China. The UN Country Team decided to take a bold approach to this challenge and, in 2002, eight UN programmes, funds and specialized agencies – International Labour Organization, United Nations Office on Drugs and Crime, United Nations Development Programme, United Nations Educational, Scientific and Cultural Organization, United Nations Population Fund, United Nations Children's Fund, World Health Organization and the World Bank, supported by UNAIDS – developed a joint, multisectoral programme to fight AIDS-related stigma and discrimination.

The Joint Programme is funded by UNAIDS Programme Acceleration Funds, amounting to US$ 675 000. These are catalytic seed funds which are channelled through the UNAIDS Secretariat in Geneva to UN Theme Groups in programme countries. A 2002 review of the UN Theme Group on HIV/AIDS in China had, although positive, suggested that members needed to move from joint analysis to an integrated action programme in order to provide more comprehensive support to the AIDS activities of the Government of China.

ILO is addressing AIDS-related discrimination in the workplace and promoting the greater involvement of people living with HIV. Injecting drug use is the main mode of HIV transmission in China, so UNODC is focusing on de-stigmatizing injecting drug users. It is also working closely with law enforcement officers and staff – for example, training them in HIV prevention and care for people living with HIV, and training teachers in the provincial police colleges in line with best international practices. UNDP ran national anti-stigma comprehensive media campaigns and UNESCO worked on raising the awareness of young people of HIV prevention and legal rights in schools and vocational centres, and established networks of young advocates and peer educators. UNFPA worked on improving access to high quality condoms in a number of regions and UNICEF worked with school children, adolescents and community leaders with the aim of reducing stigma and ensuring they have correct knowledge about HIV. However, in 2007 stigma continues to be a major challenge for people living with HIV in China.

154

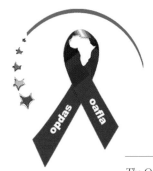

The Organisation of African First Ladies against HIV/AIDS (OAFLA) is an innovative advocacy initiative to combat AIDS in Africa. The organization was founded in July 2002, with the support of UNAIDS and the International AIDS Trust. At this meeting, 37 first ladies signed an agreed Framework of Action, and by 2007, some 40 first ladies from across the African continent were part of the organization, whose seven-member Steering Committee was, at the time of writing, presided over by the First Lady of Zambia, Maureen Mwanamasa.

The Organisation of African First Ladies against HIV/AIDS (OAFLA) founded in July 2002.

The goal of OAFLA is to make a unified contribution to combating the impact and consequences of AIDS in Africa. Through coordinated advocacy, OAFLA members work to raise awareness, advocate HIV-prevention initiatives, promote treatment, care and support programmes, reduce stigma and discrimination, and develop partnerships with international organizations and local partners. The organization focuses its attention predominantly on women, children, youth and people living with HIV.

Since its inception, UNAIDS has supported the organization, providing technical support towards the development of the Plan of Action and the advocacy and communication strategy, as well as funding for the functioning of Secretariat. At country level, UNAIDS Country Coordinators and Regional Support Teams aim to provide communication support and technical assistance as and when required, for example in relation to the continent-wide campaign mentioned earlier.

This bond with UNAIDS was reaffirmed through the signing of a Memorandum of Understanding in 2005 on strengthening commitment for enhanced collaboration between OAFLA and UNAIDS, an understanding to which UNICEF is also a full partner.

OAFLA has proved to be an innovative and effective initiative, as the African first ladies are in a unique position to use their profile and power for continued high-level advocacy and action.

Continuing partnerships

In strengthening its work at country level, UNAIDS has promoted and supported the establishment of partnership forums led by governments and bringing together the community and private sectors, as well as international organizations. These forums contribute to coordinating the development and implementation of National Strategic Plans on AIDS.

By June 2003, there were 11 partnership forums in Asia and the Pacific, 20 in Africa and 12 in Eastern Europe and Central Asia. Civil society, in those countries at least, is playing a larger role in the way their governments are responding to the epidemic.

What do activists expect from UNAIDS and the UN system at country level? Zackie Achmat from South Africa's Treatment Action Campaign (TAC) explained his viewpoint.

"So a Country Representative has a greater responsibility in managing conflict and trying to avoid conflict wherever possible. Geneva does not need to play the diplomatic game in the same way".

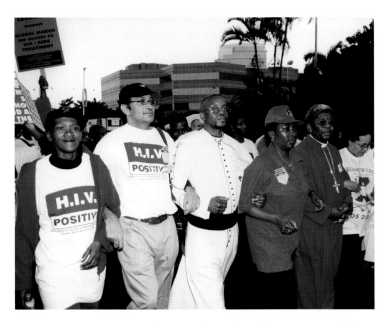

Zackie Achmat (second from left) from South Africa's Treatment Action Campaign demonstrates with Archbishop Njongonkulu Winston Hugh Ndungane of Cape Town (second from right) at the 13th International AIDS Conference in Durban, South Africa.
Panos / Gisele Wulfsohn

"We do not expect the UN office to be an implementing agency in our country, we expect it to be a facilitator – although we do not think that it is doing enough publicly to bring people together. I think the relationship has improved tremendously and I think Mbulawa Mugabe [UNAIDS Country Coordinator] has been very skilful in maintaining a relationship with us and holding a relationship with government, without treading on either's toes but making sure that what needs to be done is getting done … With Geneva we have a relationship where we can push them to do more because they can say things that our country representative cannot say, because our Country Representative is here all the time and has to traverse real abnormalities concerning local practice both in relation to us and in relation to government. So a Country Representative has a greater responsibility in managing conflict and trying to avoid conflict wherever possible. Whereas Geneva, when there is a conflict, can take a principled position because they are not here, and I think that's how we approach it. Geneva does not need to play the diplomatic game in the same way. So our relationship with UN international, or Geneva, is very different [from] the country office".

Achmat continued: "As activists, our job first and foremost is that we create a movement in our countries where … we hold our governments accountable. We cannot expect the UN to hold our countries accountable if we cannot do it ourselves. It's like I say to anyone who is a fag or a dyke – if you cannot come out to your mom and dad to say that I am gay or a lesbian how can you expect the government to treat you equally? There is no use in screaming at the UN, we need to know that we can use the UN and that the UN has a mandate to protect life and to protect rights and so on and that we should use. We do not use it enough in an appropriate manner".

The UNAIDS Secretariat and some of its Cosponsors have supported networks of people living with HIV in many countries, in various ways. UNDP supported 10 countries (Burkina Faso, Burundi, Chad, Côte d'Ivoire, Ethiopia, the Democratic Republic of Congo, Niger, Rwanda, Togo and Zambia) in reviewing laws and administrative measures to prevent stigma and discrimination against people living with HIV. It also supported a number of AIDS nongovernmental organizations to strengthen their governance structure (so often a weakness of underfunded nongovernmental organizations) and strategic planning process, including the Society for Women and AIDS in Africa.

156

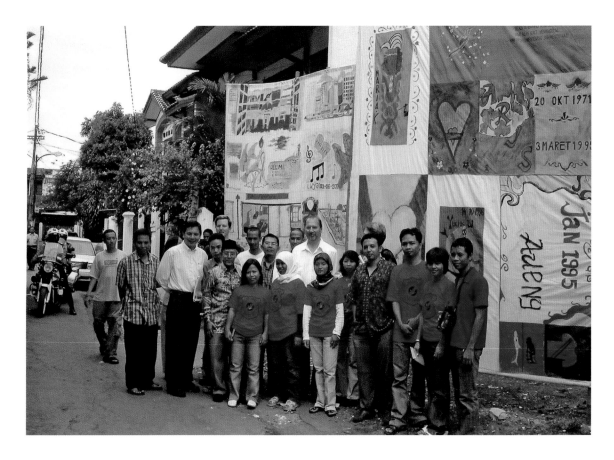

UNAIDS has funded the Andean International Community of Women living with HIV/AIDS (ICW) Project, aimed at strengthening the capacity of HIV-positive women in five countries. Women have met officials and ministers, as well as other women in similar circumstances, and have received training on leadership, advocacy and sexual and reproductive health and treatment. 'The project has put HIV-positive women at the centre of the AIDS response, linking them with relevant actors'[13].

In 2003, Jane Wilson, the UNAIDS Country Coordinator in Jakarta, was wondering how she might better apply the Greater Involvement of People living with HIV/AIDS (GIPA) principle and increase the involvement of HIV-positive people within UNAIDS. At the time, the UNAIDS office in Jakarta offered office space to a new nongovernmental organization called PITA that supported parents of drug users living with HIV. 'Pita' is an evocative name: it means 'ribbon' in Indonesian, but it also refers to Michelangelo's *Pietà*. Linked to the image of a mother compassionately holding the body of her crucified son, the name is meant to highlight the care and understanding that people living with HIV deserve.

Both organizations decided to dedicate a large community room within their shared office for the use of people infected or affected by HIV. Members of the community immediately began to see this space as a safe haven: soon, there were back-to-back bookings for counselling

UNAIDS Executive Director Peter Piot with UNAIDS Country Coordinator for Indonesia Jane Wilson and staff member Victor Mari Ortega, meet members of Yayasan Pelita Ilmu, a nongovernmental organization, 2003. UNAIDS

---

[13] UNAIDS (2004). *Executive Director's Report to the 16th Meeting of the UNAIDS PCB*, December. Geneva, UNAIDS.

and discussions on HIV-related matters. One morning, Wilson arrived at the office to see a group of fathers of injecting drug users around the table sharing their concerns, and she felt that the room was taking on a life of its own.

Some of the HIV-affected individuals who had been using the room eventually became UNAIDS staff members, demonstrating UNAIDS' recognition of their extraordinary experience and how much they could contribute to UN work.

The Global Fund opens for business

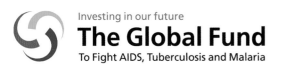

On 28 January 2002, the Board of the new Global Fund to Fight AIDS, Tuberculosis and Malaria had its first organizational meeting in Brussels.

By that time, the major decisions about the type of organization, and its way of working, had been taken. But in the previous few months, the disputes between the range of stakeholders involved were reminiscent of those that took place during the setting up of UNAIDS.

There were disagreements about where the new Global Fund would be based. Several European Union member states wanted it to be housed in Brussels; others preferred Paris or Geneva. Geneva was eventually chosen because WHO, UNAIDS and other members of the UN family were there. Ironically, given this decision, the most serious disagreement had been about whether the Global Fund should be part of the UN.

Like former UN Secretary-General Kofi Annan, UNAIDS Executive Director Peter Piot had been convinced from the late 1990s that a special funding mechanism was needed for AIDS because the normal system [of overseas aid] could not generate the amounts of money needed. Both he and Annan had fought hard to get the Global Fund established.

The Global Fund was not housed within the UN because, according to Marta Mauras, who was at the time Director of the Office of the UN Deputy Secretary-General, "... the donors were only going to accept such an instrument if it was partly controlled by them".

Kathleen Cravero, now Assistant Administrator at UNDP, explained: "There was very much the view that the Global Fund was necessary because the UN hadn't worked ... If the UN could 'solve' AIDS, it would already have done so. UNAIDS is fine as a policy and advocacy group but it doesn't really have the muscle or the money to get the job done, so let's create this huge fund. This really was an undercurrent, although not explicitly stated, which is why it would not have been in UNAIDS from the outset".

Ben Plumley, Director of the UNAIDS Executive Office until March 2007, added, "I don't think the UN family was at peace enough with itself [to have those resources inside the UN] ... Nonetheless, we have, in the donors, an acceptance that a good proportion – not enough, by any means, but a good proportion – of donor aid should [flow] through a multi-lateral mechanism".

At some meetings there had been downright hostility towards the UN. Piot recalled: "... So at some point in the negotiations, one G8 [Group of Eight] donor said, 'Well, why should we have the UN here? Why don't we replace the UN by somebody from a pharmaceutical company?' I mean ... that was the level of hostility against the UN system".

Furthermore, Mauras believes that civil society, which was very involved, did not want "a United Nations kind of outfit". They wanted, "... a private-public formula, where donors and recipient countries as well as organized civil society and the UN had a seat at the table".

Defining roles as a new actor emerges

Piot and his colleagues had to be politically pragmatic, and they worked hard to get the Global Fund up and running, despite the view from many that it would be the end of UNAIDS. Piot always smiles when this is said: "The death of UNAIDS has been announced so many times". UNAIDS fought hard to ensure a strong and equal voice for the developing countries in the Global Fund.

An important problem, recalled Mauras, was that "the creation of a global funding outfit should not enter into competition with all the other agencies, especially UNAIDS. In other words, it should truly be a funding mechanism searching for additionality, plus it should not enter directly into operations".

When the planning phase for the Global Fund was completed in mid-December 2001, it was clear that the Global Fund was a financing mechanism, not an implementing or techni-cally oriented body. It would raise and transfer funding to programmes in countries but it would not design, set up or run the programmes.

Plumley stresses that there was always the expectation from some people (possibly not at first within the Global Fund) that "... entities like UNAIDS and others will really drive the policy agenda, continue to advocate and be there to support this mechanism".

The Global Fund is a partnership between governments, civil society and the private sector. Its Board includes representatives of governments (an equal number of donor and devel-oping countries), plus two nongovernmental organization seats and two private sector donor seats. Each constituency is responsible for selecting its representatives. WHO, UNAIDS and the World Bank, the Global Fund's trustee, have non-voting seats on the Board. There is

UNAIDS fought hard to ensure a strong and equal voice for the developing countries in the Global Fund.

also a seat for a person affected by one of the three diseases. The Global Fund depends on teams of people (the Country Coordinating Mechanisms) in each country to review and submit proposals for funding and, once a proposal is accepted, to oversee the establishment and running of the programme. Unlike the International Monetary Fund or the World Bank, the Global Fund does not lend money nor does it place economic conditionality on the funds. Proposals must be 'owned' by the countries and therefore specific to their needs.

From when it was created, tension and competition between the Global Fund and UN agencies inevitably arose. These relationships have greatly improved today.

"It's very clear that the programmes the Global Fund finances could never get anywhere unless there are partners like WHO, UNAIDS and others on the ground who help countries to be successful".

The process of developing the Global Fund, in such a short space of time and with a number of difficult and tense meetings, was, stressed Andrew Cassels, who represented WHO in the negotiations, an example of a good working relationship between WHO and the UNAIDS Secretariat. "There was an element of competition but on the whole it worked pretty well".

Bernard Schwartländer, formerly Chief Epidemiologist at UNAIDS, became Director of WHO's HIV/AIDS Programme in 2001 and in 2003 joined the Global Fund as its Director for Performance Evaluation and Policy. He has followed the interaction between the three partner organizations and has seen a substantial evolution in the relationship.

"There have always have been some tensions and difficult institutional issues challenging the collaboration between the Global Fund, WHO and UNAIDS. I think these tensions were amplified by initial uncertainty about roles and responsibilities and an initial perception that there would be a competition for resources. … It also became clear that rather than competing for resources, the three institutions are interdependent and the Global Fund programmes are crucial to the realization of both UNAIDS and WHO policies and targets. Now the partners' tremendous effort is being recognized by the Global Fund and its recipients and I believe the three institutions mainly work together to solve their challenges".

After a year or more, the relationship between the Global Fund and UNAIDS improved. Schwartländer observed: "Now, I think what has come much to the forefront is the recognition that the Global Fund is nothing without its partners and also the Global Fund is a unique opportunity for all the partners because, for the first time, the partners have the money or there is money in countries to do what UNAIDS and what WHO always wanted to do. On the other side, it's very clear that the programmes the Global Fund finances could never get anywhere unless there are partners like WHO, UNAIDS and others on the ground who help countries to be successful. I think that was always the intention when the Global Fund was created".

The Global Fund's form, function and overall effectiveness are still issues for discussion and disagreement, for example, whether combining the three diseases was the right decision. The impetus behind the Global Fund clearly came from the AIDS world.

But Richard Feachem, the first Executive Director of the Global Fund, disagreed: "The three diseases are a natural fit for the Global Fund. For all three, there was clear evidence that additional financing for the implementation of existing tool and strategies could have a significant impact on the burden of disease ... The challenge was where to draw the line. There are many other scourges from leishmaniasis to diarrheal diseases that need and deserve increased attention and financing".

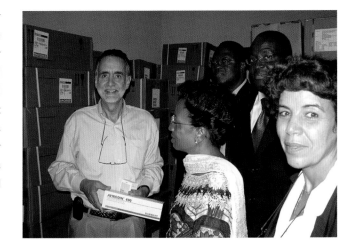

Richard Feachem, the first Executive Director of the Global Fund with UNAIDS Country Coordinator for Benin Yamina Chakkar.
UNAIDS

First funding proposals to the Global Fund

At the end of January 2002, the Global Fund approved its first call for funding proposals; the initial grants would be made in April. At this point, the Global Fund had US$ 1.9 billion committed but far more resources were needed.

It was announced that the Global Fund would finance plans developed through country partnerships in severely affected countries as well as in areas with growing epidemics. Its approach would be integrated and balanced, covering prevention, treatment and care and support in dealing with the three diseases. Proposals would be funded rapidly, with a minimum of red tape but with enough safeguards to make sure funds were used responsibly and effectively.

In February 2002, UNAIDS stressed the funding gap that existed – and therefore the high expectations it had of the new Global Fund[14]. AIDS programmes needed to spend US$ 10 billion every year to ensure an adequate response to the epidemic (though it was not expected that this would be raised solely by the Global Fund). The goal could be reached only through major increases in allocations from national governments, greater support from the private sector and increases in international assistance through the Global Fund, bilateral funding programmes and international organizations.

During 2002, such resource mobilization would increase rapidly, but not rapidly enough, and extra funding would cause more challenges to countries as well as UNAIDS.

Piot made it clear to staff that the new Global Fund brought various new opportunities and risks "but should be a dynamic incentive for UNAIDS to do its job right". It also had to be made clear to donors that the Global Fund was there to mobilize additional resources,

---

[14] UNAIDS (2002). *Fact Sheet*, February. Geneva, UNAIDS.

not to replace existing disbursements. Total international (donor) spending on AIDS and sexually transmitted infections in 2000 was estimated to be US$ 396 million according to figures reported to the Netherlands Interdisciplinary Demographic Institute, but US$ 521 million according to what was reported to the Development Assistance Committee of the OECD[15]. According to a Futures Group assessment: 'A warranted conclusion may be that year 2000 donor assistance was almost US$ 600 million'[16].

UNAIDS had also been working with relevant partners, such as the World Bank, on other ways to release more resources. At the Monterrey International Conference on International Conference on Financing for Development, Marika Fahlen, then UNAIDS Director of Social Mobilization and Strategic Information, highlighted debt relief efforts as an important additional mechanism to slowing down the spread of HIV, as long as the monies freed up by debt relief were channelled into national AIDS programmes.

In the same speech, Fahlen described some of the developmental impacts of AIDS on countries. Botswana, one of the worst affected countries, estimated the government would lose 20% of public revenue by 2010 due to the economic impact of AIDS. Zimbabwe's life expectancy between 2000 and 2005 was estimated to be 26 years lower that it would have been without AIDS. In Haiti, where prevalence had risen to 6%, life expectancy had dropped by six years for the same reason.

By July, the Global Fund had received over 400 proposals and the new Executive Director, Feachem, a public health official and academic who had worked at the World Bank, was brought in to assist. During 2002, with two rounds of funding, grants totalling almost US$ 1.5 billion had been approved for two years, covering 154 programmes in 93 countries. The first US$1 million was disbursed in December 2002. By July 2003, over US$ 70 million has been disbursed[17].

Desmond Johns, Head of the UNAIDS New York office when the Global Fund was created, commented: "If the Global Fund worked as intended, if it could truly serve as this major conduit to get resources to countries with minimum overheads and a lot less bureaucracy – and to the extent that they have succeeded in doing that – this should be recorded as the success story of the Fund".

Plumley took a more optimistic view than some of his former colleagues. "You could argue that the Global Fund in 2001 is not a huge success for UNAIDS, because it is the creation of a new multi-lateral financing mechanism, outside the UN. But I don't see it that way … [it is] a way of channelling the needed new resources into AIDS. Who [fought] for those resources? UNAIDS did …".

[15] UNFPA (2004). *Financial Resource Flows for Population Activities in 2002*. New York, UNFPA.
[16] McGreevey W, Bertozzi S, Gutierrez J-P, Izazola J-A, Opuni M (2002). 'Current and future resources for HIV/AIDS', in *State of the Art: AIDS and Economics*. International AIDS Economic Network for IAEN symposium, Barcelona, Spain, June.
[17] The Global Fund to Fight AIDS, Tuberculosis and Malaria (2003). *The Global Fund Annual Report 2002/2003*. Geneva, The Global Fund.

UNAIDS report causes waves in China

In June 2002, UNAIDS issued a report entitled *HIV/AIDS: China's Titanic Peril* which warned that China was heading for an AIDS epidemic of 'proportions beyond belief'. The report compared Chinese leadership to the officers on the Titanic who refused to believe the fact that the ship was sinking until it was too late[18].

At the end of 2001, it was thought that 400 000 people in China were infected with HIV, up from 27 000 in 1991 (subsequently these estimates were revised downwards). The report said that this number may only represent the 'tip of the iceberg': unless swift countermeasures are taken, the number of infected people in China could easily soar to 10 million by 2010, placing China on the brink of a catastrophe 'that could result in unimaginable suffering, economic loss and social devastation'.

The UN report added unusually severe criticism of the Chinese Government for its response to the disease[19]. It blamed China's slow response on a lack of commitment and leadership by government officials, 'dramatically insufficient' funding for AIDS programmes, and a 'crumbling public health care system'. It said that the Chinese Government had not done enough to educate the public; many Chinese still erroneously believed that HIV could be contracted through mosquito bites or by shaking hands.

The report emphasized 'the mostly hidden HIV vulnerability conditions' that could cause the epidemic to explode in China, and warned that China's predominantly medical response to the epidemic cannot continue. "If this government wants to do something, it has the power to do it", said Siri Tellier[20], who headed the UN Theme Group that produced the report with Emile Fox, then UNAIDS Country Coordinator.

Joel Rehnstrom served as UNAIDS Country Coordinator in China between 2003 and 2007. He explains that although the 'Titanic' report was not well received by the Chinese Government, there has since then been a great change in the way AIDS is viewed and dealt with in China. With continued advocacy efforts from UNAIDS as well as visits from the Secretary-General, the UN helped to bring the consequences of inaction on AIDS to the Chinese Government's attention. Piot highlighted lessons that could be learnt from dealing with SARS (Severe Acute Respiratory Syndrome) between November 2002 and July 2003 to lever an effective AIDS response in China.

On World AIDS Day 2003, Premier Wen Jiabao publicly shook hands with HIV-positive patients in Beijing, promising "they would have the love and care of the entire nation". This closely broadcast event marked the recent shift in the Chinese Government's response to AIDS.

---

[18] Pan P (2002). 'China faces Titanic AIDS crisis'. *Washington Post*, 28 June.
[19] Ibid.
[20] Ibid.

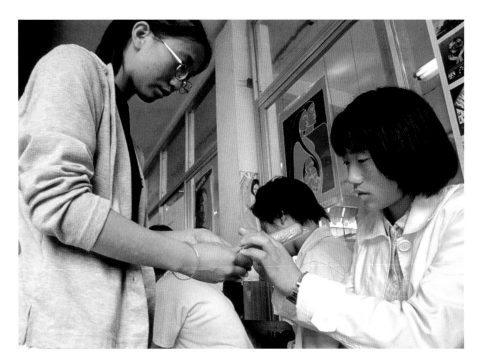

Attitudes to AIDS in China have changed greatly. Here young students in Bejing are learning how to use condoms.
UNAIDS/K.Hesse

After a meeting in June 2005 with Wen, Piot was the first UN official to address the powerful Central Party School of the Chinese Communist Party, which distributed his speech among its membership. According to Plumley, UNAIDS now has "an extraordinarily privileged relationship with the Chinese government", and "is well on its way to helping build provincial responses to AIDS".

Further moves to expand access to antiretroviral treatment

More resources became available for antiretroviral treatment when, in March 2002, the Board of Directors of the World Bank endorsed Multi-Country HIV/AIDS Programme for Africa (MAP) funding for antiretroviral procurement as part of comprehensive AIDS programming.

Also in March, in an effort to assess the quality of HIV medicines, and after years of lobbying by UNAIDS Secretariat, WHO published the first list of HIV medicines to meet WHO recommended standards: the Access to Quality HIV/AIDS Drugs and Diagnostics project. In the same month, WHO also published the first edition of the WHO treatment guidelines for resource-limited settings[21] that included simplified schemes for treatment and clinical diagnosis. They made the first mention of the "3 by 5" target – that is, the aim to treat three million people with antiretrovirals by the end of 2005.

---

[21] WHO (2002). *Scaling up Antiretroviral Therapy in Resource-limited Settings: Guidelines for a Public Health Approach* (1st edition). Geneva, WHO.

164

Schwartländer, Ian Grubb and Jos Perriëns from the Global Fund and WHO[22], have written that the list of essential drugs and the WHO treatment guidelines are well-accepted standards today. 'However, we can easily forget how bold and controversial these steps were at the time. For example, the US National Institutes of Health (NIH) had provided a grant to WHO to produce the simplified treatment guidelines. When NIH did not want to fully subscribe to the approach proposed, WHO took the unprecedented step of returning the funds to NIH'.

Around this time, the lead responsibility for HIV treatment within UNAIDS moved from the UNAIDS Secretariat to WHO. Piot commented that this was when WHO finally started taking up its role fully within the UNAIDS Programme. It was also the beginning of a difficult process to agree on a rational division of labour among the Cosponsors and the Secretariat. Even in 2007, there was still a lack of clarity between WHO and UNICEF over responsibility for mother-to-child transmission.

June saw the publication of the progress report on the Accelerating Access Initiative (AAI); it showed that one significant achievement was to lower prices for antiretroviral treatment[23]. Africa was able to increase significantly the number of people treated, both within and outside the framework of UN-brokered supply agreements within the AAI. About 35 500 people were being treated with antiretrovirals supplied by six companies by the end of March 2002 – a fourfold increase in 18 months. Still, according to the AAI final report, too few patients had benefited and generic producers had not been sufficiently involved[24].

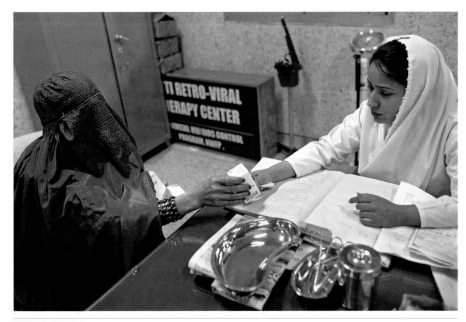

More resources became available for antiretroviral treatment when the World Bank endorsed funding for drug procurement as part of comprehensive AIDS programming.
UNAIDS/J.Moore

---

[22] Schwartländer B, Grubb I, Perriëns J (2007). 'The 10-year struggle to provide antiretroviral treatment to people with HIV in the developing world'. *The Lancet*, 368.
[23] WHO/UNAIDS (2002). *Accelerating Access Progress Report, 2002*. Geneva, WHO/UNAIDS.
[24] Ibid.

By the end of the AAI, perceptions had changed. Providing large-scale care and treatment was now shown to be feasible in the developing world.

Not everyone would be so unreservedly enthusiastic about the results. According to Jamie Love, Director of Consumer Project on Technology: "Accelerating Access Initiative (AAI) played a negative role because it was an attempt to undercut the real important work that was to be on generics. It was a public relations mechanism; it was a way of trying to force developing countries to buy premium, high-priced products which undercut the economies of scale of the generics market. So it was really designed to keep prices higher for AIDS patients instead of lower. It was really the wrong thing to do".

By the end of the AAI, perceptions had changed. Providing large-scale care and treatment was now shown to be feasible in the developing world. The inclusion of the possibility of purchasing antiretroviral drugs within the scope of the Global Fund and the availability of World Bank financing for care and treatment were further evidence of the changed attitude of donors to financing the purchase of antiretrovirals[25]. 'Globally, governments, the UN system, bilateral donors, the Global Fund, and civil society increasingly were focusing on treatment and care as part of their commitment to scaling up the global AIDS response'[26]. This was all preparing the way for a far more ambitious project the following year.

There were mounting demands for access to treatment in low- and middle-income countries and increasing evidence that antiretroviral therapy could be provided effectively in places without Western-style health services – examples include Médecins Sans Frontières clinics in South Africa, the work of Partners in Health in Haiti and UNAIDS' two initiatives on Drug Access and Accelerating Access. The evaluation of the Drug Access Initiatives in Côte d'Ivoire, Senegal and Uganda[27] clearly establishes that antiretroviral therapy can be successful in Africa. 'Virologic and immunologic outcomes, adverse events, and estimated survival are similar among patients in African DAIs [Drug Access Initiatives] and ART [antiretroviral therapy]-treated patients in Europe and the USA'.

Support from other donors was urgently needed to ensure technical support for programmes, sustainability rather than a project approach to treatment, and to strengthen health systems.

But until late 2002, the donors, with the exception of France and Luxembourg, were reluctant to talk about treatment financing for people with HIV in developing countries. The "3 by 5" goal was received very critically by the donors in 2003.

---

[25] Ibid.
[26] UNAIDS (2004). *Global Report 2004*. Geneva, UNAIDS.
[27] Katzenstein D, Laga M, Moatti J-P (2003). 'The evaluation of the HIV/AIDS Drug Access Initiatives in Côte d'Ivoire, Senegal and Uganda: how access to antiretroviral treatment can become feasible in Africa'. *AIDS*, 17, July.

The Barcelona conference

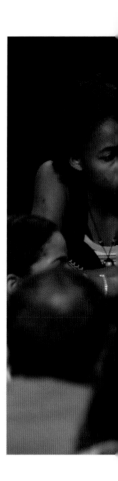

In July 2002, the 14th International AIDS meeting was held in Barcelona and access to treatment was a priority topic. At the opening ceremony, Piot told an audience of thousands that it was now clear that the AIDS epidemic was still in its early stages – and the response was at an even earlier stage. He told them: "Ten billion dollars annually is all that it will take for a credible minimum response to the epidemic. Yet that sum is three times more than is available today …".

Piot explained that treatment was now technically feasible everywhere in the world and warned against viewing prevention and care as competing priorities. He then presented a road map of what was required to keep the promises made on AIDS (at UNGASS). "So, let's make the AIDS response truly political. Let's bring forward today world leaders who keep their promises on AIDS, are rewarded with our trust, and those who don't, lose their jobs to those who will".

Gro Harlem Brundtland, Director-General of WHO at the time, made a significant announcement at the conference: "We are aiming for three million people world-wide to be able to access ARVs [antiretrovirals] by 2005 – around half of those who will need such treatment. The current total of people in low-income countries on treatment is around 230 000 and over half of these are from one country, Brazil. It is a promising start, but we have much further to go".

Some donors might not have entirely endorsed these sentiments, but the activists, out in force, certainly did. They were calling for more access to treatment.

'… your advocacy has to be that the current level of funding is shamefully inadequate and suggests some evidence of planned failure through underfunding … "thanks, but not nearly enough" should be the standard response to donors' miserly donations … the Fund has to become the major player for a coordinated, universal access response to these global pandemics'[28].

The Network of People Living with HIV in Asia urged national governments to accord them a greater voice in policy, decision-making and all other aspects of the responses against the epidemic. When Tommy Thompson, US Secretary of Health and Human Services, came on to speak, he was jeered and heckled. Activists stormed the stage with banners accusing the USA of the 'murder and neglect' of people living with AIDS.

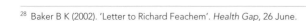

28 Baker B K (2002). 'Letter to Richard Feachem'. *Health Gap*, 26 June.

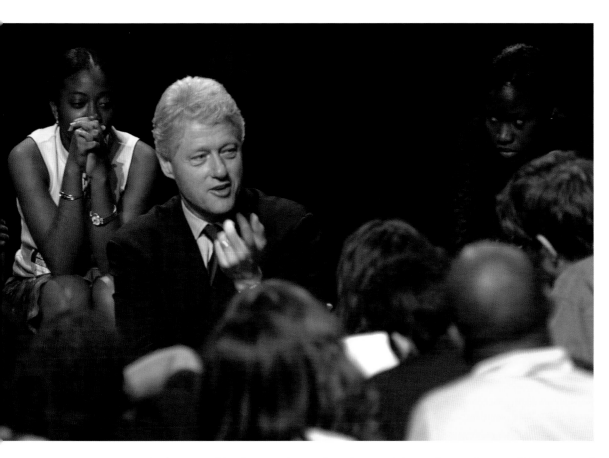

*Former US President
Bill Clinton talking to
young people during the
recording of MTV'S
'Staying Alive Forum' at
the International AIDS
Conference in Barcelona,
2002 MTV*

Partly inspired by the speeches at Barcelona and the evidence of successful antiretroviral therapy programmes in Africa, in October 2002, the Dutch Government organized a meeting of donors (together with WHO and the UNAIDS Secretariat) in Amsterdam on 'Integrating HAART [highly active antiretroviral therapy] in care, support and treatment'. This was a turning point for the donor community in terms of resistance to spending money on the widespread use of antiretroviral therapy – though not for all.

Schwartländer recalled: "Peter Piot and myself as the Director of WHO's HIV Department had been invited and we tried to move the treatment access in developing countries agenda forward. The donors saw only the problems. Pushing an agenda that the donors hate carries substantial risks. You may actually undermine your own resource-base".

He continued: "In that meeting, the Canadians actually put forward their global strategy on HIV/AIDS, which didn't mention [the] word treatment. Yet about a year later, the Canadians were the single biggest donor that saved and carried forward the '3 by 5' initiative by financing it in the WHO".

Some reflections on success in order to move ahead

The Executive Director's report to the 13th PCB meeting, held in Lisbon in December 2002, spelt out some of the major successes in the response to the epidemic in recent years (as well as responding to the *Five Year Evaluation Report*). These included:

- The mobilization of senior political leadership on all continents, raising the profile of the epidemic in national, regional and global forums, most notably through the UN Secretary-General's leadership in mobilizing new partners

- National Strategic Plans developed through a participatory process in virtually all affected countries, with a tripling of the number of high-level national AIDS councils or commissions in the past three years

- A nearly sevenfold increase in international resources targeted at AIDS in Africa to approximately US$ 1 billion

- The establishment of new funding mechanisms, notably the World Bank's Multi-Country HIV/AIDS Programme for Africa (MAP) and the Global Fund to Fight AIDS, Tuberculosis and Malaria

- That the Security Council had taken up the issues of AIDS in Africa, and HIV prevention in UN peacekeeping operations

- That the UN General Assembly held a Special Session on HIV/AIDS, resulting in clear agreement among Member States on strategies and approaches, and a set of ambitious and measurable goals and targets

- An order-of-magnitude reduction in the price of AIDS drugs for developing countries.

As the report rightly concludes, 'these are not UNAIDS achievements; they are global achievements'. The Programme had a major role to play in each of them (though some critics would question how great a role) but – and this is key – 'none of them could have been accomplished without the concerted efforts of the much larger and still rapidly growing coalition that now comprises the "global AIDS movement"'.

The purpose of taking stock of these successes was not self-congratulatory, but 'to remind us that the most significant challenges we are facing today are largely a result of those successes'. Over the next five years, the UNAIDS Secretariat and Cosponsors would struggle to meet these challenges and to ensure the sustainability of the successes.

'These are not UNAIDS achievements; they are global achievements. None of them could have been accomplished without the concerted efforts of the much larger and still rapidly growing coalition that now comprises the "global AIDS movement"'.

2003 – a year of the significant progress in funding

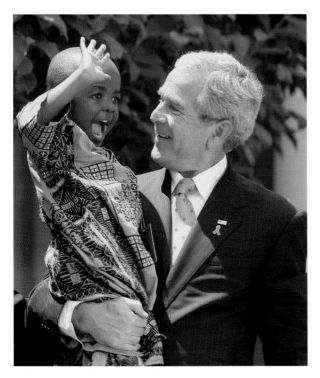

When UNAIDS was first established, the global actions and resources addressing the epidemic were roughly one tenth of what they were in 2003. 'To be successful in containing the progression of the epidemic, another 10-fold increase in the global effort will be required by the end of this decade … While this increase is not inevitable, it is no longer seen as wishful thinking'[29].

Nor was it, as yet more resources were forthcoming. In January 2003, US President George W Bush, in his State of the Union address, announced the launching of the U.S. President's Emergency Plan for AIDS Relief (PEPFAR). It aimed to spend US$ 15 billion over five years, a target representing a huge leap forward in international funding for AIDS. Some US$ 10 billion of this was new funding. Although Piot was disappointed that more of the money would not go multilaterally to the Global Fund, he believes that this was one of the most crucial moments in the history of the epidemic so far: "… [when] the most powerful person in the world puts 15 billion dollars on the table, it completely changes the landscape".

It was a significant moment in the history of AIDS, especially given the limited action of previous US Governments in relation to AIDS in the developing world. And other leaders would follow, including British Prime Minister Tony Blair, who pledged £1.5 billion (approximately US$ 3 billion) over three years in July 2003. A 2002 briefing note to Piot stated that the White House was strongly influenced to opt for higher spending levels after receiving UNAIDS' unpublished analysis of optimal spending allocations among major donors.

Michael Iskowitz, former Director of the US Office of UNAIDS, commented: "Despite a sometimes contentious relationship between the US Administration and the UN overall, there has been a very solid working relationship between UNAIDS and this administration. UNAIDS has contributed to the implementation of PEPFAR with some very tangible results, particularly in the area of coordination".

Ambassador Randall Tobias, the first US Global AIDS Coordinator, explained that although UNAIDS had nothing to do with the design of PEPFAR, "… once those decisions were made, the existence of UNAIDS has been very critical to the development of PEPFAR and

US President George W Bush holds Baron Mosima Loyiso Tantoh in the Rose Garden of the White House in May 2007, after delivering a statement on PEPFAR. White House photo by Eric Draper

"The existence of UNAIDS has been very critical to the development of PEPFAR and the implementation [of its work]. UNAIDS has played a very important role on the technical side of providing data that [are] universally accepted …".

[29] UNAIDS (2002). *Executive Director's Report to the 13th Meeting of the UNAIDS PCB*, December. Geneva, UNAIDS.

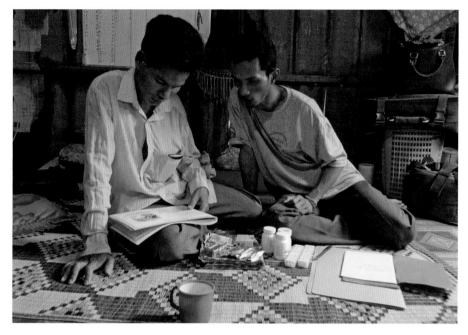

Many people in developing countries were not fortunate enough to receive antiretroviral treatment. The '3 by 5" campaign did make a difference, eventually providing treatment to about one and a half million people. UNAIDS/O.O'Hanlon

the implementation [of its work]. UNAIDS has played a very important role on the technical side of providing data that [are] universally accepted …".

UNAIDS data from countries, he says, provide credibility and a "certain legitimacy that comes from the seal of approval, so to speak, of UNAIDS on a number of things".

UNAIDS used its network of Country Coordinators to facilitate the launch of PEPFAR, gathering strategic information about the status of treatment programmes to help PEPFAR's decision-makers.

PEPFAR represented a radical innovation in the way the US Government's AIDS funding is coordinated to ensure optimal use of resources by many different agencies. A third of the money was earmarked for existing bilateral programmes in 75 countries and the remaining two thirds was for new programmes, including the Emergency Plan Worldwide which focuses on 15 countries heavily burdened by AIDS (Botswana, Côte d'Ivoire, Ethiopia, Guyana, Haiti, Kenya, Mozambique, Namibia, Nigeria, Rwanda, South Africa, Tanzania, Uganda, Viet Nam and Zambia). Each of these was to have a national coordinating authority responsible for coordinating the country's response to AIDS.

PEPFAR aimed to provide antiretrovirals to two million people by 2008; to prevent seven million new infections, and to provide care and support to 10 million HIV-infected individuals and children orphaned by AIDS.

There was no shortage of controversy surrounding PEPFAR's policies. Congressional rules governing how PEPFAR funds could be used for HIV prevention have been the source of substantial international criticism. In addition, US Government funds could not lawfully be used for needle exchange programmes for injecting drug users. Perhaps most controversial was the requirement that 33% of PEPFAR prevention money be spent on abstinence-only programmes. Yet PEPFAR is also the world's largest funder of condoms.

The "3 by 5" initiative promotes access to treatment

Once PEPFAR's treatment targets had been announced, 'whether and how WHO should further advance the treatment agenda therefore loomed as an important challenge for Lee Jong-wook (the new Director-General of WHO). That Lee unequivocally embraced the treatment agenda is now part of his legacy'[30].

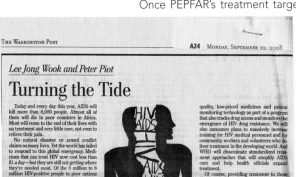

THE WASHINGTON POST

A24 MONDAY, SEPTEMBER 22, 2003

Lee Jong Wook and Peter Piot

Turning the Tide

In September 2003, Lee joined with Piot and Feachem to launch the "3 by 5" ('Treat 3 million by 2005') initiative, which had first been announced at the 2002 Barcelona AIDS conference by Brundtland, Lee's predecessor. The aim was to treat half of those in need of treatment in developing countries[31]. This was presented as an achievable (though many thought unlikely) target, given increased resources, on the way to the ultimate goal of universal access. It also heralded a significant scaling up of WHO's work on AIDS, including a much larger department, more country-based staff focusing on the epidemic and strong leadership from Lee, as well as the directors of the HIV/AIDS Department, Paolo Teixeira followed by Jim Yong Kim.

Washington Post op-ed article by Lee Jong-wook and Peter Piot, September 2003, announcing the "3 by 5" initiative. WHO/UNAIDS

But to succeed in scaling up access to treatment, "business as usual will not work", Lee stated at the launch of "3 by 5"[32]. Countries had to act faster and, in some cases, differently, but they needed support from the global community.

Such support was rather slower in coming than had been hoped for. Some people felt uncomfortable with such a time-bound target. Donors were slow to provide funding because they felt they had not been fully consulted and that a consensus on the initiative had not been reached. It took time to involve donors in the initiative, explained Kim, who was Director of WHO's HIV/AIDS Department from 2004-2005. "The donors felt "3 by 5" put too much pressure on them, that it set too high a target; they felt they should have been consulted. I tell you if we'd consulted on it, almost all of them would have said 'Don't do it' and, indeed, many of them opposed the initiative all the way along … it was frankly my personal lack of familiarity with the donors and my background as an activist that made me push it through

---

30 Schwartländer, Grubb, Perriëns (2007).

31 In 2001, partners within UNAIDS and other organizations had calculated that, under optimal conditions, three million people living in developing countries could be provided with antiretroviral therapy and access to medical services by the end of 2005. However, there was then little support for acting on this from governments or donors.

32 WHO (2003). Press Release, 22 September. Geneva, WHO.

... Looking back, I think there's little question that without that target the Ministers of Health would not have felt pressure to actually deliver on anything. I think it was most important that the UN asked Ministers of Health and governments to actually perform and be held accountable for outcomes".

This meant that it was several months before the planned new staff could be recruited in countries. 'While WHO could only support the implementation efforts of its Member States, time was lost in disputes over ownership and the feasibility of achieving the target, rather than the action needed'[33].

Interestingly, at the 15th PCB meeting in June 2004, although the PCB welcomed the greatly increased focus on treatment, as exemplified by the "3 by 5" initiative, it stressed that '... prevention must remain a cornerstone of a comprehensive response, not only to prevent new infections but also to reduce stigma and discrimination'. There was a growing concern, not only among PCB members, that prevention had been side-lined by the focus on treatment.

Monitoring and evaluation

Monitoring and evaluation are crucial to determining whether funding is being used effectively and whether programmes are reaching target populations and accomplishing their objectives.

Monitoring and evaluation are crucial to determining whether funding is being used effectively and whether programmes are reaching target populations and accomplishing their objectives. It supports the information needs of partners such as the Global Fund and PEPFAR. However, there was evidence that efforts at monitoring and evaluation were being hampered by a lack of technical capacity and resources[34]. In September 2003, UNAIDS published its first *Progress Report in the Global Response to the HIV/AIDS Epidemic*, the follow-up to the 2001 UN General Assembly Special Assembly on AIDS, and it reported that 75% of the 103 reporting countries felt they did not have the capacity to report reliably on indicators such as HIV workplace policies, coverage of antiretroviral therapy and access to prevention of mother-to-child transmission services. Only 43% of these countries had a national monitoring and evaluation plan.

Consequently, UNAIDS has established a Monitoring and Evaluation Unit within the Secretariat as well as in the World Bank (the Global Monitoring and Evaluation Team), as part of the effort to strengthen countries' capacity to track the epidemic. This was also the result of a recommendation from the *Five Year Evaluation of UNAIDS*.

Paul De Lay runs the Secretariat's Evaluation Department and he explained that it has three functions. The first is to help countries develop their monitoring and evaluation systems. More than 40 full-time Monitoring and Evaluation Advisers and their teams provide technical assistance to countries and Regional Support Teams, and support the coordination and capacity building of national monitoring and evaluation systems. The advisers' role is to work with governments, civil society and UN system counterparts to strengthen national capacity in

---

[33] Schwartländer, Grubb, Perriëns (2007).
[34] UNAIDS (2004). *Global Report 2004*. Geneva, UNAIDS.

monitoring and evaluation. In general, they function as mentors to colleagues in national AIDS authorities to facilitate the implementation of a unified monitoring and evaluation system.

The Evaluation Department's second main line of activity is to work with a wide range of partners to harmonize and reduce the number of global monitoring and evaluation indicators. This is achieved through the UNAIDS-initiated Monitoring and Evaluation Reference Group, made up of about 80 members from many countries and institutions.

The Evaluation Department's third line of activity consists of global reporting, for example, on progress towards the Declaration of Commitment, on global and national resource tracking, and on specific initiatives such as universal access.

De Lay, reflecting on recent progress, said, "the capacity of monitoring and evaluation systems at country level has been assessed in 2007 and shows steady and dramatic improvement. Nearly 150 countries have provided national reports on the UNGASS indicator that include not only epidemiologic data but also information on changes in risk behaviour, the policy environment, national funding for AIDS, and the coverage of prevention and treatment services. Furthermore, there is much more a sense of country ownership of the collection analysis and reporting of the data. Setting national targets is also part of a monitoring and evaluation process which will help countries better define what is meant by 'universal access' and will provide clear, quantitative guidelines for what progress should be expected".

Indeed, UNAIDS monitoring and evaluation information has proved its value and credibility in that it now serves the needs of new partners, such as the Global Fund and PEPFAR.

In a speech he made in Berlin in September 2007, Piot said: "Six years ago there were over 300 indicators to measure AIDS programmes by donors. Now we are already at around 50. Our ambition is to go below 20 so that every donor uses the same ones. It will save transaction costs in a huge way for the developing countries".

The World Food Programme becomes the ninth Cosponsor

On 16 October 2003 – World Food Day – the Rome-based World Food Programme (WFP) became the ninth Cosponsor of UNAIDS. It is the world's largest humanitarian agency and focuses on responding to HIV through a range of food aid programmes.

- **Prevention:** Through its school feeding programmes, including take-home rations, some of the most vulnerable children are encouraged to attend school. Education is a key factor in preventing HIV, especially for girls. WFP has also linked up with UNICEF, UNFPA and governments in 18 countries to integrate HIV prevention into school feeding programmes, so children are doubly protected.

- **Care and support:** WFP provides nutritious food for many people living with HIV, including many receiving antiretroviral treatment. Good nutrition is an important aspect of treatment; without it, many people find it hard to continue on treatment. It also provides food in many countries to tuberculosis patients in hospitals, thus encouraging them to remain until they are cured, and take-home rations for their families.

- **Mitigating the impact:** many poor households caring for people with AIDS or headed by orphaned children, receive food aid from WFP. In Mozambique, WFP supports chronically ill people and their families through home-based care as well as providing food to day-care centres.

- **Food for training:** Food assistance helps older orphans and children living on the street learn some marketable skills, food production, literacy and life skills.

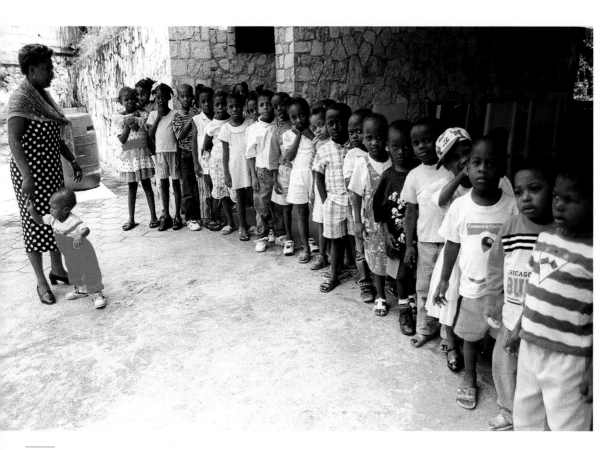

*Haitian AIDS
orphans queueing
outside their classroom
at La Maison Arc
du Soleil (Rainbow
House), 1999. It was
established outside the
capital, in Boutilier, by
Plan International.
AFP/Getty Images/
Thony Belizaire*

Haiti

Haiti is the poorest country in the Western hemisphere. About 65% of its population
live below the poverty level and the country has had a violent political history – 13
governments within two decades. However, in relation to its HIV epidemic, the
news is not all bad, even though Haiti is the worst hit country in terms of prevalence
outside sub-Saharan Africa. Haiti has the highest prevalence of HIV in Latin America
and the Caribbean. According to the UNAIDS 2007 *Global Report*, 3.8% of all adults
are living with HIV.

At the onset of the epidemic in the early 1980s, Haiti was one of the so-called '4-H'
club: 'homosexuality, heroin-injecting drug use, haemophilia and Haiti'. Stigma and
fear badly affected tourism, a key source of income to the country, in those first few
years. They also kept the infection underground, which facilitated a gradual spread
from urban to rural areas.

In 1982, 13 health professionals from Haiti founded the Haitian Study Group on Kaposi's Sarcoma and Opportunistic Infections (GHESKIO). This early initiative has, over the years, developed and grown from a focused research group to a number of centres offering not only clinical and laboratory services related to HIV, tuberculosis and other sexually transmitted infections but also broader primary and reproductive health-care services. These centres merge testing and counselling with prevention of mother-to-child transmission services. The centres are supported by the United Nations Population Fund, working with the Ministry of Health.

UNAIDS established a presence in Haiti in March 2001, with Maria Tallarico as the first Country Programme Adviser. The main challenges she encountered upon arrival were practical, logistical and political: no electricity, no running water, roadblocks and a great deal of political insecurity and instability following the election of President Jean-Bertrand Aristide. Tallarico, with other (United Nations) partners and development organizations, addressed the situation as best as she could. She recalls the strength of the collaborative environment of the time, both within the UN (the Pan American Health Organization was Chair of the Theme Group at this time) and among other partners, including donors such as the United States of America. Tallarico felt that in spite of the difficult circumstances, Haiti was an inspiring place to work because of the many brilliant minds she encountered, such as Jean William Pape, one of the founders of GHESKIO, and Paul Farmer, who was among the first to provide an integrated package of prevention, treatment and support through Partners in Health.

The year 2002 was a busy one. The National Strategic Plan was completed, the first Global Fund proposal was submitted and an in-depth assessment of the Theme Group was performed. The UN Theme Groups of Haiti and the Dominican Republic jointly developed an integrated work plan on migration and HIV, a unique collaboration between two Theme Groups. The UNAIDS focus at this time was on improving surveillance, expanding access to testing and counselling, and promoting care and support and the empowerment of women. Although USAID was by far the biggest donor on AIDS in the country, the coordination and facilitation role of the UN system, especially in a situation of political instability, was explicitly called for both by national and international (donor) partners in the response to AIDS.

The business sector played a key role in visualizing the economic impact of the epidemic on the country, and there was concrete and strategic support from the country's major enterprises in raising funds for nongovernmental organizations and for people living with HIV.

Raúl Boyle succeeded Tallarico as UNAIDS Country Coordinator, serving from January 2003 until August 2005. In his opinion, though Haiti was an incredibly

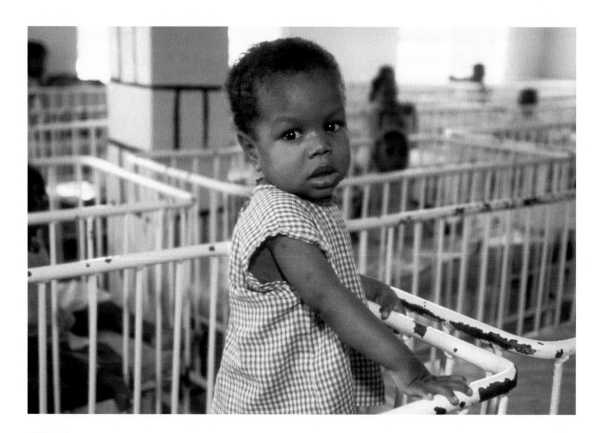

Haiti has the highest prevalence of HIV in Latin America and the Caribbean. UNAIDS/PAHO/ A.Waak

difficult country to work in, the challenging circumstances led, paradoxically, to better and greater collaboration among and between the UN agencies. To paraphrase his words, if the problems are so clear, and so serious, everyone sees the need to assist and tries to do it in the best way possible, which is through working together. Making sure that one's agency's logo appears upfront becomes much less important.

An essential element in such collaboration is a UN Resident Coordinator, who takes on a personal commitment to HIV within the Country Team and puts it on the agenda consistently. An equally committed Theme Group Chair is also important: during Boyle's time, this Chair was UNFPA.

The UNAIDS office's particular achievements at that time included working with, and strengthening, the associations of people living with HIV. Three different groups existed and, by bringing these and several other related organizations together to assist in the creation of a network or platform, their visibility was strengthened and they became a much more credible forum in consultation and collaboration with the UN, donors and nongovernmental organizations. Boyle also emphasized the role of UNAIDS as a trusted partner, building up the confidence, especially among vulnerable groups and people living with HIV, that UNAIDS was there to assist and support them.

The UN's role as a source of technical support and as key partner to the various ministries was stressed by the Haiti's First Lady, Mildred Aristide, during a visit by Kathleen Cravero, then Deputy Executive Director of UNAIDS, in April 2003. Both Tallarico and Boyle mentioned Mildred Aristide as a committed leader on AIDS in general, and of the Global Fund's Country Coordinating Mechanism (CCM) in particular. In the meeting with Cravero, Mildred Aristide acknowledged that the government faced challenges of coordination and she indicated the need for a more multisectoral response.

Haiti also provides some clear examples of how Programme Acceleration Funds (PAF) really can kick-start action or programming, or funding, in overlooked or sensitive areas. Examples include the creation of the Network of People living with HIV, and support for an association of men who have sex with men. As this association became more involved in the Network of People living with HIV, it developed both capacity and credibility. This led to an increase in recognition among development partners of the need to address this group, and to the inclusion in the Global Fund proposal of a programme targeting men who have sex with men.

For Boyle, the greatest confirmation of the trust and confidence in UNAIDS came in 2004. When Aristide was removed from power, Mildred Aristide, who had chaired the CCM until that time, could no longer perform this function. As an interim solution, the CCM members agreed that UNAIDS was the most appropriate partner to chair the CCM.

The Theme Group was chaired by the UNFPA representative, Hernando Clavijo, who was a strong collaborator. As a Cosponsor, UNFPA was at the forefront of the response, as demonstrated by the agency's support to the GHESKIO centre in Port au Prince. The centre provides counselling and testing, as well as care and support for victims of sexual violence.

That both HIV and violence against women were high on the agenda is exemplified by the inclusion of both areas in the flash appeal that went out to the international community in 2004 after the overturning of Aristide's government. Throughout the appeal, UNFPA and UNAIDS collaborated with the Ministère à la Condition Féminine (the Ministry of Women's Affairs) and nongovernmental organizations to raise awareness on AIDS, women and sexual violence. Again, UNFPA and the Theme Group Chair played a critical role in this, while these efforts were in part supported by PAF.

As a good example of advocacy, and as one of the main achievements of 2005, Boyle mentioned the production of the film, *Le Président a-t-il le SIDA? (Does the President have AIDS?)*, by Haiti's most well-known film-maker Arnold Antonin. A number of very popular Haitian stars participated in this movie. UNAIDS was instrumental in advocating the production of the film, in mobilizing resources from the UN agencies and bilateral donors and in providing technical advice to the filmmaker. The film was first shown in commercial cinemas before being shown in schools and open-air screenings in towns and rural areas throughout the country.

Haiti managed to submit a sound proposal for the first round of the Global Fund and, with Ghana, was one of the first two countries to receive disbursements from the Fund. Boyle felt that UNAIDS, through Tallarico, played a key role here, by being a strong advocate, providing information and strategic advice on the process and facilitating the involvement of all partners. Tallarico herself emphasized the importance of the functioning of the CCM in a difficult environment, since lack of transparency was one of the major obstacles during the Aristide administration. The CCM came up with an innovative mechanism to safeguard accountability and transparency to counter the doubt that a troubled country such as Haiti could manage the almost US\$ 67 million that would be coming its way. This mechanism made Haiti one of the best examples of a functioning CCM.

Through an equally successful fifth round proposal, Haiti now receives almost US\$ 117 million through the Global Fund. The second proposal was prepared under very difficult circumstances. In Boyle's view, this illustrates the strength of the joint efforts by the UN and other development partners, in particular, the US President's Emergency Plan for AIDS Relief (PEPFAR) that became operational in Haiti in 2004 through the CCM.

Surveillance estimates over the years have shown a decreasing prevalence of HIV, predominantly in urban areas, from 9.3% in 1993 to 3.7% in 2003-2004. The national estimate currently stands at 3.8%, down from 5.9% in 1996. Although many challenges remain, and Haiti is still a poor country, the response to HIV is making good progress. The collaboration of civil society, the UN, donors, the government and other partners continues.

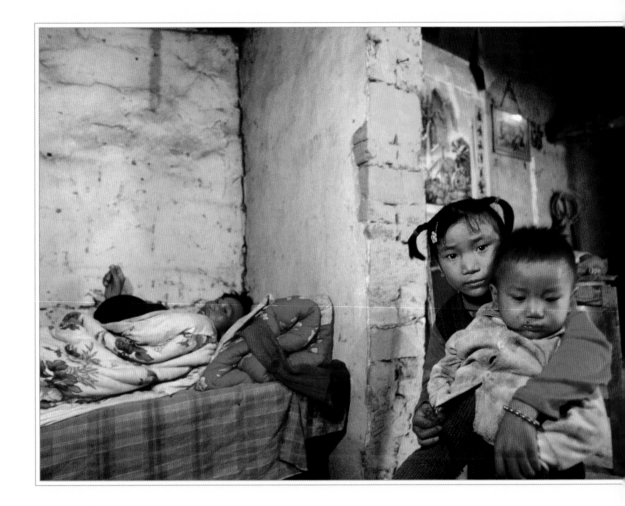

The challenges of the
AIDS epidemic are still
enormous. There are
many children like these
in their home in Henan
province China, who are
caring for dying parents.
Panos / Qilai Shen

Chapter 7:
Making the money work, 2004–2005

UNAIDS had undoubtedly become a significant player in the AIDS world; now the doors of prime ministers, presidents and ministers of finance were open to it.

By the end of 2003, UNAIDS estimated that 30.9 million people were living with HIV. In that year, 3.0 million were newly infected and 2.0 million people died.[1] In 2004, US$ 6079 million was spent globally on AIDS and in 2005, the figure was US$ 8297 million.

By the start of this biennium, there had been a huge increase in funding for tackling AIDS. From around US$ 300 million a decade earlier, global resources for AIDS in 2005 were estimated to be US$ 8.3 billion[2]. While this was only about 70% of the US$ 12 billion per year that UNAIDS estimated was needed to finance a comprehensive response by 2005[3], it was still a considerable increase.

The majority of the new funding came through the US President's Emergency Plan for AIDS Relief (PEPFAR), the Global Fund to Fight AIDS, Tuberculosis and Malaria and the World Bank's Multi-Country HIV/AIDS Programme in Africa (MAP). The two latter programmes are funded by the major donor countries. However, not to be ignored was the fact that an estimated 33% of all AIDS spending in low- and middle-income countries in 2005 came from the developing countries themselves[4].

UNAIDS' advocacy work had contributed to this huge increase in funds. Donor countries, although not entirely uncritical of the organization were keen to work with UNAIDS and, in particular, welcomed its monitoring of the epidemic and information on policies and programmes.

The AIDS movement had become huge. 'A' list celebrities, mainly from the United Kingdom and the United States of America, regularly visited AIDS projects in low-income countries and proudly displayed their red ribbons as well as their white 'Make poverty history' wristbands. People working in other areas of health and development could, and did, feel undermined and overlooked.

Jon Lidén, Director of Communications with the Global Fund, observed: " UNAIDS has made AIDS cool … The fact that so many celebrities have been engaged with AIDS and [that] AIDS has been adopted by the culture industry has, I think, helped tremendously to de-stigmatise AIDS".

---

[1] *2007 AIDS epidemic update*, November 2007.
[2] UNAIDS (2007). *Global Report 2007*. Geneva, UNAIDS.
[3] UNAIDS (2004). *Fact Sheet 2004: Funding for AIDS*. Geneva, UNAIDS.
[4] UNAIDS (2005). *Global Resource Availability for AIDS 2005*. Geneva, UNAIDS.

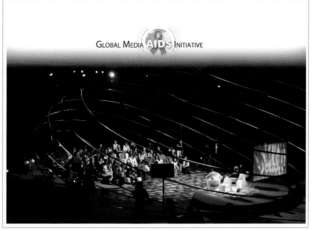

"But isn't it interesting how we have had the emergence of celebrity leadership in the vacuum of political leadership?" commented Stephen Lewis, former Special Envoy of the Secretary-General for HIV/AIDS in Africa, somewhat controversially. He then pointed out that celebrities may be raising consciousness but "… ultimately, it is governments and the UN [United Nations] that have to make the difference".

In January 2004, Kofi Annan, the United Nations Secretary-General, launched the Global Media AIDS Initiative.

He continued: "I mean, Bono himself said, 'I go to the Foreign Relations Committee in the United States when they're discussing the appropriation in the Senate and I tell them what's going on', – and he actually used this phrase – 'and their eyes mist over'. I tell them how much more is required and I leave, and they cut the budget'".

From its beginnings, UNAIDS recognized and harnessed the power of the media in the fight against the epidemic. Working with MTV has been one of the organization's most successful partnerships. Media companies have used their creative and technical resources to produce public service announcements and to weave themes and stories about HIV into their programmes, whether current affairs or 'soaps'. A new initiative would create a huge expansion of such activities.

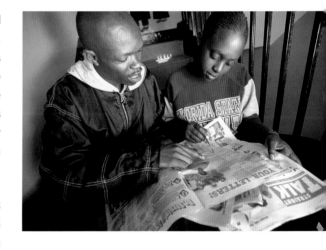

In January 2004, Kofi Annan, the United Nations Secretary-General, launched the Global Media AIDS Initiative (GMAI) to underscore the importance of the media in responding to the AIDS global crisis. He asked all major media companies to commit to using their resources to expand public knowledge and understanding about HIV. Executives from more than 20 media corporations across 13 countries attended the launch and committed their companies' resources to raising the level of public awareness and understanding about AIDS. Bill Gates, Chairman of Microsoft Corporation, was the keynote speaker.

In Kenya, young people aged 15 to 19 produce the newspaper Straight Talk for their peers on all aspects of sexual health including HIV prevention and testing
UNAIDS/G. Pirozzi

This initiative was conceived by UNAIDS and the Kaiser Family Foundation (a United States-based, non-profit, private operating foundation focusing on health issues). In April 2004, Bill Roedy, Vice-Chair of MTV Networks and UNAIDS Goodwill Ambassador, was appointed Chair of the GMAI Leadership Committee. He said: "If education is currently the only vaccine available to us, then the global media industry has in its hands the means to deliver that vaccine.

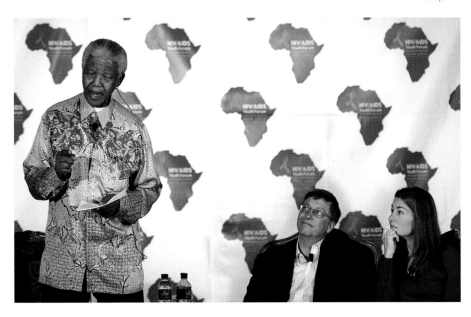

If we harness our immense communications power, with all the creativity and innovation at our disposal, the impact will be felt far and wide". Since 2007, Dali Mpofu, the Chief Executive Officer of the South African Broadcasting Corporation, has been the new Chair of the GMAI.

Partnership is key to the GMAI – an unprecedented initiative for an industry that normally thrives on competition. In 2004, Gazprom-Media began working with Transatlantic Partners against AIDS, a Moscow-based nongovernmental organization, and the Kaiser Family Foundation to establish the Russian Media Partnership to Combat HIV/AIDS. This coalition now includes more than 50 leading media and consumer goods companies. Another partnership that has grown out of the GMAI is the African Broadcasting Media Partnership on HIV/AIDS. Recently, this African partnership committed its members to dedicating 5% of all airtime to HIV-related programming and messages.

Raising levels of awareness and educating people about prevention of HIV infection was as essential in 2004 as in any other year of the epidemic's life.

By the end of 2005, more than 130 companies from 69 countries had become involved with the GMAI, with the result that numerous new campaigns were launched and existing programmes expanded.

Raising levels of awareness and educating people about prevention of HIV infection was as essential in 2004 as in any other year of the epidemic's life. Despite some progress in lowering prevalence rates and increasing numbers of people on antiretroviral treatment, HIV had taken a firm hold in many countries and was growing in others.

The challenge of the new funding: 'too many cooks'

At global and country level, there was a particular sense of urgency about using the new financial resources effectively. If the available funding failed to produce sound results in scaling up prevention and treatment, it would not be easy to convince donors of the need to continue investing.

UNAIDS coined the phrase 'making the money work'. This was the major challenge. There was the perception that only a brief window in time existed in which to do this – to convince politicians, for example, of the sustainability of the response – and thus the urgency.

If the available funding failed to produce sound results in scaling up prevention and treatment, it would not be easy to convince donors of the need to continue investing.

But 'making the money work' was no easy task for most countries. Many of those applying for or receiving funds did not have what some economists call the 'absorptive capacity' to use them. They lacked the personnel to process funds and ensure their distribution, the planners and policy makers to make the necessary proposals based on the right technical know-how and, in particular, they suffered from extreme shortages of staff on the ground – doctors, nurses, community workers, programme managers and others. The lack of capacity of some countries to absorb aid assistance was not a new problem, but it had never been satisfactorily resolved. The increased funds for AIDS made the countries' absorptive capacity problem even more obvious.

Donors could not profess ignorance of such problems, and in fact, in some instances, they have exacerbated them by requiring these hard-pressed countries to execute programmes according to their own rules and to report regularly – again according to donor-specific standards – on the programmes or projects they were funding. For instance, some countries might have 10 donors, and so would have to produce 10 different reports.

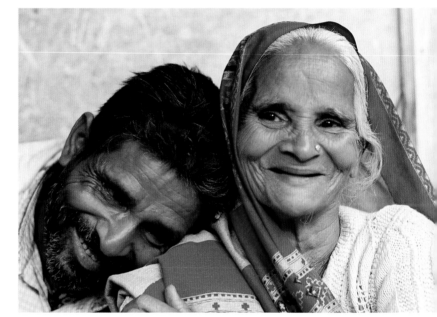

Despite the great hike in AIDS funding, family care is still essential in all affected countries
UNAIDS/W.Phillips

Every year donors would visit countries and, yet again, require specific work to be done. In one year, for example, Tanzania might receive 2,000 donor delegations and aid missions, all of whom would expect to be met by top officials, and the Minister of Finance would have to supply 10 000 reports[5]. Donors would impose reporting requirements that were overwhelming for small countries. For example, the island of Saint Vincent (population 117,000) was asked to monitor 191 indicators, and Guyana, 169 indicators. Time and money was wasted in duplicating tasks to meet the demands of a multiplicity of public and private agencies. The same time and money could have been spent on extending prevention programmes, support and treatment for people living with HIV and on eradicating serious gaps in many national responses to AIDS, such as surveillance to identify people most at risk.

[5] United Nations Millennium Campaign website, 2007. *Harmonization of Aid: Why Does Harmonization Matter So Much?*

Kristan Schoultz, former UNAIDS Country Coordinator in Kenya and now Director, Global Coalition on Women and AIDS, described the problem: "A country like Kenya receives a lot of international attention, and the National AIDS Control Council staff could be completely burdened, from eight o'clock in the morning until five o'clock in the afternoon, by consultant visits. And often, those consultants, who would all have been brought in by different partners, would be looking at very similar things. So, clearly, when you think about it, the better idea is [to say] 'Why don't you donors bring a team together? Let's not have so many missions'. It's extraordinary when you actually talk to colleagues in the NACC [National AIDS Control Council] how much time they spend being very gracious and very polite to external visitors, when indeed they should be thinking about policies and strategies and moving the response forward".

Mary Kapweleza Banda, Malawi Minister of State responsible for HIV/AIDS, pointed out: "At the country level, governments are struggling to fight the AIDS epidemic, while rushing to respond to conflicting and often repetitive donor requirements"[6].

Towards better coordination

This is not just a question of bureaucracy gone awry; such chaos impedes attempts to save lives, to plan prevention programmes and reach more people with antiretroviral treatment".

This lack of coordination (or 'harmonization', the term more often used in development circles) had been a recurrent theme at a number of high-level meetings. In 2002, the UN Conference on Financing for Development in Monterrey, Mexico, concluded that the best way to use aid effectively was through processes led by the countries themselves.

The Monterrey Consensus, as the meeting's final agreement is known, expanded on this and provided a framework for international cooperation on development. Various subsequent meetings built on this agreement. In February 2003, the High-Level Forum on Harmonization issued the Rome Declaration committing donors, recipient countries and bilateral and multi-lateral institutions to harmonize their policies and procedures. Then in April 2004, in Paris, the Development Cooperation ministers and agency heads of the Organisation for Economic Co-operation and Development (OECD) Development Assistance Committee agreed a statement promising to 'turn the principles of harmonization and alignment – agreed at the Rome High-Level Forum in 2003 – into reality on the ground'. A year later, both low- and high-income countries joined with multilateral organizations and international aid organizations to endorse the Paris Declaration on Aid Effectiveness. However, the history of development is littered with such declarations, so only time would tell if this one would have any effect.

UNAIDS was determined to push for coordination in AIDS work and responded to the call for reducing transaction costs and duplication. Working with the Global Fund and the World Bank, the UNAIDS Secretariat initiated consultations in various African countries as well as at global level. Peter Piot, UNAIDS Executive Director, explained: "There was really a chaotic

---

6   UNAIDS (2004). Press Release, 25 April. Washington, DC, UNAIDS.

situation in Africa. Donors used separate reporting standards, different coordination committees, advisory groups and so on. This is not just a question of bureaucracy gone awry; such chaos impedes attempts to save lives, to plan prevention programmes and reach more people with antiretroviral treatment".

The relationship between various stakeholders in Tanzania.

Reports came back to Geneva describing the high costs of poor coordination, and the need to eliminate isolated project funding, so common in the majority of affected countries, in order to scale up the national response

Graphic from The "Three Ones" in Action: Where We Are and Where We Go from Here, illustrating the complex relationships between stakeholders in one country- Tanzania (UNAIDS)

to AIDS and to reduce the heavy administrative burden on countries. In many countries, too, advisers found that different government departments, as well as donors, had differing policies and programmes for the epidemic: '… they engage in parallel financing, planning, programming and monitoring. "The right hand does not know what the left is doing" would apply, except there are many hands involved'[7].

Bernadette Olowo-Freers, UNAIDS Country Coordinator in Tanzania, said: "This is the partnership mapping. It is precisely because of such a colourful picture [see above] that the Development Partners decided to support the Paris Declaration vigorously and the General Budget Support".

Michel Sidibe, now Deputy Executive Director, Programme, UNAIDS, explained: "When we saw this graph, we realised that it would be better if the countries had a more consolidated framework within which to work. In fact, three major challenges led us to that conclusion. First, we realised that the priority setting was fragmented. Two, we realised that the procedures for using the resources were not aligned with national priorities. Three, the monitoring of progress was not consistent and was generally based just on satisfying the requests of donor-countries. All of this was slowing implementation down".

The consultations on the need for better coordination were facilitated by Sigrun Mogedal, who had been Chief Technical Adviser for Social Sector Development at the Norwegian Agency for Development Cooperation in the late 1990s, then State Secretary for International Development in the Royal Norwegian Ministry of Foreign Affairs. She became a Senior Policy Adviser to UNAIDS in 2003. One of her (many) strengths was that she had worked in develop-

---

[7]   UNAIDS (2005). *The "Three Ones" in Action: Where We Are and Where We Go from Here.* Geneva, UNAIDS.

ment and health even though, in her own words, she "was not an AIDS expert". Thus she was able to bridge the gap between the 'development people' and the 'AIDS people', to take a cool, hard look at the barriers to countries' working effectively against AIDS and to reflect on how UNAIDS and partners might dismantle these barriers.

Mogedal noted the huge bureaucratic burden on government officials who had to meet the extra targets and guidelines created by the UN Millennium Development Goals and the Poverty Reduction Strategy Papers, all complicated by the different approaches taken by donors. Some donors, for example, were much less likely to collaborate with the public sector but preferred to work through international and national nongovernmental organizations.

She also explained that the purpose of National AIDS Councils, the creation of which had been encouraged by UNAIDS, the World Bank and then the United Nations General Assembly Special Session (UNGASS) through the Declaration of Commitments, was "very little understood" in many countries. There was also a tension between the Councils and ministries of health: "They were somehow outside the development framework".

Sidibe worked closely with Mogedal. He explained that it was very clear that without a "consolidated, inclusive and nationally owned plan – that is, a plan owned by all the actors, not just the government – it's impossible to make the money work for everybody. Without such a plan the money is not aligned to national priorities".

The next step was a review of the necessary steps for reaching national-level coordination of the AIDS response; this was conducted at the International Conference on AIDS and Sexually Transmitted Infections in Africa in Nairobi in September 2003. Consensus was reached on a set of guiding principles to be agreed by all players involved in countries' response to the AIDS epidemic.

Initiating the "Three Ones"

When the report of this consultation arrived on Piot's desk, his reaction was: "It was pretty long and complicated and I put it aside several times, [thinking] this is one of those incomprehensible reports which we specialize in". After reading the report, it was clear to him that three principles were of key significance. There should be:

- one agreed HIV/AIDS action framework, a nationally devised strategic plan that provides the basis for coordinating the work of all partners and ensures national ownership
- one national AIDS coordinating authority (such as a National AIDS Council) with a broad-based, multisectoral mandate
- one agreed country-level monitoring and evaluation system.

Piot dubbed these the "Three Ones" – inspired, he said, by reading a book on old Chinese propaganda posters and wishing to simplify the usual UN jargon.

Donor and host countries, bilateral and multilateral institutions and international nongovernmental organizations all endorsed these principles at the Consultation on Harmonization of International AIDS Funding on 25 April 2004 in Washington, DC. The meeting was co-hosted by UNAIDS, the UK and the USA[8].

Mogedal stressed the need to 'drive agreement' at this meeting around three key concepts: the rationale for **exceptional** AIDS action, national **ownership**, and **accountability** (who is accountable and to whom).

Piot emphasized the importance of "having all the donors in the one tent", even if they took different approaches to their work. Ambassador Randall Tobias, then US Global AIDS Coordinator, said after the meeting: "The agreement reached today will help all partners to exercise their comparative advantage in a manner that will enhance and not constrain our collective response"[9].

National ownership is defined so as to include government, civil society and other national stakeholders, who are providers and/or beneficiaries of the AIDS response[10]. Piot also explained that "when we say one authority, that does not only include the government sectors but also civil society". Some governments do not seem to have understood this and therefore civil society has been suspicious about being excluded.

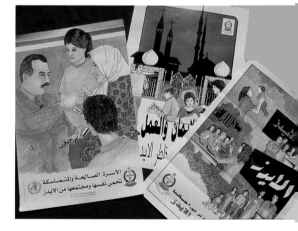

Arabic leaflets on AIDS awareness
UNAIDS/G.Pirozzi

Until recently, donors were rarely held to account for their performance, and their commitments were not monitored. The Paris Declaration marks the commitment of all development partners to strengthening mutual accountability mechanisms – both donors and country partners have expressed their intent to enhance their respective accountability to their citizens and parliaments for their development policies, strategies and performance.

In addition to providing timely, transparent and comprehensive information on aid flows so as to enable partner authorities to present comprehensive budget reports to their legis-

---

[8] The countries attending the meeting were Australia, Belgium, Brazil, Canada, Côte d'Ivoire, Denmark, Finland, France, India, Ireland, Italy, Japan, Luxembourg, Malawi, the Netherlands, Norway, South Africa, Sweden, the UK and the USA. Organizations present were the UNAIDS Secretariat, UNDP, WHO, the World Bank, OECD/Development Assistance Committee, ICASO and GNP+.

[9] UNAIDS (2004). Press Release, 25 April. Geneva, UNAIDS.

[10] UNAIDS (2005). *Making the Money Work Through Greater UN Support for AIDS Responses. The 2007–2007 Consolidated UN Technical Support Plan for AIDS*. Geneva, UNAIDS.

latures and citizens, donors have committed to reforming and simplifying donor policies and procedures to encourage collaborative behaviour and progressive alignment with partner countries' priorities, systems and procedures.

"The history of development is the history of re-branding the same ideas again, and again, and again".

The UK Secretary of State for International Development, Hilary Benn, also welcomed the agreement: 'The UK, as the world's second largest bilateral donor on HIV/AIDS, is firmly committed to the 'Three Ones' principles for harmonizing the efforts of donors in support of developing countries. This approach … will be adopted in the UK's new strategy for tacking HIV/AIDS globally'[11].

Some people, explained Julia Cleves, then Senior Policy Adviser to the UNAIDS Executive Director, view the "Three Ones" as just a snappy title for an old concept, or a repackaging of old ideas – but, said Cleves, "the history of development is the history of re-branding the same ideas again, and again, and again".

However, addressing the 15th meeting of the Programme Coordinating Board in June 2004, Piot stressed that the "Three Ones" concept "is not another buzzword or slogan but rather a fundamental principle by which to govern the response at national level. Taken singly, these principles are not new, but when applied simultaneously and consistently upheld by all stakeholders, they hold the key to effective and sustainable national responses".

Board members made it clear that governments, donors and other partners would have to play their part in ensuring that the principles were adhered to. 'The "Three Ones" should be viewed as an "urgent special case" in light of the exceptionalism of AIDS and the current boost in the number of actors and volume of funding involved'[12]. They also stressed the importance of country ownership of plans: '… it was essential to respect this process and not impose plans from outside'[13].

Country ownership is essential because the AIDS epidemic is so diverse and affects different groups of people in different countries. One of the barriers to tackling AIDS effectively is that some donors – but not all – may be reluctant to fund proposed programmes, for example, harm-reduction programmes or antiretroviral therapy. So part of the delicate balancing act UNAIDS and the rest of the UN team have to perform when supporting countries in their response to the epidemic is to ensure that the "First One" – the National AIDS Framework – reflects the real needs of the response in that country and that donors truly 'buy into' it. Thus it is essential that development agencies incorporate progress on the "Three Ones" in their staff performance indicators. For example, in April 2005, the Office of the US Global Coordinator and the UNAIDS Secretariat held a bilateral meeting to evaluate success to date in implementing the "Three Ones" and to explore how to accelerate this progress most effec-

[11] Ibid.
[12] UNAIDS (2004). *Executive Director's Report to the 15th Meeting of the UNAIDS PCB*, 23–24 June. Geneva, UNAIDS.
[13] Ibid.

190

tively – particularly in those countries receiving substantial US aid. However, most donor agencies have not yet included promotion of the "Three Ones" as a performance indicator for their staff.

Putting the "Three Ones" into action

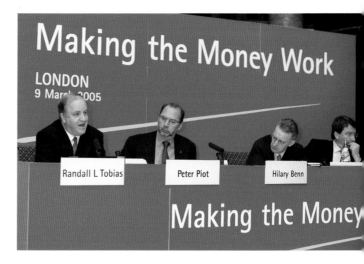

In March 2005, a high-level meeting took place in London on 'Making the money work: the "Three Ones" in action', involving representatives of governments, donors and international organizations. The meeting was co-hosted by the UK Department for International Development (DFID), France, the USA and UNAIDS. Unfortunately, attempts at harmonizing the meeting were to some extent undermined by the behaviour of several groups.

For some months before the meeting, a reference group of experts, brought together by the UNAIDS Secretariat, had worked on two models for future resource needs. As Achmat Dangor, then Director of Advocacy, Communication and Leadership at UNAIDS, explained, one model described the funding that would be needed to achieve the level of coverage required by the UNGASS goals – "the aspirational goal which is the maximum amount of money available with few constraints".

Making the Money Work meeting in London, March 2005, co-chaired by US Global AIDS Coordinator Ambassador Randall L. Tobias, UNAIDS Executive Director Peter Piot, UK Secretary of State for International Development Hilary Benn, and France Minister delegate for Cooperation, Development and Francophony Xavier Darcos. Astonleigh Studio

The second model described what resources could realistically be spent, taking into account low-income countries' limited ability to implement programmes. These papers were circulated to the three donor co-hosts of the meeting and the Cosponsors and recognized later that it should have been more widely circulated.

As Dangor explained, a debate on the substantial issues of resource needs for AIDS and on countries' capacity for implementation was going to be difficult: "The miracle is that we were still able to extract one vital thing, and that was a mandate to pursue country-level harmonization, because it gave birth to the Global Task Team."

Paul De Lay, from the UNAIDS Secretariat' Evaluation Department and now Director of Evidence, Monitoring and Policy, said that many UNAIDS staff perceived the meeting as a real challenge: "There was a lot of hostility from all different groups. Some of our own Cosponsors seemed to be turning against us, and some in civil society were turning against us...also, we can argue and fight all we want in an internal forum but not in such a public, destructive way". Others felt donors had not been supportive.

Piot commented that when he suggested that spending money wisely in development is not always easy, "immediately an email circulated accusing me of being 'a puppet of the donors'".

Indeed, as people reflected on the meeting, memories of the early days of the organization surfaced. Piot said that it provided a good example of how the slightest mistake by the Secretariat could be amplified and exploited. It also revealed how a technical issue – estimating resource needs for AIDS – "is eminently political, and a calm debate is very difficult, if not impossible, because there is a lack of trust amont he various stakeholders". An important role for the UNAIDS Secretariat is, and always has been, creating and maintaining this trust: it is vital, if effective work is to be achieved.

However, despite the bitter clashes before and during the meeting, a key outcome was established – the Global Task Team on Improving Coordination among Multilateral Institutions and International Donors. The Global Task Team, co-chaired by Sidibe and the Swedish AIDS Ambassador, Lennarth Hjelmaker, was composed of senior representatives from 24 low-income and developed countries, civil society groups, regional bodies, the Global Fund and UN organizations. In addition to the establishment of the Global Task Team, the London meeting tasked the UNAIDS Secretariat in collaboration with relevant partners to refine the methods for estimating resource needs on AIDS.

A technical issue – estimating resource needs for AIDS – "is eminently political, and a calm debate is very difficult, if not impossible, because there is no trust among the various stakeholders".

Facilitated by the UNAIDS Secretariat and with representatives from all stakeholders, the new team was asked to develop a set of recommendations on improving the institutional architecture of the response to the epidemic.

Sidibe explained: "The purpose of the London meeting was to rethink the architecture of the response at the country level, and the Global Task Team has been instrumental in this. It was a major task [in the 80 days' time-frame given to them] to look at what was not working, why it was not working and how we could make sure that the recommendations would help to implement the principles of the 'Three Ones' effectively".

The Global Task Team speedily developed recommendations presented to UNAIDS' PCB in June 2005[14]. The main aim of all these meetings was to ensure that as many people living with HIV as possible received treatment and support as well as providing nationwide prevention programmes, so there was a real urgency behind the process.

Piot believes that the Global Task Team recommendations are probably the most advanced agreements on multilateral reform. For many years, various working groups, governing boards and suchlike – both within the UN and among development organizations generally – have talked about coordination and division of labour. But, said Piot: "… many of the

---

[14] For the full Global Task Team recommendations, see http://data.unaids.org/Publications/IRC-pub06/JC1125-GlobalTaskTeamReport–en.pdf.

reform proposals were exclusively donor-driven and the developing countries were hardly included in their development and would understandably not be very supportive. But the Global Task Team's recommendations had been pushed by a real mix of donors and developing countries. The recommendations were endorsed by the governing bodies of all the Cosponsors and the Global Fund, and have provided the basis for UNAIDS' work".

Sidibe explained the importance of the Global Task Team: "[It ensures] country ownership of the AIDS programme, including civil society… by placing the country's costed and evidence-informed plan at the centre of all our actions. … The GTT [Global Task Team] helps us to think about the alignment of resources to national priorities, and it dealt with the critical issue of division of labour among UN agencies. Also, the Global Task Team clearly spells out the concept of mutual accountability … the joint responsibilities of donors, multilaterals and UN agencies in terms of dealing with development".

Sidibe continued: "The GTT [Global Task Team] has been spearheading UN reform and demonstrating that we can really start with a concept of a joint team … It is a turning point for UNAIDS … positioning the organization as a central instrument for change".

"The GTT [Global Task Team] has been spearheading UN reform and demonstrating that we can really start with a concept of a joint team … It is a turning point for UNAIDS … positioning the organization as a central instrument for change".

Supporting the "Three Ones" in countries

It would have been much harder for UNAIDS to support countries in implementing the "Three Ones" had not this initiative roughly coincided with the expansion of staff in countries. Roger Salla N'tounga, UNAIDS Country Coordinator in Ethiopia, explained that strengthening UNAIDS country staff was essential to promoting the "Three Ones". "If our responsibility is to help a country make the money work, we need to scale up our way of working, to reinforce our offices and those of Cosponsors. With the current [i.e. before 2004] staffing, people were working 48 hours a day".

Between 2004 and 2005, the UNAIDS Secretariat increased the number of international country-level professional staff by 61 members. UNAIDS Country Coordinators were now full members of the UN Country Teams. In 2005, the UNAIDS Secretariat decentralized its management and set up Regional Support Teams in all regions, replacing existing Inter-Country Teams, to provide management support to the UNAIDS Country Coordinators and UN Theme Groups on AIDS. Many of the functions carried out by the Secretariat in Geneva were transferred to these teams. The Secretariat also greatly expanded its investment in monitoring and evaluation, including the Country Response Information System (CRIS)[15], social mobilization and support to the Global Fund.

---

[15] As a software programme developed to address countries' problems in improving monitoring and evaluation, CRIS provides the platform for a database to support monitoring and evaluation and provides countries with the ability to store and analyse data and to exchange data with those from other systems. A prototype based on CRIS has been developed for PEPFAR. CRIS has been catalytic in supporting development of monitoring and evaluation systems in developing countries.

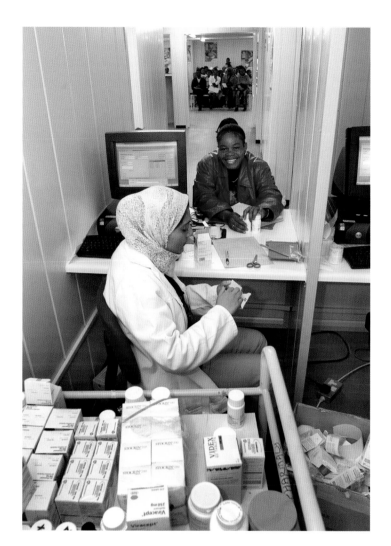

Since 2004, UNAIDS has placed 41 monitoring and evaluation advisers in its country offices, as well as six regional monitoring and evaluation focal points in the Regional Support Teams. The advisers work directly with national monitoring and evaluation staff and they usually have an office in the national structure responsible for AIDS monitoring and evaluation.

George Tembo, a Team Leader in the UNAIDS Country and Regional Support Department, explained: "It's UN reform in action … as a UN system we are working together in a more coordinated, structured way without duplicating, and in cognizance of the fact that we have the least amount of resources at country level. But we are the ones who have the trust of most of the national partners. We can serve as effective brokers and facilitators".

It was now clear to the Global Fund, for example, that the UNAIDS Secretariat and its Cosponsors such as the World Health Organization could play a vital part in supporting countries to prepare

A dispensary providing antiretrovirals in Botswana where free antiretroviral treatment has been available for several years. UNAIDS/E.Miller

proposals to the Fund and other bodies for resources. During the first four funding rounds of the Global Fund, the UNAIDS Secretariat provided an estimated US$ 5.3 million in technical support for developing national proposals. An analysis of the third and fourth funding rounds indicates that proposals receiving technical support from UNAIDS were four times more likely to be funded than proposals from countries without UNAIDS support[16].

The UNAIDS Secretariat, the Global Fund and WHO worked on developing an early-warning system for identifying poor-performing (Global Fund) grants, and a technical assistance strategy for Global Fund HIV proposals and grants. It is crucial that countries do not 'fail' with Global Fund funding, especially if that funding is paying for antiretroviral therapy, because of the implications for sustainability and adherence to treatment.

[16] UNAIDS (2005). *From Advocacy to Action: a Progress Report on UNAIDS at Country Level.* Geneva, UNAIDS.

Progress in countries

How are countries doing in terms of the "Three Ones"? By the end of 2005 and early 2007, there was clear improvement in establishing these new principles. Most countries had achieved the "First One" – that is, a national AIDS action framework or National Strategic Plan. For example, the Lao People's Democratic Republic has developed a new National Strategy and Action Plan on HIV/AIDS and sexually transmitted infections for 2007–2010, with the support of UNAIDS. The Plan prioritizes prevention and care activities in terms of specific groups such as sex workers and their clients, drug users, mobile populations, vulnerable youth and men who have sex with men. It also prioritizes provinces and districts based on selected vulnerability criteria such as areas with high HIV prevalence and high population density, areas that are tourist and business centres offering high levels of entertainment, as well as areas that are on crossroads or have highly mobile populations[17]. It aims at a 90% reach for prevention programmes targeting vulnerable groups, and nearly 100% coverage of treatment and care for people in need.

Unlike in the Lao People's Democratic Republic, few country plans are specific about priorities, and approximately 40% of plans are neither costed nor budgeted[18]. This obviously limits their usefulness in providing overall guidance to all who are working in those countries on programmes for AIDS. External donors are less likely to ensure the work they fund meets a country's priorities when these are only vaguely presented.

By the end of 2005, 85% of countries reported having established the "Second One" – one national coordinating authority for the AIDS response. Moreover, according to a UNAIDS survey, 81% of countries have additional coordinating mechanisms on AIDS[19]. For example, the Global Fund's Country Coordinating Mechanisms (CCMs), while providing much needed funding, can lead to a confusion of roles when it comes to policy making: 'In some countries the CCM makes de facto policy decisions through funding decisions related to investment in some areas and not others. The UNAIDS survey also states that in 32% of the countries surveyed, the national AIDS authority does not play a significant role in the CCM'[20].

There has been an improvement in the state of monitoring and evaluation – the "Third One" – in many countries, though, in 2005, more than 40% of countries rated national monitoring and evaluation efforts as average or below average. More countries have a dedicated monitoring and evaluation budget and share monitoring and evaluation results with UN agencies, bilateral agencies and other partners. But 'much more progress on data-sharing is needed to maximize evidence-based decision-making'[21].

Inevitably, the road to harmonization, to achieving the "Three Ones" in every affected country, is a tough one. UNAIDS' role is not an easy one.

[17] National Committee for the Control of AIDS (2005). *National Strategic and Action Plan on HIV/AIDS/STI 2007–2010.* Geneva, UNAIDS, July.
[18] Buse K, Sidibe M, Whyms D, Huijts I, Jensen S (2007). *Scaling up the HIV/AIDS response: From Alignment and Harmonization to Mutual Accountability.* Briefing Paper, Overseas Development Institute, London, August.
[19] UNAIDS (2007). *Effectiveness of Multilateral Action on AIDS. Report to the 18th Meeting of the UNAIDS PCB,* June. Geneva, UNAIDS.
[20] Ibid.
[21] Ibid.

Challenges to the "Three Ones" and the United Nations Consolidated Plan to 'Make the Money Work'

Documents such as this by the African Council of AIDS Service Organizations, the International HIV/AIDS Alliance and the International Council of AIDS Service Organizations, were developed to help encourage the involvement of civil society groups in the coordination of national AIDS responses.

Inevitably, the road to harmonization, to achieving the "Three Ones" in every affected country, is a tough one. UNAIDS' role is not an easy one. Mogedal said that it is very hard for UNAIDS to drive change in countries "… because of the way it's hooked into the UN system. If they have a Resident Coordinator in UNDP that wants to drive these kinds of changes along with them, then they're able to do that but, if not, they will be a voice in the wilderness".

Salla N'tounga raised another challenge: "It is very difficult to convince countries that if they really want to mobilize all the sectors, the coordinating body has not to be in a ministry like the Ministry of Health but at a higher level. We have succeeded in having these National AIDS Commissions established but in most of those countries we still face a conflict between the former unit at the Ministry of Health and the new National AIDS Commission".

Ben Plumley, Director of the UNAIDS Executive Office at the time, commented: "The biggest challenge – and it's not resolved – is that, while donors have in principle agreed to implement the 'Three Ones', the behaviour of their country teams – and indeed of other outside stakeholders in-country – hasn't necessarily been adapted fast enough. Another issue is how the 'respect for the leadership of national governments to implement AIDS strategies' has been interpreted. To some, they mean ownership and direction from Ministries of Health, with minimal engagement of other sectors either inside or outside government: to others – and this is what is so exciting about the 'Three Ones' – they mean a genuinely multisectoral engagement with civil society. It remains a significant challenge to build this kind of genuine multi-stakeholder ownership of the 'Three Ones'. To this day, one sees continued scepticism, including from some activist groups and national civil society groups, who fear that the 'Three Ones' may just be an excuse to exclude them from the national response".

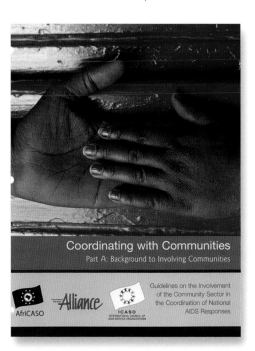

Coordinating with Communities
Part A: Background to Involving Communities

AfriCASO   Alliance   ICASO
INTERNATIONAL COUNCIL OF
AIDS SERVICE ORGANIZATIONS

Guidelines on the Involvement
of the Community Sector in
the Coordination of National
AIDS Responses

With the arrival of the Global Fund and the "Three Ones", the capacities of civil society – such as nongovernmental organizations and community-based organizations – are often fully stretched. In the International Council of AIDS Service Organizations (ICASO) report *NGO Perspectives on the Global Fund*, the point is made that 'civil society representatives do not automatically come to the table with the knowledge and skills to participate fully in policy-making; decision-making; priority setting; and programme design, implementation and monitoring'.

Indeed, some countries have not fully involved civil society in national AIDS authorities. In Mozambique, for example, a recent "Three Ones" assessment revealed that a large percentage of prevention and care activities are implemented by civil society but financed by government. But, according to this assessment, 'civil society representatives frequently do not feel empowered to disagree with government or other partners' opinions in the multisectoral coordination meetings, as this may influence the process of selecting projects for financing'[22].

Countries also differ in their attitudes to various sectors of civil society. In Eastern Europe, for example, networks of people living with HIV seem to be well represented in coordinating AIDS authorities but representation from other communities of people at high risk of exposure to HIV such as injecting drug users, are absent – probably a reflection of the stigma, discrimination and legal oppression such people have to contend with. In Barbados, on the other hand, even though the legal status and stigmatization of men who have sex with men is still a problem in society, representatives of this community and other populations at higher risk of exposure to HIV have been included in the national HIV/AIDS Commission.

Some senior development figures are optimistic about the long-term effects of the "Three Ones". Mogedal commented: "AIDS has always been demanding quicker, broader, better, more creative responses, so ... if we're able to go that road [of the 'Three Ones'], the AIDS response infects the development response. Then I think there is hope. And of course there is hope. We celebrate so many people staying alive ... we celebrate some of the countries being able to level off the epidemic".

Tobias stressed the importance of the "Three Ones": "I have been talking with Development Ministers and Finance Ministers around the world about the need to take that concept and expand that to all development assistance and use that whole concept as a vehicle for the way in which we are all focusing our education programmes and health programmes".

Thus, many countries require technical support to improve the governance framework in which the national AIDS response is planned and executed. In August 2005, the UN launched a Consolidated Technical Support Plan to 'Make the Money Work', which provides, for the first time, a unified and consolidated UN-sourced technical support plan to address implementation bottlenecks (in contrast to the presentation of piecemeal, parallel and sometimes competitive plans and appeals in the past). The Plan aims to support key actions to put the "Three Ones" principles into practice. It includes elements to support the development of inclusive national ownership, the formulation of evidence-based AIDS plans, support for national AIDS coordination authorities, and the strengthening of national monitoring and evaluation systems.

Furthermore, the Plan aims to strengthen health systems to ensure the scale-up of quality treatment and prevention services. Multilateral and bilateral partners have been seeking long-term sustainable solutions, such as the human resources for health initiative described below.

Many countries, particularly in Africa, struggle because they do not have the right people, or the right number of skilled people, to do the work.

[22] UNAIDS (2007). *Executive Director's Report to the 18th Meeting of the UNAIDS PCB*, June. Geneva, UNAIDS.

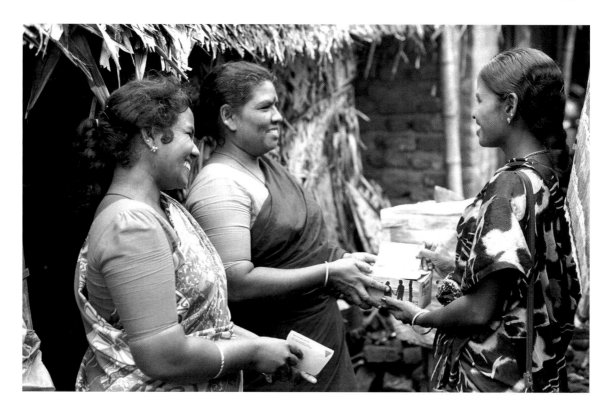

The chronic lack of human resources

A strong national AIDS framework and a national AIDS authority are necessary, but not enough, for an efficient use of resources. Many countries, particularly in Africa, struggle because they do not have the right people, or the right number of skilled people, to do the work. The WHO 2007 World Health Report revealed an estimated shortage of almost 4.3 million doctors, midwives, nurses and support staff worldwide[23]. This report also observes that the African region suffers more than 24% of the global burden of disease but has access to only 3% of health workers and less than 1% of the world's financial resources[24].

The lack of skilled health workers is a serious problem in most low-income countries. Large numbers emigrate to richer countries where ageing populations are outstripping the numbers of indigenous health workers (partly because insufficient numbers are being trained in rich countries). The Kenyan Ministry of Health estimates that the country is losing about 20 nurses per week or more than 1000 nurses per year to countries such as Australia, the UK and the USA. Other destinations include Botswana and Namibia.

Others leave the public sector for the richer pastures of the private sector in their own country (including programmes run by international nongovernmental organizations, development agencies and research institutes). In some countries – for example, Kenya – there is a limit on the number of nurses that can be recruited in the public sector. This partially relates to

[23] WHO (2007). *Working Together for Health. World Health Report*. Geneva, WHO.
[24] Ibid.

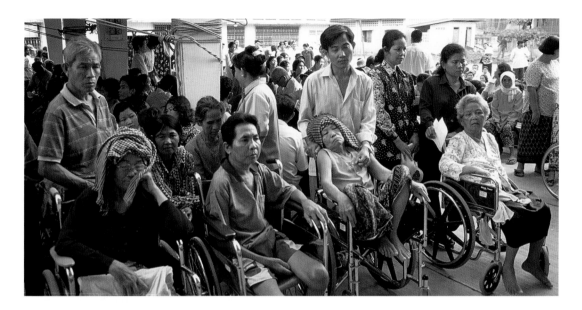

government budget ceilings and available allocations, but can also (in Kenya) be traced back to an employment embargo instituted in 1993 by the Directorate of Personnel Management, largely in response to pressures of structural adjustment programmes that required large cuts in public spending[25]. So despite the desperate need for their skills, several thousand nurses are unemployed.

Hospitals and clinics face severe human resource challenges. Here in Phnom Penh, hundreds of people wait outside the Centre of Hope clinic. There are only 22 beds for in-patients. Lotteries have to be drawn every morning for any available space. UNAIDS/ S.Noorani

Another reason for the shortages is the impact of AIDS on the workforce. In Zambia[26], for example, AIDS-related deaths account for a large percentage of nurses and doctors lost to the country – 68% of nurses and clinical officers, compared with 23% due to resignation and 9% due to retirement. Countries such as Zambia do direct public health sector employees who are positive to public clinics for treatment, but 'Zambian nurses tell us that stigma makes HIV-positive staff reluctant to report for treatment at their own institutions'[27].

Donors could help by recognizing that helping to meet countries' needs for human resources is 'perhaps the single greatest contribution they could make and that demonstrating their impatience with the lack of capacity is counter-productive'[28]. Often, donors are reluctant to invest in fair salaries and benefits or training, yet these are vital to providing prevention and treatment programmes nationwide. Donors' reluctance often springs from a concern that by investing in improved salaries in one sector, they may be distorting the labour market and be unable to sustain the necessary funding. Judges, teachers, agronomists and many other professions are equally poorly paid in many countries.

[25] ALMACO Management Consultants Ltd, in collaboration with the African Medical and Research Foundation (2005). *Budget Ceiling and Health: the Kenya Case Study.* Wemos Foundation, Amsterdam, October.
[26] Feeley R, Rosen S, Fox M P, Macwan'gi M, Mazimba A (2004). *The Costs of HIV/AIDS among Professional Staff in the Zambian Public Health Sector.* Central Board of Health, Zambia/USAID.
[27] Ibid.
[28] UNAIDS (2005). *Making the Money Work. Where We Are and Where We Go from Here.* Geneva, UNAIDS.

Special human resources programme in Malawi

In an effort to resolve the human resource crisis in Malawi, in 2004, the Ministry of Health, with the support of its development partners, put together a plan called 'The 6-Year Emergency Human Resources Relief Programme'. This programme includes the expansion of health workers' training institutions and the retention of health workers in the public sector, through improving their remuneration package and providing incentives to health workers operating in underserved areas. By October 2005, this US$ 273 million programme had been fully funded[29].

"This problem stared us right in the face. It wasn't just a brain drain of skilled workers, it was a brain haemorrhage".

The Malawi Government had been well aware of the scarcity of health workers and the effect on the country's response to AIDS, and had documented this. But the plan to tackle the problem emerged only after Piot made a joint visit to the country with Suma Chakrabarti, the Permanent Secretary at DFID.

As Piot explained: "This problem stared us right in the face. It wasn't just a brain drain of skilled workers, it was a brain haemorrhage". Human resources clearly had to become a top priority, even though the visit was intended to focus on harmonization and the "Three Ones"; otherwise how could Malawi effectively use all the funding pouring into the country?

But who would provide the funding? Erasmus Morah, who was UNAIDS Country Coordinator in Malawi until July 2007, explained: "The UN family, UNAIDS, was able to devise a strategy in collaboration with DFID. ... DFID said, 'We will put $100 million to this plan if UNAIDS could use its position to get the Global Fund to put in another $100 million'. We took on the challenge and we did just that. We immediately advocated and supported the technical reprogramming of about $40 million of the existing resources. When Round Five of the Global Fund came around, we also marshalled the arguments and provided the technical support for Malawi to apply".

"Under the leadership of the National AIDS Commission, we brought in WHO consultants and contributed UNAIDS staff such as David Chitate, the Monitoring and Evaluation Adviser. We sequestered them with the government counterparts for about a week. A month later, *Voilà!*, Malawi became the only country globally that received assistance ($65 million) for health system strengthening and human resources for health. So, that totalled just over the US$100 million DFID talked about".

By providing money for training and human resources, DFID broke some taboos. But the result is that the Emergency Human Resources Programme has shown encouraging signs of early success.

---

[29] *Malawi HIV and AIDS Monitoring and Evaluation Report, 2005* (2005). Follow-up to the Declaration of Commitment on HIV and AIDS (UNGASS). Office of the President and Cabinet, Malawi, December.

Salary top-ups of more than 50% have improved retention and recruitment of health professionals, and the schools will increase their output of health professionals by 50% – double the number of nurses and triple the doctors in training. Morah commented: "We've never been able to attract all the graduating nurses, but the last class that graduated, about 43, all of them joined the Ministry of Health, unlike before, where they would get, maybe, one-third if they're lucky or just a handful".

An innovative source of technical assistance: technical resource facilities

Technical support has been a long-standing and unresolved problem in international cooperation on development. Most developing countries lack the number of people needed with the technical expertise in many areas of AIDS work, and look to the UN and to consultants

A child watches his mother on a antiretroviral drip in a hospital in Tigray, Ethiopia.
Panos/Pep Bonet

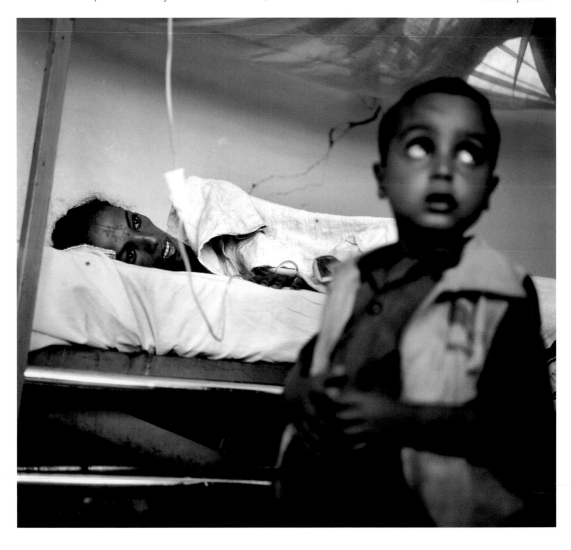

from the developed world for support, especially with the increase in funding. The use of external consultants is not an ideal solution, as it does nothing to build the skills of local people and takes money out of the country. Nor do experts from the North necessarily understand the specific needs and complexities of the South.

Staff in the UNAIDS Secretariat did some hard, lateral thinking and produced an innovative and well-targeted solution – regionally based Technical Support Facilities. These facilities provide high-quality technical assistance for the strategic planning, implementation, management, and monitoring and evaluation of national HIV/AIDS programmes.

The idea was to expand UNAIDS' cooperation with already existing regional networks and institutions, in order to enable an enhanced, nationally owned and cross-regional support system. Four such facilities have now been set up in Southern Africa, West and Central Africa, Eastern Africa and South-East Asia and the Pacific since 2005.

The UN Consolidated Plan to 'Make the Money Work' contributes to the development of regional technical support capacity and South-South cooperation.

The role of UNAIDS in these Technical Support Facilities is to ensure quality, to do training and exchanges to strengthen local experts' skills and to provide core and seed funding. These facilities are innovative insofar as they are more culturally appropriate to each specific country and build in-country capacity using local and regional expertise; in that sense they have helped to 'redefine' the traditional paradigm of development, whereby the North provides aid to the South. In Latin America and the Caribbean, UNAIDS partners with the Technical Horizontal Cooperation Group, Brazil's FIOCRUZ (one of Brazil's and Latin America's largest biomedical research institutes), Mexico's National Institute of Public Health and the Regional HIV/AIDS Initiative for Latin America and the Caribbean.

A better coordinated United Nations effort

In December 2005, Annan wrote to all UN Resident Coordinators directing them to establish a Joint UN Team on AIDS, with one joint programme of support, as recommended by the Global Task Team. It was an unprecedented directive to the whole UN system, aimed at strengthening its work in countries including support for the "Three Ones". Annan wrote: 'The Team should consist of the operational level staff working on AIDS, including those currently working at the Technical Working Group. The Team should work under the authority of the UN Resident Coordinator System and the overall guidance of the UN Country Team, and be facilitated by the UNAIDS Country Coordinator'.

This decision by the Secretary-General, commented Piot, showed once again how AIDS and UNAIDS have triggered a new way of doing business.

Every country's UN Joint Programme on AIDS should include a defined UN Technical Support Plan with a clear set of deliverables and detailed collective and individual accountability of the UN Country Team to enhance national responses to AIDS.

The directive also reflected the agreements made in August 2005 on the division of labour among UN agencies, funds and programmes. This agreement identified individual Cosponsors or the UNAIDS Secretariat as the Lead Organization within a particular UNAIDS technical support area, that would act as the single entry point for government and other stakeholders asking for UN support. This was another step on the road to coordinating UN support in countries.

Although the division of labour is not fully activated in all countries, or even at global level, it was, according to Piot, "… an amazing agreement and shows the real progress UNAIDS has made. At the beginning, in 1996, I would have thought it was possible because it seemed the obvious action to take, and I didn't know what I know now about how agencies work together. But five years ago I would have thought such an agreement was impossible". Thus, as UNAIDS approached the end of its first decade, some of the early challenges had been met but many more were yet to be overcome.

Kenya – an early proponent of the "Three Ones"

In the mid-1990s, in Kenya as in many other countries, stigma and denial about AIDS were strong, there was limited engagement beyond the health sector, and considerable advocacy was still needed to engage political leaders and foster high-level political commitment. However, by the late 1990s, things were beginning to change. The drive for a comprehensive, multisectoral response began in earnest when, in 2000, Kenya embarked on its US$ 50 million, five-year, World Bank-supported, Multi-Country HIV/AIDS Programme for Africa (MAP) project, one of the first on the continent. With the initiation of MAP, the national coordinating authority was established in the Office of the President, and efforts to engage communities and key government sectors were initiated. Government, civil society, development partners and other stakeholders started to come together with new unity in purpose.

Helen Nyawira and her team of Youth Ambassadors teach their peers HIV/AIDS awareness, Kenya. Sven Torfinn/Panos.

Kenya's collaboration with the United Nations Children's Fund (UNICEF) on including HIV education in the curriculum of teachers' training colleges was an early example of multisectoral programming. In a number of (such) areas, UNAIDS

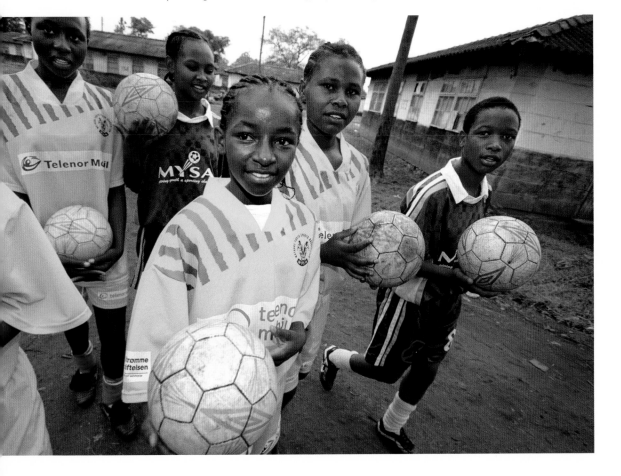

Programme Acceleration Funds were used to kick-start new processes or programmes, scale up promising initiatives such as prevention of mother-to-child transmission programmes, or strengthen ongoing activities such as sentinel surveillance.

Kenya has a long history of activism and civil society involvement in the country's general development, and undoubtedly this contributed to the early engagement of civil society in the national response to AIDS. For example, the Kenya NGOs AIDS Consortium was a leader in the area of nongovernmental organizations networking in the early 1990s. Today, the Consortium is one of several strong nongovernmental organization networks actively contributing to the national response in Kenya, but it continues to provide capacity enhancement and information networking for a wide range of civil society organizations.

Faith-based organizations (particularly mission health facilities) have been active in the health sector response to AIDS in Kenya for decades although, at times, engaging religious bodies in discussion around issues such as the promotion of condoms and life skills education has been a challenge.

In the mid-1990s, Kenya had an estimated HIV prevalence of 10% in adults. This had dropped to 6.8% by 2003 and is currently estimated at 6.1%[1], although there are significant regional variations; levels of 15% have also been recorded[2]. Gender disparities also need to be taken into account: prevalence among women is almost double that of men, and among girls aged 15–19 years, prevalence is six times higher than among young men in that age group[3]. Nonetheless, Kenya is one of the few countries in Africa with a sustained decline in prevalence, although this is not a country-wide occurrence, and the reasons for it are varied. They include behaviour change such as increased condom use and reduced number of sexual partners, but prevalence will also have lowered due to the demographic impact of AIDS: higher death rates[4]. Though this suggests that the many prevention and behaviour change campaigns and programmes have made an impact, Kenya has had and is still facing some major challenges.

Internally, corruption has plagued the National AIDS Control Council (NACC), leading to the prosecution and eventual imprisonment of its director in 2003. The UNAIDS Country Coordinator at this time, Kristan Schoultz, recalled this as a particularly difficult period as the confidence of both the public and the donors hit a serious low.

[1] UNAIDS (2007). *Global Report 2007*. Geneva, UNAIDS.
[2] Ministry of Health (2005). *AIDS in Kenya: Trends, Interventions and Impact*. Seventh edition. Nairobi, Government of Kenya.
[3] Ibid.
[4] UNAIDS (2005). *AIDS Epidemic Update, 2005: Briefing notes for Kenya visit, 16–17 January 2007*, prepared by Kristan Schoultz.

In response to this challenge, a broad-based group of stakeholders, including government, donors, the UNAIDS family and civil society, attempted not only to revamp the image of NACC and of the national response, but also to put in place a process of realignment and restructuring. This process took about 18 months and, according to Schoultz, was perhaps the foundation of Kenya's relative success in donor harmonization. It was decided, with government at the helm, to conduct a joint institutional review of NACC. Through this critical experience, Kenya started to understand and appreciate the concept of donor harmonization and support for the national response, probably even before UNAIDS and the global community were starting to focus on it and certainly before the "Three Ones". The process of realignment and restructuring resulted in a streamlined NACC, in the government taking some hard decisions about human resources and staffing patterns and in the beginnings of a new process for national strategic planning.

Kenya was one of the first countries to initiate the concept of a Joint AIDS Programme Review (JAPR) – 'joint' meaning a review undertaken by all stakeholders. By 2007, Kenya had held four JAPRs and this process, now somewhat institutionalized, deserves close attention. It has enabled the Kenyan Government, through NACC, to be in the driving seat of the review process. NACC, as the single national coordinating authority, convenes stakeholders to review the single national strategic framework and to use one monitoring and evaluation framework to do so.

As Schoultz said, "this has been very exciting for me, personally, and I would say that the UN system played a very strategic role in all of that. The UNAIDS Secretariat was requested by partners to help conceptualise the strategic planning process, and how to make the JAPR process a useful tool, leading to better programming. And that is, indeed, what it is used for now; and the new National Strategic Plan in Kenya, which was developed a couple of years ago, has an annual results framework built into it which is reviewed at every annual JAPR process. So, the National Strategic Plan is a results-based document, it's used as a monitoring tool, as a management tool for the national response and, while the process could certainly be more rigorous, I think that it's been a good example of broad stakeholder consensus around the direction of the national response. In addition, and importantly, the JAPR process provides a forum for discussion of mutual accountabilities. While NACC and other government bodies use the forum to report back to the community on achievements and challenges, the forum is also useful for providing feedback to donors and other development partners regarding how their own contributions might be strengthened".

At the same time, Schoultz does not want to paint too rosy a picture and acknowledges that there still are tremendous challenges in the country. Kenya has experienced absorption and capacity issues related to its very large Global Fund grant, and there have been struggles arising from the broad range of partners in the country, including some partners that bring very big money, such as the US President's Emergency Plan for AIDS Relief (PEPFAR). Largely as a response to that, the UNAIDS Secretariat has worked very closely with NACC to develop a harmonization process. NACC convenes a newly established harmonization Task Force which brings a full range of stakeholders to the table. Stakeholders include donors and civil society, which also has harmonization needs.

While the Task Force is new and is still experiencing teething problems, Schoultz is convinced that it will emerge as an important mechanism with regard to NACC's effectiveness in coordinating the many different development partners present in Kenya. "Some partners didn't expect, for example, the United States Government to come to that table but they have come, they are there, they want to participate. And what we have found was that, if you just get people to sit around the table and constantly reinforce the concept of the 'Three Ones', [not simply] paying lip service to it, but really reinforcing it, partners do respond … I think that that's been a very valuable tool, that the whole concept of the 'Three Ones' has been very valuable, to Kenya and to the Kenyan Government and in helping to really lead the way for the national response".

In terms of the practical effects of harmonization, Schoultz gives the example of coverage of counselling and testing throughout the country. "There are so many duplications of effort, and … so many gaps as well. So, it's looking at a specific area such as counselling and testing in the country, and realising – just by sitting down together and looking at a map of the country and saying, 'Where do you support counselling and testing?' – … that everybody is in half of the country, and nobody's in the other half, and then readjusting. Key partners did this in Kenya, and counselling and testing services coverage is consequently far more rational now than it was five years ago. It's a question of pragmatic decision making".

A harmonized approach to development partner initiatives can contribute to a stronger and more cohesive national response. Schoultz commented: "I think that, certainly in Kenya, we've benefited greatly from the UNAIDS Secretariat's own efforts to bring joint missions, high-level missions, to the country. Our Executive Director came with Suma Chakrabarti, Permanent Secretary at DFID (the UK Department for International Development), Bjorn Skogmo, Deputy Secretary-General of Norway's Ministry of Foreign Affairs and Gerard Byam, Director, Operational Quality and Knowledge Services at the World Bank, in a joint mission, and the benefits of that … kind of visit are enormous. Not only does it send a very strong signal that, 'We are all in this together and we are coming here to work with you, Kenya', but it also assures that the leadership of these organizations … from the

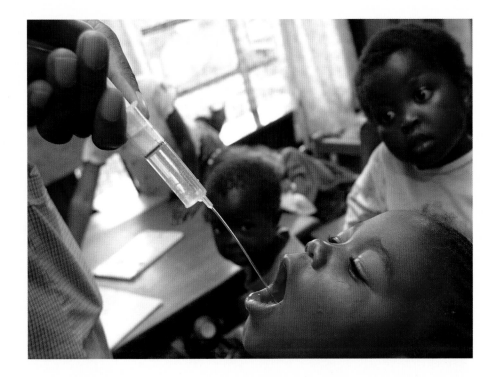

Charles aged 9, receives
oral antiretroviral therapy
in the Grace Childrens'
Home, Nairobi.
Corbis /
Radhika Chalasani

global level, actually talk with each other, understand each other's ways of work and programmatic concerns. So it is a PR [public relations] event, and certainly if you plan them well, you can have some very effective focused messages coming out from such a group. But I think that the benefits are more than that in terms of … helping global leadership understand … the reality on the ground".

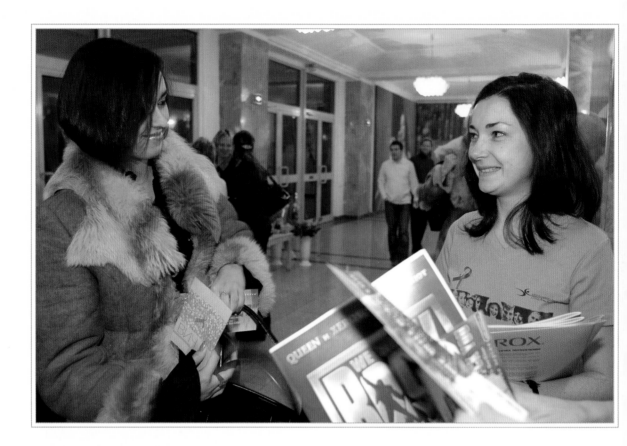

*By 2004 it was very clear that the focus on treatment
has overshadowed prevention. It was essential to
strengthen prevention and public education programmes,
like this one in Moscow.*
UNAIDS/J. Spaul

CHAPTER 8:
Improving the focus on prevention and key populations, 2004–2005

While the story of treatment is a dramatic tale of activists, 'big bad pharma', demonstrations and court cases, prevention is not a 'sexy' topic, and has not received the same media attention.

Every day, UNAIDS' staff in Geneva and in country offices were struggling to deal with the urgency and the long-term nature of the epidemic. At the same time as working on advocacy and policy issues, they had to be prepared for troubleshooting – from interruption in the antiretroviral drug supply to the jailing of gay AIDS educators. Every day, a broad range of issues jostled for their attention. There would always be clear priorities, and 'making the money work' was a major one for this biennium. But there was also a decision to focus more on policies and programmes that had been sidelined, if not actually neglected – not only by UNAIDS, but by the 'AIDS industry' as a whole.

Thus, during 2004 and 2005, the UNAIDS Secretariat and Cosponsors highlighted the fact that the focus on treatment had tended to sideline the importance of prevention, as well as overshadow the problem of the growing numbers of infected women.

Prevention gains ground

Since the announcement about the successful research findings on antiretroviral therapy at the 1996 Vancouver International AIDS Conference, it was inevitable that the spotlight would be on treatment rather than prevention. While the story of treatment is a dramatic tale of activists, 'big bad pharma', demonstrations, court cases and, to some extent, a happy ending, prevention is not a 'sexy' topic, and has not received the same media attention.

William Easterly, who was a Senior Research Economist at the World Bank for 16 years[1], has criticized the donors for concentrating on treatment rather than prevention: 'The rich-country politicians and aid agencies get more PR [public relations] credit for saving the lives of sick patients, even if the interests of the poor would call for saving them from getting sick in the first place'. Ironically, until recently, the same donors – with the exception of France and Luxemburg – refused to fund antiretroviral therapy and put all their money into HIV prevention.

Indeed, although antiretroviral therapy had reduced AIDS-related sickness and death in many countries, there were still nearly 2.9 million HIV infections estimated in 2004[2]. These infections could have been averted had effective prevention programmes been in place. It was estimated that a comprehensive HIV prevention package could prevent 29 million (or 63%)

---

[1] Easterly W (2007). *The White Man's Burden: Why the West's Efforts to Aid the Rest Have Done So Much Ill and So Little Good.* New York, Penguin Books.
[2] UNAIDS/WHO (2004). *AIDS Epidemic Update, 2004.* Geneva, UNAIDS.

of the 45 million new infections expected between 2002 and 2010[3]. Given the growth of the epidemic, treatment will not be sustainable, even with increased access to antiretroviral therapy, unless prevention programmes are intensified.

HIV prevention programmes are still failing to reach the populations most at risk. Only 9% of men who have sex with men received any type of prevention service in 2005, ranging from 4% coverage in Eastern Europe and Central Asia to 24% in Latin America and the Caribbean. Fewer than one in five injecting drug users received HIV prevention services, with especially low coverage (10%) in Eastern Europe and Central Asia where drug use accounts for the rapid expansion of the epidemic[4]. Although many epidemics are concentrated among sex workers and injecting drug users, only a small number of countries have prevention programmes for sex workers, and those projects that do exist rarely reach large numbers of people.

In Cambodia, India and Thailand, prevention efforts with these groups, as well as with men who have sex with men, have paid off. In other areas, for example, in parts of Latin America, there is still not enough data and information about at-risk groups and their behaviour.

The lack of prevention programmes for these key populations, and the discrimination they often face, is a denial of their human rights as well as a challenge to the public health of the whole community. In parts of Eastern Europe, for example, HIV has spread from users of drugs to their sexual partners. In this way 'specific' epidemics become 'generalized'. The UNAIDS Secretariat and the Cosponsors are working with governments and other partners to combat the stigma and discrimination faced by particular groups of people.

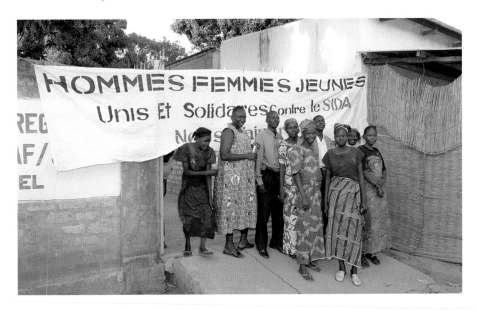

Chad women with banners, public AIDS awareness meeting
UNAIDS/H. Vincent AVECC

3 Stover J, Walker N, Garnett G P et al. (2002). 'Can we reverse the HIV/AIDS pandemic with an expanded response?' *The Lancet*, 360 (9326).
4 UNAIDS (2004). *Global Report 2004*. Geneva, UNAIDS.

"Prevention is challenging because you have to deal with social norms and behaviours".

Thus, UNAIDS began developing a strategy in order to place prevention 'more centrally on the global AIDS agenda'[5]. 'Prevention for all' was a major policy issue for UNAIDS during the 2004–2005 biennium.

The challenges to expanding prevention

The subject of HIV prevention is controversial and disturbing. In most societies, there is strong cultural resistance to discussing sexuality, especially sex between men and commercial sex, and the use of drugs. Social conventions and taboos get in the way of saving lives. In countries where sex work and injecting drug use are illegal, it is not easy to provide prevention programmes for these key populations. This reluctance has not been confined to countries in the developing world. In Margaret Thatcher's United Kingdom, the first *National Survey of Sexual Attitudes and Lifestyles* (Natssal 1990), a major research project into people's sexual behaviour, was denied public funding, and was funded independently instead[6]. The Roman Catholic Church still does not condone the use of condoms, although in 2007 the Vatican was considering moves towards a revised policy.

Prevention efforts are severely hampered by stigma. Stigma and discrimination against people living with HIV and gender inequality were, experts agreed, the two biggest challenges to HIV prevention in South Asia and Africa. Noerine Kaleeba, founder of The AIDS Support Organisation in Uganda and formerly Partnerships and Community Mobilization Adviser at UNAIDS, said: "Even in Uganda, though we've come a long way, there's still very, very subtle stigma that continues to hinder people from accessing care".

Thoraya Obaid, Executive Director of the United Nations Population Fund, commented: "I think the issue of prevention sometimes falls off the table because it is much easier to emphasize treatment: treatment is concrete, whereas prevention is harder to measure … Prevention is challenging because you have to deal with social norms and behaviours".

There had been relatively little information on how treatment affected prevention in developing countries, but research done in 2004 using epidemiological modelling suggested that treatment makes prevention more effective and prevention makes treatment more affordable[7]. There is also increasing evidence from many locations that the push to expand treatment has led to an expansion of testing and counselling. In one district in Uganda, the introduction of antiretroviral therapy led to a 27-fold increase in numbers of people seeking testing and counselling. When the Global Fund's first substantial grant to Haiti scaled up treatment for people living with HIV, tens of thousands sought testing and coun-

---

[5] UNAIDS (2004). *Executive Director's Report to the 16th Meeting of the UNAIDS PCB*, December. Geneva, UNAIDS.

[6] Results from the first Natssal were published in the book *Sexual Attitudes and Lifestyles* by A Johnson, J Wadsworth, K Wellings and J Field (Blackwell, Oxford, 1994).

[7] Salomon J A, Hogan D R, Stover J, Stanecki K A, Walker N, Ghys P D, Schwartländer B (2005). 'Integrating HIV prevention and treatment: from slogans to impact.' *PLoS Medicine*, 2, (1, e16) January.

selling. Obaid highlighted that an adequate response to AIDS requires that treatment and prevention have equal focus. "We always need to emphasize that an effective response is prevention, treatment and care; we need an integrated and comprehensive package, and we need to emphasize this package as a whole".

Having made the decision to develop a new strategy on prevention, the UNAIDS Secretariat chose to work with the Bill & Melinda Gates Foundation Working Group on Prevention, rather than setting up another reference group. The collaboration between UNAIDS and the Foundation has turned out to be a very productive one.

A major policy breakthrough on HIV prevention

Work started on a major policy document on HIV prevention. For many months, Secretariat staff worked with Cosponsors and Programme Coordinating Board members to negotiate the final draft, which contained strongly worded positions on harm reduction for injecting drug users and on sex workers. PCB members worked as advocates within their own countries, negotiating informally with various groups, and civil society had an input. Achmat Dangor, former UNAIDS Director of Advocacy, Communication and Leadership, explained that UNAIDS acted as a facilitator, as in other processes, bringing people together and "agreeing to act on what they feel comfortable with".

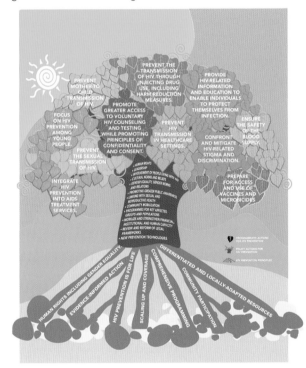

The prevention tree – UNAIDS HIV prevention guidelines

Purmina Mane, formerly Director of the Policy, Evidence and Partnerships Department at UNAIDS, explained: "We organized consultations with civil society to get their inputs. Civil society also organized itself to create lobby groups to pressure their own governments to ensure that the evidence was reflected adequately in the document. So we had microbicide groups, vaccine groups, harm reduction groups, women's groups, people living with HIV; their inputs were substantial. Of course, managing all these inputs was quite a challenge".

It was a very political process. A major challenge was to reach a consensus on harm reduction and needle exchange to prevent HIV transmission among injecting drug users. Peter Piot, UNAIDS Executive Director, explained that for several months he did not speak out about this issue because if he had, "it would have allowed the many opposing countries to mobilize against this". He discussed the various issues with each board member and

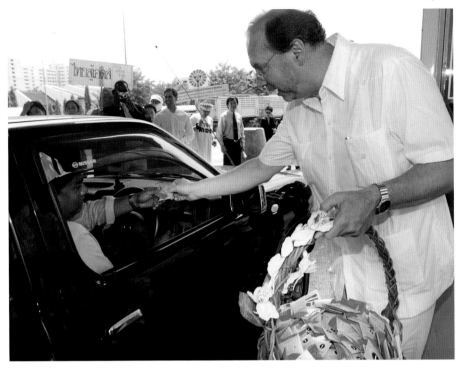

UNAIDS Executive Director Peter Piot distributing condoms during the International AIDS Conference in Bangkok.
Getty/Pornchai Kittiwongsakul

eventually all except the Russian Federation and the United States of America agreed to harm reduction. "China changed their policy; that was a big coup".

The draft new paper on prevention of HIV was presented to and, after fierce debate, endorsed by the 17th PCB in June 2005. For the first time there was an internationally agreed comprehensive policy on HIV prevention. "This is a true milestone in the response to AIDS", explained Piot, "and UNAIDS was clearly fulfilling its role as the world's reference point in AIDS policy".

Ben Plumley, Director of the UNAIDS Executive Office until March 2007, explained that this was really "a big success, generating approval from the PCB for the UNAIDS HIV prevention policy was profoundly significant for the global AIDS movement – to my mind, as important as the ground-breaking agreements on reduced ARV [antiretrovirals] pricing in 2000. The policy is truly comprehensive and reaffirms the importance of developing ABC and harm reduction strategies. Not all PCB members were comfortable with every aspect—the USA stands out[8], given its policy of not funding harm reduction programmes in international assistance. However, the key achievement was the building of consensus around UNAIDS work on those most sensitive and politically charged of HIV prevention issues".

As Piot explained, there are many 'turf wars' on prevention among academic HIV prevention experts and among different agencies; "with the approved prevention policy we now have an agreed menu of what to do".

---

[8] When the Prevention Paper was agreed at the PCB meeting in June 2005, the USA made a statement that it could not fund needle and syringe programmes because such programmes were inconsistent with current US law and policy. The PCB noted the statement, and that this external partner cannot be expected to fund activities inconsistent with its own national laws and policies.

The 'feminization' of the epidemic

The numbers of women becoming infected with HIV had been increasing in every region since before 1996. In 1997, 48% of adults (15+) living with HIV were women[9]; by 2004, nearly half of all adults (15+) living with HIV between 15 and 49 years of age were women – in Africa, the figure rose to 59%[10]. Currently, infection rates among women are rising faster than among men. In the Russian Federation, one of the worst-affected countries in Eastern Europe, women accounted for an increasing share of new cases – up from one in four in 2001 to one in three only one year later[11]. Globally, in 2004, about 5000 women were being infected every day.

Ensuring that women's prevention needs are met has been particularly challenging.

Ensuring that women's prevention needs are met has been particularly challenging. Obaid explained: "The concept of ABC: 'abstain, be faithful and use condoms' is not sufficient. For instance, if women are married, they cannot abstain; they might be faithful but their husbands who may not be faithful and refusing to use condoms will bring HIV into the home. So we promote women-controlled prevention methods such as the female condom and microbicides and women's rights to counter the inequality, discrimination and violence they face and that fuel the pandemic. Again, this is the challenge that we face – that of changing mindsets and behaviours".

From the early days of the epidemic, women's vulnerability to HIV had been recognized. In 1990, the World Health Assembly of the World Health Organization (WHO) had urged states to 'strengthen the involvement of women by including in national AIDS committees a representative of women's organizations'. Under pressure from feminist organizations, the International AIDS Conference of 1992 (held in Amsterdam), for the first time, gave the position of women a central place in the AIDS response[12]. UNAIDS and others had emphasized that gender inequality and the low status of women remain two of the principal drivers of the epidemic. Much later, at the United Nations General Assembly Special Session (UNGASS) on AIDS in 2001, Member States had agreed that gender equality and women's empowerment were fundamental to ensuring an effective response to AIDS and specific pledges had been made, such as promoting women's rights. However, despite some progress, women's concerns were too often sidelined or just ignored by those working on AIDS.

Keeping the Promise: An Agenda for Action on Women and AIDS

A UNAIDS Initiative
The Global Coalition on Women and AIDS

---

[9] UNAIDS (2004). *Global Report 2004*. UNAIDS, Geneva.
[10] Ibid.
[11] Ibid.
[12] *Global AIDS News 1992*, No. 3; in John Iliffe (2007). *The African AIDS Epidemic: A History*. London, James Currey.

Sigrun Mogedal, who is currently the Norwegian Government's Ambassador for HIV/AIDS, commented: "I've started to say 'look back at Beijing and Cairo'[13]. If we had done what we said then, the local communities would be much more resilient to AIDS. We have a series of missed opportunities, we've somehow known what we needed to do with women's vulnerability, with the link between reproductive health (at that time, not AIDS because we hadn't come to grips with it yet) … and how important it was for women to choose and to be empowered to protect their own sexuality and so on. So I feel that the history of AIDS is sort of a parallel history, demonstrating the missed agenda, the missed opportunities in the development agenda [for women]".

Stephen Lewis, former Special Envoy of the Secretary-General for HIV/AIDS in Africa since 2001, has consistently pressed the international community to focus more on women. He asked: "Where are the laws that descend with draconian force on those who are guilty of rape and sexual violence? Where are the laws that deal with rape within marriage? Where are the laws in every country that enshrine property and inheritance for women? Where are the laws that guarantee equality before the law for women in all matters economic and social? In short, where are the laws, which move decisively towards gender equality? … Whole societies are unravelling, as parts of Africa are depopulated of their women".

In early 2004, a major new initiative – the Global Coalition on Women and AIDS (GCWA) – was launched by a number of partners led by UNAIDS[14]. The aim was to draw attention to the failure of countries, when planning and implementing AIDS prevention programmes, to address the factors that put women at risk for HIV. The coalition stressed the need to focus on women's economic, biological and social vulnerability, to secure women's rights, to invest more money in AIDS programmes that work for women and to 'allocate more seats at the table for women' in, for example, the forums where AIDS strategies are discussed. It has brought together key actors from the UN, governments and civil society to promote greater attention to the needs of women and to empower them to take control of their lives.

The coalition adopted the slogan 'To make women count, count women', based on the fact that 'we measure what we value'. UNAIDS and WHO published all the available evidence and data on women and AIDS in the 2004 *Epidemic Update*, and WHO agreed to collect data disaggregated by sex and age in the "3 by 5" initiative.

At the 16th Meeting of the UNAIDS PCB in December 2004, Piot warned that though the focus on women, gender and AIDS was extremely critical, it was not popular everywhere. Neither did such a focus mean that UNAIDS would neglect the issues surrounding men who have sex with men, including the discrimination and violence faced by them. PCB members voiced

---

[13] In 1995, the UN Fourth World Conference on Women took place in Beijing, China, and, in 1994, the International Conference on Population and Development (ICPD) was held in Cairo, Egypt.

[14] Convening agencies include the Global Campaign on Education, UNICEF, the International Center for Research on Women, the United Nations Food and Agriculture Organization, the United Nations Development Fund for Women, WHO, the International Women's Health Coalition and UNFPA.

their support for the GCWA. Obaid called for efforts to empower women and promote their rights. She quoted a representative of women living with HIV who said: "What will kill us more than AIDS is despair. Please give us hope".

The coalition was welcomed as a much-needed initiative but there was concern that like similar bodies, it might produce more words than action. Marta Mauras, who had left the Office of the Deputy Secretary-General for the Economic Commission for Latin America and the Caribbean, said: "I think the Global Coalition of Women still has to find its way. What it's done for now [is] to create ... a very important network throughout the world ... [but] now comes the litmus test, 'so fine, now what about it, we have this network, we have some very prominent people attached to it and what are we going to do about it?'" However, Mauras stressed that the coalition has highlighted, notably at the Bangkok AIDS Conference in 2004 and Toronto in 2006, the very important work being done on inheritance rights and property, and on violence against women.

Kaleeba also said: "I think it is a good start but, like all global initiatives, it still needs to be localized". She explained that countries need their own national plans and projects, specific to the needs of their women, such as shelters for abused women.

However, by 2005, the GCWA had begun to provide catalytic funds to United Nations Theme Groups in a number of countries, to strengthen the gender components of National AIDS Strategies, and to promote the inclusion of women's groups in civil society forums on AIDS.

Country programmes for women

The growing impact of the epidemic on girls and women had become increasingly obvious in Kenya, explained Kristan Schoultz, who was UNAIDS Country Coordinator in Kenya from July 2003 to April 2007. As well as being part of Kenya's surveillance data, the 2003 demographic and health survey included a module on AIDS and on gender violence: this revealed very high levels of violence towards women and "incredible rates of rape, violent rape, and assault". She explained: "What the Global Coalition on Women and AIDS brought to us in Kenya was the language and the tools to start focusing on sexual violence as one of the key modes of HIV transmission".

The UN Theme Group in Kenya has, with the help of UNAIDS Programme Acceleration Funds, supported a joint UN advocacy programme on women, girls and AIDS. As Schoultz explained, this has brought together women involved in AIDS with others involved in more traditional "women in development" programmes. "What was striking to us was how these two groups of women had not been collaborating, that the machine that is the national response to AIDS was not interacting with those dealing with women and development

"What will kill us more than AIDS is despair. Please give us hope".

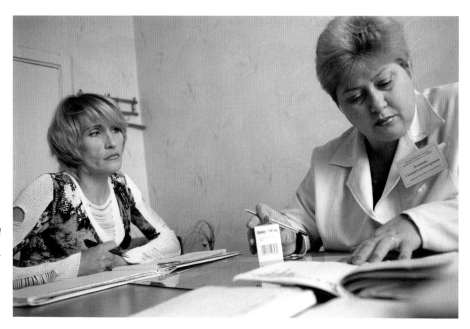

The rates of HIV have soared in many Eastern European countries. Olga, the mother of five children, is collecting her antiretroviral drugs from a clinic in Odessa, Ukraine.
WHO/V.Suvorov

issues. That was surprising because Kenya has a very strong tradition of activist women and women's organizations. But we did what UNAIDS does best, we brought these two women's groups to the table". The focus of the joint initiative is on violence against women, property and inheritance rights, and access to services and information; studies in all three areas have been undertaken. The study on violence against women has, for example, led to the strengthening of the effort to address this issue at the policy-making level, including the development of a National Action Plan on women and violence which includes attention to AIDS.

Most importantly, the issue of women and AIDS is a priority in key national documents such as the Joint HIV/AIDS Programme Review (JAPR). At the same time, Kenyan media have been covering issues related to violence against women, its links to HIV and property and inheritance rights.

UNAIDS and seed funds from the GCWA have also played an important role in catalysing advocacy and action in Papua New Guinea.

On 25 November 2005, International Day for the Elimination of Violence Against Women, UNAIDS Papua New Guinea and World Vision mobilized hundreds of women to march for national action against domestic violence. The women put together a petition to the Prime Minister and marched through the streets of Port Moresby, the capital. The media flocked to report the event, and so women nationwide became aware of what was going on.

Nii-K Plange, former UNAIDS Country Coordinator in Papua New Guinea, described the ripple effects of this march: "… women leaders from outside Port Moresby began to call our offices asking us to help them organize marches in provincial towns. They wanted to hold

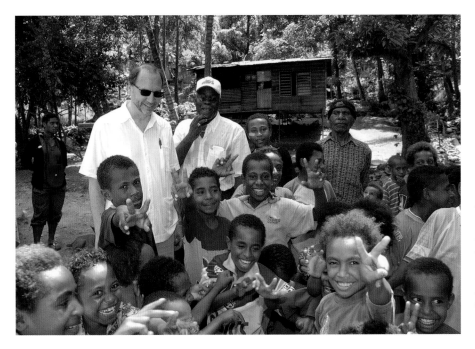

UNAIDS Executive Director Peter Piot and Nii-K Plange, former UNAIDS Country Coordinator in Papua New Guinea, during a visit to Papua New Guinea in 2005.
UNAIDS

these on World AIDS Day, and needed money to bring women in from the villages and stay overnight so they could march in the towns".

He recalled: "All this was a stage-setting venture. I wanted to create a context within which gender-based violence and the links with HIV would become major issues for national dialogue. I knew that UNAIDS and the UN Theme Group on HIV/AIDS could have called for government action on violence against women, but I felt the impact would be greater if we could get local women to initiate the calls, with the UN coming in later to provide the support".

Although Papua New Guinea has laws against violence against women, Nii-K feels they need to be better implemented. He described domestic violence as "rampant", and explained that the situation for women is exacerbated by the disconnection between traditional norms and "modern lifestyles", combined with poverty, unemployment, and a lack of decision-making power in the household. More and more women are becoming infected with HIV: women aged 15–25 are three times more likely to be infected than men.

Working closely with Dame Kidu, Minister for Community Development, Nii-K began to look for ways to make the AIDS response work better for girls and women. Kidu agreed with Nii-K's strategy of bringing women's groups together to advocate on HIV and violence, but realized that most members had no advocacy experience. The two agreed to find out more about what women felt they needed, and to provide them with the requisite skills so they could advocate more effectively. But for this to happen, they required money.

The GCWA provided funds to UNAIDS Papua New Guinea to run a series of workshops in selected provinces to learn more about women's concerns about development, HIV and gender based violence, and to help them devise ways to address these issues. The GCWA also funded the production of a training manual.

"Slowly, things are changing", noted Nii-K, "this summer, there was a case where a senior bureaucrat was actually jailed for ten years for raping his sister-in-law. Gradually, you're beginning to see issues relating to women and the way they have been dealt with in the law slowly coming up in the newspapers. It's a first little step, but at least it's a step in the right direction".

It is too early to see what results the GCWA will bring. Undoubtedly it is important to bring together all the players but, at country level, far more work is needed to protect women from infection and support those who are living with HIV or who are caring for sick relatives and orphans. The efforts of UNFPA and others to integrate AIDS into reproductive health services is an important contribution, but this needs to be done on a much larger scale. Women facing violence need refuge, and governments need to legislate for women's property and inheritance rights.

Chinese migrant workers waiting at a station. Prevention programmes need to focus on selected communities such as migrant workers. ILO/UNAIDS/ J.Maillard

Women who are living with HIV tend to be more stigmatized than men. This explains their reluctance to be tested, including when pregnant. Most countries (82%) have a policy in place to ensure women's and men's equal access to prevention and care. In reality, however, social, legal and economic factors impede women's ready access to vital services[15].

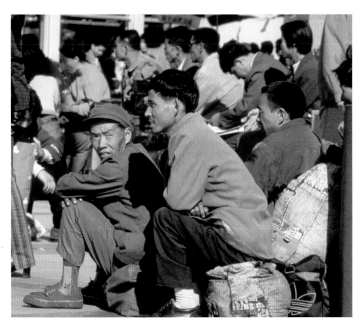

Obaid commented: "We need to understand cultures in order for us to understand how to work with communities and people not only at the national level but also at the community level. We need to support them, through their own community-based systems, so that they would be empowered to take care of themselves, to advocate for prevention, to insist on reproductive health and HIV services that are available, accessible and affordable, and to lead in fighting stigma and discrimination".

As Piot said at the 2007 launch of the GCWA's new Agenda for Action, "the ultimate criterion to judge all AIDS programmes is 'Does this work for women and girls?'"

---

[15] United Nations (2007). *The Declaration of Commitment on HIV/AIDS: Five Years Later. Report of the Secretary-General.* United Nations, Geneva.

A 10th Cosponsor joins the programme

In June 2004, the Office of the United Nations High Commissioner for Refugees (UNHCR) joined UNAIDS as its 10th Cosponsor. In its work with refugees and others (for example, internally displaced person and asylum seekers), UNHCR is at the forefront of combating HIV among a particularly vulnerable group of people. The very fact that UNHCR became a UNAIDS Cosponsor made a strong statement to the international community. The agency was better able to advocate for the provision of HIV services to displaced populations. Paul Spiegel, the Head of UNHCR's HIV Unit, explained: "In all major global documents on AIDS, there is now at least a mention of conflict-affected or displaced persons where there wasn't before. So [joining UNAIDS] has been a huge advocacy tool because it's brought us to the table and allowed us to advocate and say, 'Hey, let's not forget about these marginalised and vulnerable groups'".

It was only in 2002 that UNHCR decided to strengthen its work on AIDS, with the support of the Centers for Disease Control and Prevention (CDC), a United States (US) Government agency, by setting up its HIV Unit. Spiegel, a physician and medical epidemiologist who had worked for 15 years in complex humanitarian emergencies, was chosen to head the new Unit.

AIDS became a policy priority within UNHCR, and the agency has now conducted over 40 assessment and evaluation missions in 17 countries, which resulted in significant additional funding to improve their HIV programmes. Staff in the UNHCR AIDS unit increased from one to eight, with five of the eight new staff members working as field-based regional HIV coordinators. The agency has prioritized the integration of refugees in the host country's HIV programmes. In some cases, refugees have remained uprooted from their home communities for up to 20 years, with only limited access to their host countries' medical or HIV services. UNHCR's actions and policies are based on the view that refugees deserve medical services equal to those of the surrounding communities, and that reaching these individuals, in an integrated and coordinated approach with their surrounding host countries, is a vital approach for ensuring HIV prevention, care, support and treatment.

"The concept that we're really pushing is for an integration of services between refugees and surrounding populations, in particular as antiretroviral therapy expands. We should not be providing parallel systems for service delivery to host populations and to refugees", explained Spiegel. From this perspective, respecting basic human rights principles and implementing an effective public health strategy strongly coincide.

Refugees are often accused of spreading HIV in their host countries. In 2004, UNHCR published important new findings, suggesting that refugees in five out of seven countries had significantly lower HV prevalence than the surrounding communities (refugees had similar prevalence to the surrounding host communities in the other two countries). The same study had also, for the first time, examined attitudes and behavioural trends among displaced populations. It revealed that refugees in camps in Africa 'have made "dramatic strides" in changing their behaviour to reduce the risks of contracting and spreading HIV'[16].

---

[16] UNHCR (2004). News Stories, 7 June. Nairobi, UNHCR.

The needs of children and orphans

UNITE FOR CHILDREN
UNITE AGAINST AIDS

By 2004, every single day, about 1500 babies were born HIV positive or were becoming infected through breastfeeding, despite proven methods of preventing transmission from mother-to-child[17]. In developed countries, the vast majority of positive pregnant women were enrolled in prevention programmes and their babies were born negative. UNAIDS had been promoting these prevention programmes from its first year yet, in Africa, only one pregnant woman out of 20 has access to prevention of mother-to-child transmission. By 2007, the global coverage of pregnant women living with HIV was 9%[18].

Yet less than half of the countries with the most acute crisis had national policies in place to provide essential support to children orphaned or made vulnerable by the epidemic.

Children living with HIV and those orphaned by AIDS (themselves often positive) were a neglected group. By 2004, an estimated 11.4 million children under the age of 18 had lost one or both parents to AIDS, 9.6 million of whom were living in sub-Saharan Africa[19]. Yet less than half of the countries with the most acute crisis had national policies in place to provide essential support to children orphaned or made vulnerable by the epidemic. There were no specific paediatric formulations of antiretroviral drugs for children, so only a small percentage of those in need were receiving treatment.

Several of UNAIDS' Cosponsors, notably the United Nations Children's Fund and UNFPA, had been working on programmes for children, including orphans, for some years. The revised version of the major publication, *Children on the Brink*, was published by UNICEF for the 2004 International AIDS Conference in Bangkok, but it was not until October 2005 that UNICEF Executive Director Ann Veneman and Piot launched, with then UN Secretary-General Kofi Annan, a global advocacy and fundraising campaign for children affected by HIV under the slogan 'Unite for children, unite against AIDS'. It was another UN system-wide initiative. The programme aims to prevent mother-to-child transmission, provide paediatric treatment, stem new HIV infections and help orphans affected by the crisis.

"Nearly 25 years into the pandemic, help is reaching less than 10% of the children affected by HIV, leaving too many children to grow up alone, grow up too fast or not grow up at all", said the Secretary-General at the launch.

Veneman said: "This very visible disease continues to have an invisible face, a missing face, a child's face". She explained that in some of the hardest-hit countries, the AIDS pandemic is "unravelling years of progress for children". She noted that concrete measures to address the impact of AIDS on children would be essential to meeting the UN Millennium Development Goals: "A whole generation has never known a world free of HIV and AIDS, yet the magnitude of the problem dwarfs the scale of the response so far".

---

[17] UNAIDS (2004). *Global Report 2004*. UNAIDS, Geneva.
[18] United Nations (2007).
[19] UNAIDS (2004). *Global Report 2004*. UNAIDS, Geneva.

Three scenarios for AIDS in Africa by 2025

'Over the next 20 years, what factors will drive Africa's and the world's responses to the AIDS epidemic, and what kind of future will there be for the next generation?' This is the central question that an innovative report – *AIDS in Africa: Three Scenarios to 2025* – published by UNAIDS in March 2005 set out to answer.

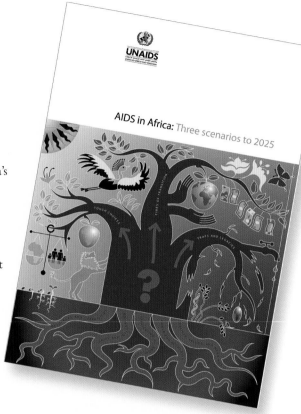

The report presents three possible scenarios for the evolution of the AIDS epidemic in Africa over the next 20 years, based on policy decisions taken today by African leaders and the rest of the world. Piot explained: "These are not predictions. They are plausible stories about the future".

Most AIDS programmes are resourced with external funds. Since commitments generally do not extend beyond five years, uncertainty remains about the level of resources that will be available in the future. The scenario 'Tough Choices' shows what is possible when there are efficient domestic policies but stagnant external aid; 'Times of Transition' describes what more efficient domestic policies and increased and high quality external aid could lead to, and 'Traps and Legacies' shows what might happen if there are inefficient domestic policies and volatile or declining external aid.

The scenarios make it clear that it is not only the extent of expenditure on AIDS programming that counts, but how well and in which context it is spent. Major increases in spending will be needed to produce significantly better outcomes in terms of curbing the spread of HIV, extending treatment access, and mitigating impact. However, more resources without effective coordination, gender equality and community participation may do more harm than good. The scenarios suggest that while the worst of the epidemic may be still to come, there is still a great deal that can be done to change the longer-term trajectory of the epidemic and to minimize its impact.

The project was conceived in 2002, when UNAIDS and Shell International Limited decided to work together to develop some scenarios that explored some of the possible long-term impacts of the AIDS epidemic in Africa, looking forward over 25 years. Other organizations were also invited to join the project, including the United Nations Development Programme, the World Bank, the Africa Development Bank, the African Union and the United Nations Economic Commission for Africa.

The project aimed to bring together a wide group of stakeholders from across Africa to create a shared and deeper understanding of the drivers, impacts and implications of the AIDS epidemic in Africa. After the project was launched in February 2003, a series of workshops was held across the African continent over 18 months. Supporting analysis and research continued throughout the project, gathered through interviews, symposia, focused research and commentary. More than 150 people, mostly Africans, have given their time, experience, knowledge and expertise to build the scenarios.

This is an excellent illustration of an action–research project: it is hoped that the very process of developing the scenarios with such a numerous and diverse group of stakeholders may lead to a more coherent and policy response across different sectors, institutions and countries.

She explained that the campaign would focus on the 'four Ps':

- reducing the **percentage** of young people living with HIV by 25%;
- covering 80% of women who need services to **prevent** mother-to-child transmission;
- providing **paediatric** AIDS treatment to 80% of children in need;
- reaching 80% of children in need of **protection** and support.

The campaign stressed that AIDS is threatening children as never before. Children under 15 account for one in six global AIDS-related deaths and one in seven new global HIV infections. A child under 15 dies of an AIDS-related illness every minute of every day, and a young person aged between 15 and 24 contracts HIV every 15 seconds.

Access to treatment

Access to antiretroviral treatment continued to be a major priority for everyone involved in the AIDS movement and the increased funding for antiretroviral treatment was beginning to take effect in many countries.

Although it was clear well before mid-2005 that the target of "3 by 5" would not be reached, all those involved could point to the initiative's transforming effects. By December 2005, data from 18 countries indicated they had met the "3 by 5" target of providing treatment to at least half of those who needed it. And people who needed treatment did not always have to travel so far to obtain it. In several countries there was a rapid expansion of public sector antiretroviral therapy services. The number of sites where people could go for treatment in Zambia, for example, increased from three in early 2003 to more than 100 in just over two years[20].

---

[20] WHO/UNAIDS (2005). *Progress report on "3 by 5"*. Geneva, WHO/AIDS.

224

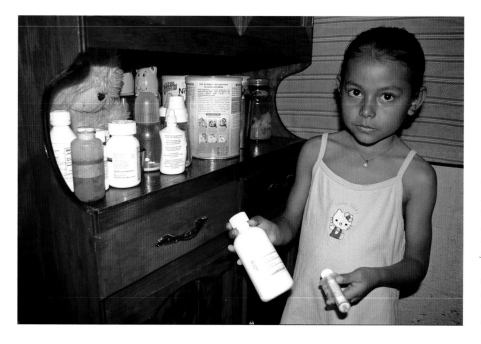

*Increasing numbers of
children are infected with
HIV and yet medication
is not specifically
formulated for children.
This Honduran girl
complains about having to
take too much.
Christian Aid /
Annabel Davis*

Thus at the end of 2005, when the actual numbers were published – 1.3 million – the general view was fairly positive. Worldwide, it was estimated that between 250 000 and 350 000 deaths had been averted as a result of increased treatment access[21].

WHO and the UNAIDS Secretariat had always considered the "3 by 5" initiative to be an emergency response, an interim milestone on the road to access to prevention, care and treatment for everyone who needs them.

On the whole, the results of the initiative received positive reviews – and praise, rather than criticism, from activists. An article in *The Economist*[22] commented: '… the initiative may have been more successful than the headline figure suggests, since part of the money has gone on infrastructure. That means building clinics and testing laboratories, but also training doctors (surprisingly many of whom, more than two decades after AIDS was identified, have still not been taught how to deal with it) and reorganizing hospital administrations. This sort of work has spin-offs beyond the treatment of AIDS'.

During the two years of the initiative there had been many achievements – not just the increase in numbers on treatment. Governments, donors and technical agencies had given higher priority to strengthening health systems, and "3 by 5" had also challenged the belief that antiretroviral therapy could not be provided where only basic health systems existed. Through a new curriculum developed by WHO and its partners – the Integrated Management of Adult and Adolescent Illness – health and community workers were trained in care that can be applied to all chronic conditions including HIV. Through such 'task-shifting', clinical teams had been expanded to include trained people living with HIV as counsellors and supporters of people on treatment.

---

[21] Ibid.
[22] *The Economist*, 1 April 2007.

Worldwide, it was estimated that between 250 000 and 350 000 deaths had been averted as a result of increased treatment access

Community-based organizations had been very involved in scaling up treatment. In Burkina Faso, for example, organizations in the community have taken the lead in providing counselling and testing, as well as nongovernmental organizations and faith-based organizations.

A major issue, however, was the potential impact on poorly resourced health services of providing lifelong treatment for a chronic health condition. Importantly, countries demonstrated their commitment to ensuring that treatment programmes were not only started but will also be sustainable over the long term. In poorer countries in sub-Saharan Africa, such as Burkina Faso and Senegal, countries increased their domestic budget allocations for AIDS.

Without the funding from three organizations – US President's Emergency Plan for AIDS Relief (PEPFAR), the Global Fund and the World Bank – the number of people receiving treatment by the end of 2005 would have been considerably reduced.

By October 2005, PEPFAR was supporting antiretroviral therapy for about 471 000 people living with HIV; approximately 60% are women and 7% are children[23]. More than 50 countries and numerous foundations and corporations have contributed financially to the Global Fund which, by December 2005, was supporting programmes providing antiretroviral therapy to 384,000 people, and the World Bank also launched a US$ 60 million Treatment Acceleration Project with initial grants for scaling up treatment access to Burkina Faso, Ghana and Mozambique in 2004 and 2005.

30-year old Sierra Leonean woman receiving antiretrovirals in a hospital dedicated to HIV patients, 2001.
Panos/ Chris de Bode

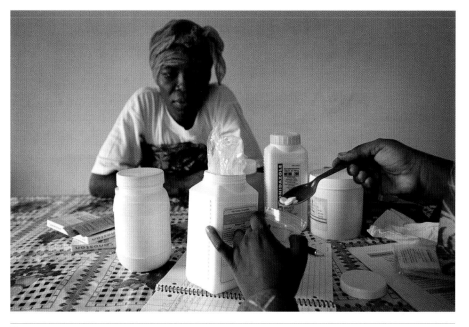

---

[23] UNAIDS (2007). *Global Report 2007*. Geneva, UNAIDS.

The contribution of the United Nations system to "3 by 5"

The "3 by 5" initiative certainly strengthened the work of WHO on HIV in countries and, stressed Jim Yong Kim, former Director of WHO's HIV/AIDS Department, put the relationship between WHO and the UNAIDS Secretariat "in very good shape". UNAIDS Cosponsors have all contributed to "3 by 5" from their relevant areas of expertise; the very existence of UNAIDS ensured that the initiative had a UN system-wide impact. The contributions of the participants are summarized below.

UNHCR has been working with governments, UN agencies and nongovernmental organizations to provide treatment for refugees on the same basis as its availability to people in the host communities. UNICEF worked to improve children's access to antiretroviral treatment and procured antiretroviral drugs and related supplies for more than 40 countries. The World Food Programme worked with WHO to design nutritional guidelines for people living with HIV and to expand their access to better food. UNDP worked to ensure countries' access to affordable medicines, with a special focus on free trade agreements on the production and importation of medicines in some regions.

UNFPA has promoted the integration of counselling and testing, prevention programmes and treatment into reproductive health services. The UN Office on Drugs and Crime has been advocating and recommending a full and comprehensive range of treatment and care services for injecting drug users, who in many countries are discriminated against and therefore do not receive treatment. The International Labour Organization promoted "3 by 5" by providing technical assistance and advisory services on workplace policies to governments and to workers' and employees' organizations and the private sector. The United Nations Educational, Scientific and Cultural Organization has contributed to developing educational materials on treatment and supporting educators through strengthened teacher training. The World Bank contributes major financial resources, as reported earlier, but also provides technical assistance, capacity building, monitoring and evaluation and other services according to a country's specific needs.

The "3 by 5" initiative brought together a wide range of players – more than 200 organizations were involved in the initiative. Zackie Achmat from South Africa's Treatment Action Campaign (TAC), speaking after attending the Global Partners' meeting in May 2004, said: "Why support "3 by 5"? This is the first time atheists like me can sit in the same room with Muslims and Christians to discuss treatment. This is the first time I see brand name pharmaceutical companies sit together with generic drug manufacturers to pursue a common goal"[24].

---

[24] WHO (2004). *"3 by 5" Newsletter*. WHO, Geneva.

The "3 by 5" initiative had an important catalysing effect at global level. In order to maintain momentum and build upon the progress, in July 2005, at Gleneagles in Scotland, leaders of the Group of Eight (G8) industrialized countries announced their intention to 'work … with WHO, UNAIDS and other international bodies to develop and implement a package for HIV prevention, treatment and care, with the aim of as close as possible to universal access to treatment for all those who need it by 2010'. This goal was subsequently endorsed by all UN Member States at the High-Level Plenary Meeting of the 60th Session of the UN General Assembly in September 2005.

228

HIV in the United Nations workplace

UNAIDS has always employed HIV-positive people and has worked over the years to establish a UN workplace programme for AIDS. But many positive people have not found the UN an accepting environment and therefore have chosen not to disclose their HIV status.

"The UN system is experiencing its own silent, internal epidemic. … If the UN were a country it would be among the top 30 countries affected by AIDS", said Kate Thomson, founder of the International Community of Women living with HIV/AIDS (ICW), at the opening of the UN Games in May 2004 (she was then working for the Global Fund). "In Zambia, a recent survey of staff working in one UN agency revealed that out of 44 respondents, over half are caring for people in their own homes – primarily orphans and the sick widows of their lost siblings – and many have up to 14 additional people in their own homes … [whom] they are supporting"[25].

The UNAIDS Secretariat has fought the battle to ensure that staff living with HIV receive antiretroviral treatment under its health insurance system. It was a tough battle, mainly with the WHO health insurance system which covers UNAIDS Secretariat staff. As a result, staff living with HIV now receive appropriate health benefits.

A major new development in 2005 was the launch of "UN+", the UN organization of employees living with HIV. The group aims to develop and improve workplace policies on HIV and to create a more supportive environment for all positive staff. 'Fear is a big issue for many staff', wrote

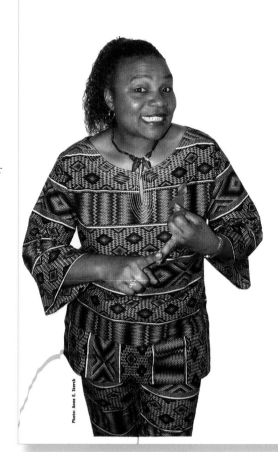

Photo: Anne E. Sterck

JANVIER ЯНВАРЬ

1月

كانون الثاني/ يناير

JANUARY ENERO

TRABAJAR POSITIVAMENTE CON LAS NACIONES UNIDAS

العمل الإيجابي مع الأمم المتحدة

WORKING POSITIVE WITH THE UN

ПОЗИТИВНО РАБОТАТЬ С ООН

TRAVAILLER POSITIVEMENT AUX NATIONS UNIES

与联合国积极地合作

UNAIDS
UNHCR·UNICEF·WFP·UNDP·UNFPA
UNODC·ILO·UNESCO·WHO·WORLD BANK

UNAIDS produced a calendar in 2006 with images of positive people working for the UN. This January image is Elizabeth Gordon Dudu, HIV/AIDS Technical Adviser, UNDP, South Africa. UNAIDS

---

25 Thomson K. *The UN against AIDS – Play Fair, Play Safe*, see www.icw.org.

Kevin Moody, a former member of the WHO HIV/AIDS Department and, since January 2007, the International Coordinator and CEO of the Global Network of People living with HIV/AIDS (GNP+), 'fear of discrimination at work and fear of losing your job'.

Members of "UN+" met with Seretary-General Kofi Annan in October 2005. "It was really one of those meetings you never want to forget", recalled Thomson, who is now Partnership Adviser at UNAIDS. The group has met since then in Amsterdam and smaller groups are being set up in countries, often with the support of UNAIDS country staff.

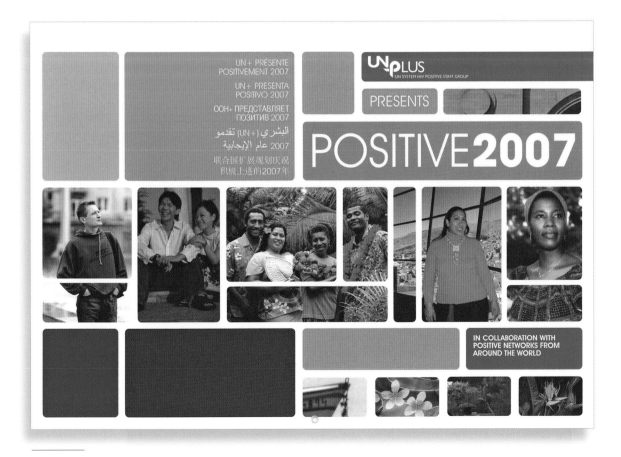

UN Plus calendar.
UNAIDS

230

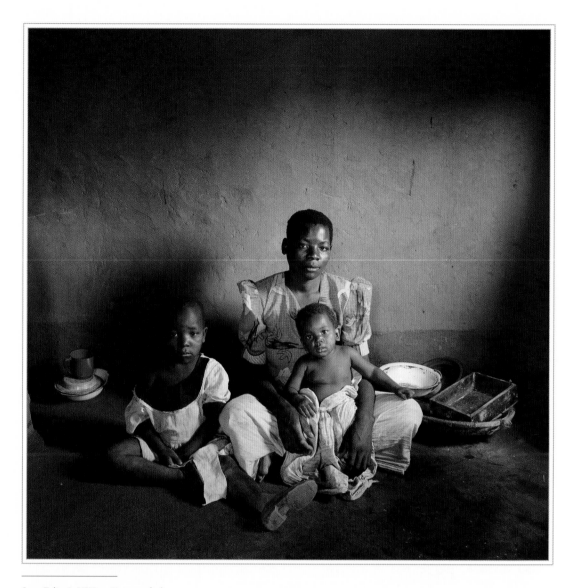

*Joyce Folias is HIV positive, cares for her
two children, one infected, the other not,
at home in Dickson Village, Malawi.
Panos/Jan Banning*

Malawi

Malawi, a sub-Saharan country landlocked by Mozambique, Tanzania and Zambia, is one of the poorest in the world. AIDS has had a particularly devastating impact on this country. Since the first case was diagnosed in 1985, an estimated 650 000 Malawians have died of HIV-related illnesses[1]. In 2007, HIV prevalence among adults aged 15–49 was 14.1%[2], and approximately 500 000 children lost one or two parents to AIDS in 2003[3]. The majority of people living with HIV in Malawi are women, estimated to be 58% of the 810 000 adults living with HIV[4]. Vulnerability to HIV remains high due to the compounded effects of poverty, low education levels, discriminatory practices against girls and women, poor farming methods and drought[5].

Nevertheless, those working in the development community share a strong sense of optimism about Malawi's capacity to respond to the pandemic. From its beginnings as a socially cohesive democracy in 1994, Malawi took deft and decisive steps to respond to AIDS. The political machinery it established for this – one consultative planning process, one coordinating authority and mechanisms for monitoring and accountability – provided a solid foundation for a participatory and well-coordinated AIDS response, and embodied the principles known as the "Three Ones" that UNAIDS would eventually uphold as a paradigm.

Malawi has also been a 'preferred development partner' from the donors' perspective. Donors have been encouraging harmonization and collaborative work in Malawi, and have also been showing their commitment to fostering country ownership of the response to AIDS. The most striking example of this occurred in 2004, when four donors moved away from project-type funding and provided support directly to the government by pooling their funds under the direct management of the National AIDS Commission[6]. The United Nations played a significant role in helping Malawi develop its political and financial arsenal against the disease.

Malawi's response to AIDS: early days

Malawi gained independence from British rule in 1964. For the 30 years that followed, President Hastings Kamuzu Banda maintained a totalitarian grip on the country[7]. Under this regime marked by political and social repression, insufficient attention was paid to

---

[1] *Malawi Country Profile*. www.Avert.org.
[2] UNAIDS (2007). *Malawi Country Profile 2007*. Geneva, UNAIDS.
[3] UNAIDS (2004). *Epidemiological Fact Sheet on HIV/AIDS and Sexually Transmitted Diseases: Malawi, 2004 update*. Geneva, UNAIDS.
[4] UNAIDS (2007). *Malawi Country Profile 2007*.
[5] Office of the President and Cabinet (2005). *Malawi HIV and AIDS Monitoring and Evaluation Report 2005. Follow-up to the Declaration of Commitment, Department of Nutrition HIV and AIDS (UNGASS)*. Lilongwe, Government of Malawi, December.
[6] *Malawi Joint United Nations Programme on HIV and AIDS at a Glance: Forging New Ways to Fight HIV and AIDS* (unpublished manuscript). Geneva, UNAIDS.
[7] *Malawi Country Profile*. www.Avert.org.

the escalating AIDS crisis[8]. A National AIDS Control Programme, established in 1989, focused mainly on blood safety and the management of sexually transmitted infections. Despite UN efforts to widen the scope of the AIDS response, the narrow, biomedical approach predominated in those early years.

In 1994, President Banda conceded power, and the first multiparty elections were held in that year. Freedom of speech was re-established and political prisoners were released[9]. It is relevant that UNAIDS arrived in Lilongwe shortly after the emergence of Malawi's new democracy, as both the nascent democracy and the respond to AIDS would be mutually reinforcing, helping to promote a culture of openness, societal self-reflection and increasing civic awareness and engagement.

When the new President, Bakili Muluzi, took office in 1994, he publicly acknowledged that the population was subject to a severe AIDS epidemic and emphasized the need for a unified response to the crisis[10]. Indeed, the narrow biomedical approach initially adopted by the National AIDS Control Programme had proved to be an ineffective weapon against the deep-rooted cultural and societal drivers of the disease. By the time the first UNAIDS Country Programme Adviser (CPA), Angela Trenton-Mbonde, had arrived in Lilongwe in 1996, the silent virus and the stigma surrounding it had already taken their toll. That same year, the National AIDS Control Programme carried out an evaluation showing that although community awareness reached about 90%, behaviour change was limited, and HIV continued to spread[11].

Mobilizing partners to join in the response to AIDS …

Trenton-Mbonde remembered that "… the Joint Programme's first major challenge was to secure the commitment of all the UN agencies to address AIDS in all of their programmes and to meet in the UN Theme Group on HIV/AIDS to discuss progress"[12].

The UN Theme Group on AIDS was initially created to coordinate UN action on AIDS in country, but soon there was to be a shift in thinking about the role of the UN: the Resident Coordinator, Terence Jones, pushed for UNAIDS' role in coordination beyond the UN, helping to position UNAIDS as 'an honest broker' in the AIDS arena generally[13].

In order to mobilize and coordinate a wide variety of partners, UNAIDS first set up an expanded UN Technical Working Group on HIV and AIDS, which soon became the national coordination forum for AIDS. To promote Malawian ownership of the AIDS response, the forum was co-chaired by the Head of the National AIDS Control Programme.

---

[8] Ibid.
[9] Ibid.
[10] Ibid.
[11] Ibid.
[12] Ibid.
[13] Ibid.

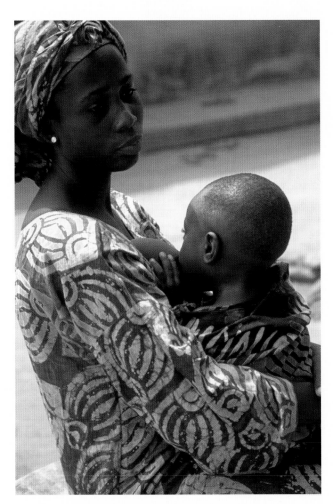

Preventing the transmission of HIV infection from mothers to their babies is a major priority in all countries. UNAIDS

UNAIDS adopted a two-pronged strategy. First, to reinforce the grassroots response, UNAIDS offered direct financial and technical support to civil society groups. This was a significant step: a few of these, such as the Malawi Network of People living with HIV, an umbrella organization for groups of HIV-positive people, would eventually play an important role in the National AIDS Commission and in the national response to AIDS.

Second, UNAIDS and the Theme Group also advocated for a stronger accountability system and more attention by the government to HIV. These efforts resulted in the creation of a government Cabinet Committee on AIDS in 1998. Led by Vice-president Justin Malewezi, a powerful AIDS advocate, and comprising all the Cabinet Ministers, the Cabinet Committee on AIDS had the mandate to build a broad-based, multisectoral, national response to the disease. From the year the Cabinet Committee was created, AIDS was increasingly mentioned in the public statements of the President, ministers and members of Parliament[14].

While the broad-based consultations that informed the development of the first National Strategic Framework in 1998 and 1999 were primarily intended as a tool for national planning, they also helped to break the silence surrounding AIDS and hence to involve a greater number of Malawians in the response to the pandemic.

… to help build political and financial momentum

It is perhaps not surprising that in 2000, the year in which AIDS attracted so much global attention through the UN Security Council Resolution, AIDS was put high on the agenda of the Consultative Group, the forum where all the donors meet with the World Bank and the International Monetary Fund to coordinate efforts for a country's adjustment and reform efforts. Malewezi, Head of the Cabinet Committee, chaired a session where he convinced donors to pledge funds for Malawi's first National Strategic Plan. Malawi made a proposal to the Global Fund in 2001 and received US$ 196 million on the first round.

[14] Ibid.

234

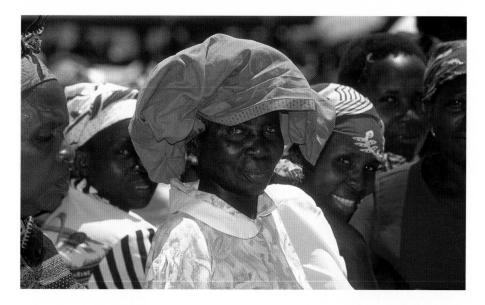

Trenton-Mbonde considered that a momentum was created in those early years: "It began with the formation of the Cabinet Committee, continued with the first Global Fund grant, and kept going with the preparations for the UNGASS. This led to national consultations, so that we could examine the issues that were to be brought to the General Assembly Special Session".

Fueling this momentum was Malawi's qualification for debt relief of US$ 1 billion in December 2001 under the enhanced Heavily Indebted Poor Countries Initiative. This initiative ensures that countries facing unsustainable debt are relieved of their burden as long as they fulfil certain conditions, such as establishing a track record of reform and sound policies, as assessed by the International Monetary Fund.

In 2002, Erasmus Morah arrived in Lilongwe as the new UNAIDS Country Coordinator, and spent the next four years supporting the Malawi Government in developing the political and financial structures necessary to respond to AIDS in a democratic and coherent manner, and in which all development partners would be held accountable for results. Morah would help to 'institutionalize' the principles of coordination, country ownership and accountability that Trenton-Mbonde had been focusing on.

Coordination and consensus

By 2004, Malawi's national response to AIDS was being planned through inclusive, consultative processes; the government had created a body to coordinate the activities and input of a multitude of stakeholders, and it had established effective systems and mechanisms for evaluation, accountability and transparency.

As a result of donor-driven requirements that were in line with the harmonization guidelines that had been endorsed in various agreements[15], Malawi established

The UN in Malawi has been working to redress the pre-existing societal inequalities that drive AIDS, such as gender-based power imbalances
UNAIDS

---

[15] These include the *Rome Declaration on Harmonization* of February 2003 and the guidelines on the coordination of AIDS interventions developed at the 13th International Conference on AIDS and Sexually Transmitted Infections in September 2003.

government structures and systems that embodied the principles promoted by the "Three Ones" before the term "Three Ones" was officially coined. In fact, Malawi's experience helped to inform the conception and development of the "Three Ones"; it was one of the two African countries that attended the 2004 Washington, DC, meeting where the "Three Ones" agreement was first signed.

In addition to its impact on the coordination effort, one of the main purposes of the "Three Ones" is to ensure country-wide ownership of the response to the disease, not only by securing the commitment of the top leaders, but also by mobilizing and coordinating grassroots activity. All "Three Ones" are designed to ensure that the government remains connected and committed to its people and their daily realities through constant, systematic dialogue and 'feedback' loops between central structures and decentralized authorities.

Created in July 2001 with the mandate to guide and oversee the development of the national response to AIDS and to enable its coordination, monitoring and implementation, Malawi's National AIDS Commission is considered one of the most effective in the region. Linking directly to both the political leadership and people of Malawi, it is generally acknowledged that the National AIDS Commission in Malawi has successfully struck the difficult balance between having a clear line of authority and securing meaningful democratic involvement in the response to AIDS. Malawi's National AIDS Commission took on different shapes and forms before it became what it is today. Some of the National AIDS Commission's transformations were required by donors, and the UN supported the Malawi Government in meeting these.

The National AIDS Commission mobilizes democratic involvement in the response to AIDS in at least three ways. First, it holds broad-based consultations to inform the development of the National Strategic Framework. Indeed, the Malawi National AIDS Commission has institutionalized the tradition of government-led Joint Participatory Reviews of the national response[16].

Second, bodies within the National AIDS Commission are representative of the population, and their decision-making processes are genuinely consultative. The National AIDS Commission's 11 board members are selected from a broad range of stakeholders, including people living with HIV, faith-based organizations, the private sector, organizations representing workers unions, women's groups, youth, traditional healers and leaders, and key government ministries including health, local government and finance. Representatives of each group are responsible for coordinating the response to AIDS in that sector. The National Youth Council coordinates youth activities; the Malawi Inter-Faith Association brings all faith communities together, and the Malawi Business Coalition against HIV/AIDS coordinates activities of the private sector.

---

[16] Office of the Pr)esident and Cabinet (2005). *Malawi HIV and AIDS Monitoring and Evaluation Report 2005. Follow-up to the Declaration of Commitment Department of Nutrition HIV and AIDS (UNGASS)*. Lilongwe, Government of Malawi, December.

The Director of the Malawi Network of People living with HIV felt that the organizations of people living with HIV were widely consulted and represented in the National AIDS Commission. He cited as an example that some concerns of people living with HIV about recruitment policies were addressed; as a result, consensus was reached that no one can be denied employment based upon their HIV status except for the military and the police force[17].

More recently, the Malawi Partnership Forum was established with the help of Emebet Admassu, UNAIDS Social Mobilization and Partnership Adviser. The Partnership Forum was created because there was a need for a single, umbrella body that brought all partners together. The Executive Director of Malawi's National AIDS Commission, Biswick Mwale, explained how these two bodies share the decision-making process: "The Partnership Forum will draw some resolutions or recommendations, which are then passed on to the Board of the National AIDS Commission for review or approval. So, once that is done, the recommendation becomes binding".

The third way the National AIDS Commission secures the meaningful involvement of the Malawian people in the national response to AIDS is by channeling funds to the local authorities or civil society groups for implementation and service delivery. Indeed, decentralization is a key element in the "Three Ones", as it is crucial for translating policies and principles into service-delivery scale-up[18]. Mwale explained: "We know that if we are going to succeed [in scaling up the national AIDS response], we need to reach out to rural communities as much as possible".

However, government capacity at the district and community level is still lacking. David Chitate, Monitoring and Evaluation Adviser at UNAIDS, explained: "Decentralization in Malawi is yet to take root as the process has been very slow. You can't really depend on the decentralized structures for effective coordination of the response because they don't have capacity and they are very weak. You can't give local authorities funds for sub-granting purposes because they don't have the financial systems; they don't have the procurement systems. The required systems are being built now, but they are still very weak and building of systems requires time". The National AIDS Commission has taken steps towards decentralization by asking international umbrella organizations to help build the capacity of the local authorities.

Greater government capacity at local levels should also help to ensure effective monitoring and evaluation processes. Malawi has made progress towards developing a national monitoring and evaluation framework aligned to the National Action Framework[19]; however, an important problem is the lack of capacity at all levels to generate quality data[20].

Given that "one of the major challenges for the [Malawi] government has been to

[17] Southern African Development Community (2005). *Putting the "Three Ones" Principles into Action: Experiences from Lesotho, Malawi, the United Republic of Tanzania and Zambia.* Gaborone, Botswana, December.
[18] Ibid.
[19] UNAIDS. *The "Three Ones" in Malawi* (unpublished report). Geneva, UNAIDS.
[20] Ibid.

… usher in the new era of democracy, good governance and rule of law"[21], it seems reasonable to hypothesize that the successful implementation of the "Three Ones" in Malawi has been helping to strengthen Malawi's democratic institutions and processes and thus to yield positive externalities beyond the AIDS sector.

"An extreme partnership"

As Malawi was developing effective mechanisms to mobilize, coordinate and monitor the AIDS response, several donors decided to pool their funds. By 2004, Malawi became the first example of a country that had pooled funding with some donors – an example of "extreme partnership"[22] in the words of the World Bank.

Pooled funding means that general programme funding is provided in a common account. These funds are available to finance any eligible programme expenditures according to a detailed, agreed financial plan that specifies which activities will be funded by 'earmarked' donors, and which will be funded by pooled donors[23].

Pooled funds have reduced reporting requirements, drastically reduced transactions costs, improved the efficiency of development initiatives and decreased the tendency of donors to dictate their terms to the country[24]. Roy Hauya, of the National AIDS Commission, said: "… the National AIDS Commission is not donor-driven anymore. Donors now ask how we want to do something instead of saying we should do this"[25].

UNAIDS played an important role in making this pooled funding happen in Malawi when, in 2004, it brought four donors together with the Malawi Government to create a basket of funds amounting to about US$ 72 million over five years.

Morah explained: "The donors wanted pooled funding and tried it but got nowhere". The donors had approached him explaining that they had tried to establish a common basket of funding but that the Malawi Government was not interested in participating. When Morah began talking with the government counterparts, he understood that they "were worried that pooled funding could readily translate to a ganging-up of the donors, which was the last thing they wanted". In the end, the government was willing to give pooled funding a try as long as the UN would facilitate the agreement. Morah was officially invited to lead the process of bringing the donors and the government counterparts together to negotiate the pool-funding arrangement.

Mwale remarked that the UN played an important role in making this partnership happen: "I think UNAIDS played a very catalytic role in resolving our own problems as a commission and with the donors. And we had endless meetings, in the night, in the

---

[21] Office of the President and Cabinet (2005). *Strategic Plan for the Department of Nutrition, HIV and AIDS.* Lilongwe, Government of Malawi.

[22] Brown J C, Ayvalikli D, Mohammad N (2004). *Turning Bureaucrats into Warriors, Preparing and Implementing Multi-sector HIV/AIDS Programmes in Africa.* Washington, DC, The International Bank for Reconstruction and Development/The World Bank.

[23] Southern African Development Community (2005).

[24] Ibid.

[25] Ibid.

afternoon, in the morning, trying to create a roadmap on how we should work together. The UN does not have a big bag of money, but they are very catalytic in terms of these issues. At the same time, I'm very appreciative of the donors themselves because they became very flexible, and they have seen the advantages of this process".

Testing and treatment scale-up

The wide consultations that were supported by the UN family to develop Malawi's National HIV Policy led to an innovative course of action on testing. Morah stated: "Everybody had an opportunity to contribute, every sector was represented and, in the end, we were able to not only come up with a good policy, but we actually developed a policy that pushed a bit on the boundaries of some of the issues".

Indeed, although the usual approach to HIV testing places the onus on the patient to ask for a test, the Malawi policy promotes the scale-up of testing by requesting the health care provider to initiate the offer of testing. It recommends a systematic offer of HIV testing to anyone who attends at a hospital ward, or an antenatal, tuberculosis or sexually transmitted infections clinic.

Morah explained that it was extremely difficult to persuade partners to agree on this policy, as some international nongovernmental organizations felt that it was too strongly reminiscent of mandatory testing.

However, when Morah started speaking to government officials about it, he did not hear a single objection. Indeed, he had made it clear that the UN would not support mandatory testing, but he also communicated his belief that a holistic interpretation of human rights, taking into account the right to life, good health, and information, would require that the offer of testing be systematic. "At the end of the day", said Morah, "the UN would like to see more people getting tested".

As a result of this new policy, Malawi has seen an acceleration of testing. The number of Malawians who are tested for HIV soared from approximately 50 000 in 2002 to more than 400 000 in 2005.

Where there is the hope and possibility for AIDS treatment, people will be willing to be tested for HIV. The year 2005, which saw an acceleration of testing, was not coincidentally the year in which antiretroviral treatment became more widely accessible in Malawi.

In 2003, UNAIDS and the World Health Organization launched the "3 by 5" global initiative, aiming to provide three million people living with HIV with antiretroviral treatment by 2005. At that time, Malawi already had a treatment programme, though its goals were less ambitious than those put forward by the "3 by 5".

Increased donor funding, as well as some key changes and innovations brought about by global efforts, made treatment scale-up possible. By 2003, the price of yearly antiretroviral

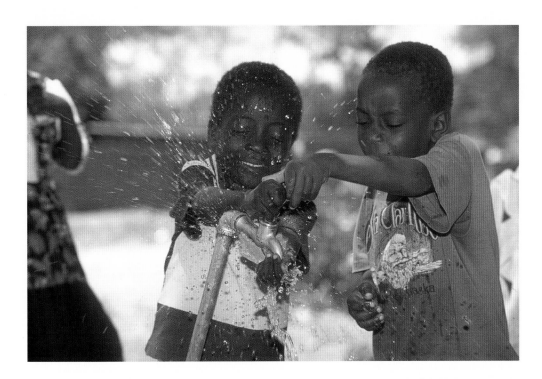

treatment had dropped tremendously in Malawi; also, in the "3 by 5", WHO introduced a simplified approach to treatment delivery which facilitated treatment access. Thus Malawi could aspire to double the number of people receiving antiretroviral medicines to 50 000. Malawi had a maximum of 4000 people receiving antiretroviral treatment in 2002. In December 2005, the number receiving antiretroviral therapy had shot up to 46 000.

Jack Phiri developed AIDS-related symptoms in 1999, and discovered he was HIV positive in 2001. Today, he receives free care and treatment. He is happy to be alive. "I have gone through the thick and the thin of it", Phiri reflected. "A lot of people were better than me and are no longer of this world. Having gone through all that I have, here I am, leading a normal life. I don't wake up one morning not knowing how I will feel that day. I can almost guarantee that it will be a nice, normal day".

"3 by 5" was only a first step in ensuring wide-scale AIDS treatment access. Today, the goal is to achieve universal access to HIV prevention, care and treatment by 2010. But in Malawi as well as many other countries in Africa, two key related challenges must be addressed in order to achieve such a far-reaching goal. These are the human resources crisis and building service-delivery capacity in the districts.

In May 2007, Mwale explained: "We have a serious human resource crisis in Malawi. As I speak now, out of the one million people that are living with HIV in Malawi, our estimate is that about 170 000 require treatment today. Yet we have only 50 000 people on treatment. It's a mammoth task, both in terms of the monies that will be required and the human resource capacity within the health sector to be able to scale to that level".

Malawian nurse Mary Ntata described the staff problem[26]: "There are enough antiretroviral drugs … but not enough staff to administer the drugs. … nurses dispense the drugs from 7am but many of those [patients] who have been waiting through the night are turned away". Diagnosis and treatment of sexually transmitted infections, prevention of mother-to-child transmission, condom distribution, counselling and treatment of opportunistic infections are not widely available to a great number of Malawians due to the lack of infrastructure and skilled health workers[27].

In order to resolve this crisis, an innovative human resources programme for the health sector was adopted and has seen encouraging results (see Chapter 7 for details). AIDS money will help to develop the health sector generally, as expanding the number of health professionals has implications not only for AIDS patients but also for those suffering from other diseases.

Malawi's exceptional response to AIDS

Malawi has been responding to AIDS in the health sector but it has also prepared plans for action in other areas. For example, Malawi's *HIV and AIDS Strategy and Plan of Action in the Education Sector* was launched in February 2005, and recently, the government has firmly placed the issues of nutrition, HIV on the national development agenda through the creation of the Department of Nutrition, HIV and AIDS in the Office of the President and Cabinet.

Furthermore, the UN in Malawi has also been assisting Malawian activists to redress the pre-existing societal inequalities that drive AIDS, such as gender-based power imbalances. Joyce Banda, an activist who has created many networks and associations to help other women achieve financial independence and break the cycles of abuse and poverty, received funding from the United Nations Population Fund at various times in her career to carry out her work. Joyce Banda has also fought for policy change. From 1999 to 2007, she, other Malawian activists and staff members at UNFPA office in Lilongwe campaigned for better laws to protect women against violence at home. In May 2007, the Malawi Government finally responded to their demands and passed the Domestic Violence Bill. Said a Malawian participant at a Committee on the Elimination of Discrimination Against Women meeting: "The Domestic Violence Bill counters once and for all the contention that what happens in a family is purely a private matter". Joyce Banda eventually became Minister of Gender and Minister of Foreign Affairs. In her closing remarks to the Committee on the Elimination of Discrimination Against Women meeting on 19 May 2007, she said that "… just a few years ago it would have been unimaginable to have a Government Ministry headed by a woman or a human rights law involving women's rights being passed in the country"[28].

---

[26] *Malawi Country Profile*. www.Avert.org.

[27] *Malawi Country Profile*. www.Usaid.org.

[28] United Nations (2007). Press Release, 19 May 2007. WOM/1560. Department of Public Information. Geneva, United Nations.

UNAIDS has helped to coordinate UN work on AIDS in Malawi, and has also moved beyond the UN to help to mobilize, technically support and improve communication among all stakeholders in the fight against the pandemic. The development partners' cooperativeness as well as the UN's combination of technical expertise and international legitimacy have enabled it to play its role effectively in Malawi. Although there is still much work to be done and progress to be made in this country, Malawi has seen notable improvements. Today, increased numbers of Malawians have access to HIV prevention services, AIDS care and treatment; the stigma surrounding HIV has decreased, and there have been recent developments including institutions, which might help to create a more equitable society.

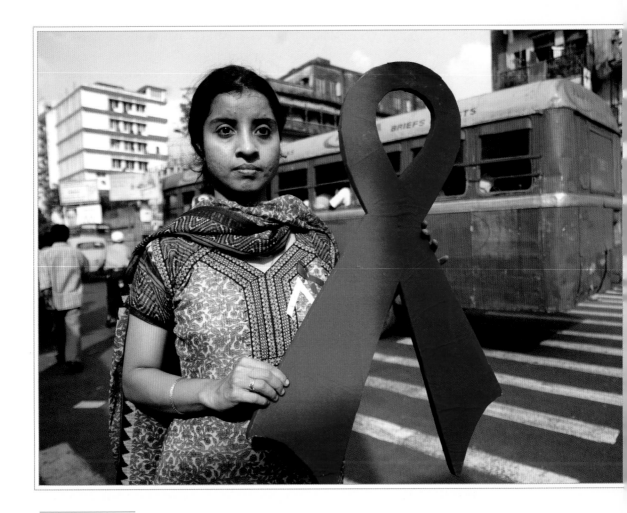

An Indian volunteer during the World
Aids Day celebrations in Calcutta,
India, 2004.
Reuters/Corbis/ Sucheta Daz

Chapter 9:
Looking to the future: the challenge of sustaining an exceptional response to AIDS

In 2005, an estimated 32.3 million people were living with HIV, of whom 2.9 million became newly infected with HIV and 2.2 million lost their lives. In 2007, the estimate of people living with HIV rose to 32.7 million, of whom 42.7 million became newly infected and 2.1 million died[1]. Global spending on AIDS in 2007 was US$ 8.9 billion.

In 2007, there were more new infections and more AIDS deaths than ever before, and there was evidence that some countries were seeing a resurgence in HIV infection rates which previously had been stable or declining.

The year 2007 marked two anniversaries: it was 25 years since the first published report of AIDS and 10 years since the announcement about the effectiveness of highly active antiretroviral therapy at the International AIDS Conference in Vancouver. But there was little cause for celebration. More than 25 million people had died from AIDS and millions of children had been orphaned. Every day, 7500 people were being infected with HIV, 5800 people were dying from AIDS-related illnesses and still only 24%[2] of those in need had access to treatment.

In 2007, there were more new infections and more AIDS deaths than ever before, and there was evidence[3] that some countries (for example, Uganda) were seeing a resurgence in HIV infection rates which previously had been stable or declining.

However, there were also some grounds for hope. For the first time since the early HIV prevention successes in Thailand and Uganda, in a number of developing countries prevention programmes were producing a return on the growing investments made in AIDS activities. Summarizing the findings of the UNAIDS *Global Report 2006*, Peter Piot, UNAIDS Executive Director, said: "2005 was the least bad year in the history of the AIDS epidemic"[4].

The latest UNAIDS data[5] revealed that the number of people living with HIV had increased in every region of the world, but there was a decline in new infections in about 10 countries. In most high-income countries, numbers of people living with HIV have risen because antiretroviral drugs keeps seropositive people alive, while at the same time other people continue to become infected with HIV.

In low- and middle-income countries, an estimated 250 000 to 350 000 deaths were averted in 2005 as a consequence of new treatment programmes[6]. There were also signs of a change in

[1] UNAIDS/WHO (November, 2007).
[2] WHO (2007). *Towards Universal Access by 2010.* Geneva, WHO.
[3] UNAIDS/WHO (2007). *AIDS Epidemic Update, 2007.* Geneva, UNAIDS/WHO.
[4] Altman L K (2007). 'Report shows AIDS epidemic slowdown in 2005'. *New York Times*, 31 May.
[5] UNAIDS/WHO (2007).
[6] WHO/UNAIDS (2007). *Progress on Global Access to HIV Antiretroviral Therapy: a Report on the "3 by 5" and Beyond.* Geneva, UNAIDS.

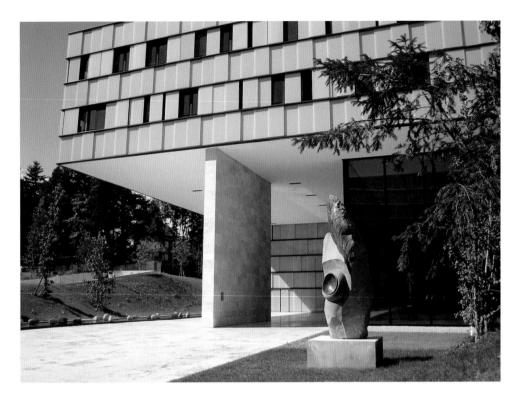

people's sexual behaviour in those countries experiencing a decline in new infections. In each of these countries, there was strong evidence that people were increasing their use of condoms, delaying the first time they have sexual intercourse and having fewer sexual partners.

But only about 10 countries were showing such results. As Piot explained: "We are only at the beginning of the epidemic in terms of impact and the challenges are enormous. Even though HIV prevalence has stabilized in many countries in sub-Saharan Africa, they have done so at unacceptably high rates and new infections are accelerating in Eastern Europe".

The year 2007 also marked the 10th anniversary of UNAIDS. After a difficult 'birth' and first few years, UNAIDS is now fully accepted as part of the United Nations 'family' and the development world generally. In a highly symbolic move, the UNAIDS Secretariat now has its own headquarters in Geneva, a new building shared with the World Health Organization, thanks to the support of the Swiss Confederation.

Piot explained: "For the first seven to eight years, I had to justify our existence almost daily. It was very destabilizing".

The future changing aspects of the epidemic will present UNAIDS and the international community with new and varied challenges as they respond to and seek to reverse the epidemic. The following pages identify some probable challenges and summarise some of the achievements of the last ten years.

The year 2007 marked the 10th anniversary of UNAIDS. The UNAIDS Secretariat now has its own headquarters in Geneva, a new building shared with the WHO, thanks to the support of the Swiss Confederation. Stone sculpture in front 'Eradication' by Zimbabwean sculptor Mike Munyaradzi
UNAIDS/N. Gouiran

Putting AIDS on the political agenda

Undoubtedly, and there is general agreement on this, UNAIDS' major achievement has been, through its advocacy and in partnership with others, to place AIDS high on the political agenda of global, regional and national leaders and powerful organizations. In 1996, no one could have foreseen that the UN Security Council would debate AIDS as a major security risk, as they did in January 2000, nor that there would be the first United Nations General Assembly Special Session (UNGASS) on a health issue – AIDS, as there was in June 2001.

"It doesn't take an over-generous interpretation of history to allow that UNGASS played a large part in bringing about the changes behind the better news..."

In low- and middle-income countries, there has been a move from denial to engagement, both nationally and in regional groupings such as the African Union, the Association of South-East Asian Nations, and the Caribbean Community (CARICOM). In nearly 40 countries, the national AIDS response is led by heads of government or state, or their deputies. AIDS is firmly on the agenda of the Group of Eight (G8), the World Economic Forum and other such bodies. More than 200 international companies are members of the Global Business Coalition on AIDS and many trade unions worldwide are actively engaged in the struggle.

Marta Mauras, former Secretary of the Economic Commission for Latin America and the Caribbean, said that she had "appreciated enormously the fact that UNAIDS, in doing its advocacy, has always been positive ... the message has always been this is a terrible problem but it has solutions. I think that's very important because it's a rallying call for people to join hands".

In rich countries, donors have become far more committed to work on HIV. Not that UNAIDS would claim it has achieved this alone. It has worked in partnership with a rather eclectic and contemporary band of players – people living with HIV and other activists, a wide range of nongovernmental organizations from tiny grassroots to international organizations, business leaders, faith-based organizations, foundations run by billionaires and former heads of state and numerous celebrities.

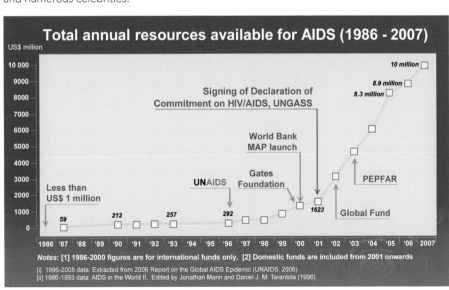

246

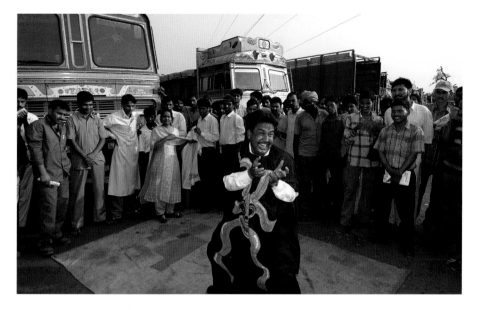

An increase in funding for the AIDS response

What has the political commitment meant in practice? First and perhaps foremost, it has led to the massive increase in funding for AIDS. Between 1996 and 2007, finance for HIV programmes in low- and middle-income countries increased more than 30-fold, from less than US$ 300 million in 1996 to US$ 8.9 billion. As *The Economist* wrote: 'Although other factors were involved, it doesn't take an over-generous interpretation of history to allow that UNGASS played a large part in bringing about the changes behind the better news …The rate at which money has been made available for AIDS (from all sources including inflicted countries as well as taxpayers of the rich world) underwent a step change in 2001'[7].

Indeed, as Piot pointed out, it was a rare example of a promise made by the General Assembly actually being honoured. The pledge was to find between US$ 7 and US$ 10 billion by 2005, and what turned up in 2005 was US$ 8.3 billion, squarely in the middle of the range.

Many developing countries have increased their own domestic funding on AIDS programmes, despite their limited resources; about a third of current spending on AIDS comes from national budgets and private payments in these countries[8]. The remaining two thirds have come from bilateral donors and multilateral institutions. In just over three years, the Global Fund to Fight AIDS, Tuberculosis and Malaria disbursed US$ 2.26 billion to grant recipients[9].

A major donor is the U.S. President's Emergency Plan for AIDS Relief (PEPFAR) which by 2007 had disbursed a total of US$ 8.4 billion and accounts for roughly half of all bilateral spending on AIDS. PEPFAR depends on UNAIDS data and policy arguments for its work. And as *The Economist* argued: '… it is hard to believe that Mr Bush would have done what he did without the prompting of events that began with UNGASS'[10].

In India, the Tata Steel Company has pioneered HIV prevention programmes including street theatre for its employees as well as truckdrivers and other communities
Panos/Helder Netocny

---

[7] 'Unhappy anniversary'. *The Economist*, 3 June 2007.
[8] UNAIDS (2007). *Global Report 2007*. Geneva, UNAIDS.
[9] The Global Fund (2007). *Investing in Impact: Mid-year Results Report 2007*. Geneva, UNAIDS.
[10] 'Unhappy anniversary'. *The Economist*, 3 June 2007.

A global reference point

There is a general consensus that UNAIDS is a vital global reference point for a wide range of data and information on the AIDS epidemic and the responses to it, as well as the tracking of resource needs.

"If there had not been a UNAIDS, there would not have been a global awareness of the epidemic. UNAIDS has also highlighted the multidisciplinary nature of AIDS, and the importance of human rights".

Keith Hansen, Health, Nutrition and Population Sector Manager for Latin America and the Caribbean at the World Bank, commented: "Very quickly the Secretariat became the accepted authoritative, legitimate voice for the UN family on AIDS. And I think we quickly realized what an advantage that was, because you wouldn't have the agencies sending mixed messages".

Michel Kazatchkine, formerly French AIDS Ambassador and now Executive Director of the Global Fund as of April 2007, commented that UNAIDS' epidemiological work has defined the areas in which countries must intervene, based on their data, and the great importance of evaluating resource needs. "If there had not been a UNAIDS, there would not have been a global awareness of the epidemic. UNAIDS has also highlighted the multidisciplinary nature of AIDS, and the importance of human rights".

Increasing access to antiretroviral treatment

Since its early Drugs Access Initiative, UNAIDS has campaigned to reduce the price of antiretroviral treatment so that it would be available to poor people in low-income countries. This and other initiatives, including the work of activists and the strong advocacy of the UN Secretary-General, have led to a major reduction in prices. UNAIDS, treatment activists and nongovernmental organizations also led the way in showing that providing antiretroviral treatment was possible in countries where health services were resource limited.

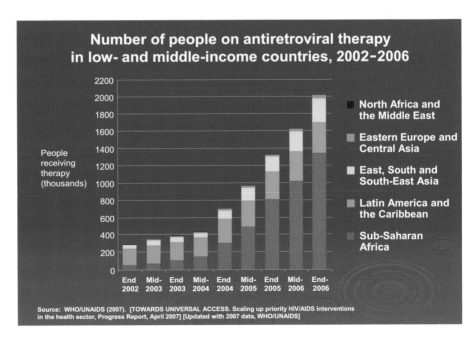

Number of people on antiretroviral therapy in low- and middle-income countries, 2002–2006

Source: WHO/UNAIDS (2007). [TOWARDS UNIVERSAL ACCESS. Scaling up priority HIV/AIDS interventions in the health sector, Progress Report, April 2007] [Updated with 2007 data, WHO/UNAIDS]

By December 2007, around 2.3 million people were being treated[11]. In addition to its Multi-Country HIV/AIDS Programme for Africa (MAP), the World Bank launched a US$ 60 million Treatment Acceleration Project in 2004-2005, with initial grants to Burkina Faso, Ghana and Mozambique. The World Bank had committed more than $2.5 billion to the responce to AIDS by the end of 2005.

Making the money work in countries

Since 2002, the UNAIDS Secretariat in partnership with its Cosponsors has focused more strongly on country-level work. Piot wrote to UNAIDS staff at the start of 2007: 'We will continue our transformation from an organization focusing on advocacy to mobilize against the AIDS epidemic to a field oriented organization that focuses on UN system support to implementation of AIDS programmes ("making the money work") while continuing the ever needed advocacy and policy activities'.

The numbers of staff in countries have increased and the UNAIDS Country Coordinators are working as full members of the UN Country Teams. In several countries, partners such as donors and civil society report a stronger UN presence.

UNAIDS developed the "Three Ones" policy, aiming to harmonize and align the work of all AIDS players in countries. Only through succeeding with this change in international development practice – ensuring that the money is where it is needed – will countries be able to 'make the money work' effectively and fulfil the commitments made at UNGASS.

UNAIDS monitoring and evaluation staff now form the largest evaluation force in the world for AIDS (and one of the largest in development in general). They play a key role in steering the response worldwide, because they provide, from a variety of sources, the accurate data that form the basis for effective planning and implementation.

UNAIDS as a pathfinder to United Nations reform

From its inception, UNAIDS has been a natural pathfinder for UN reform. When the UN was founded more than 60 years ago, the world was a very different place and the UN's systems were, to some extent, established to respond to different global concerns.

In the early days of the epidemic, AIDS challenged the way the UN worked and the aim of creating UNAIDS was to change this. UNAIDS, it has often been said, was not about 'business as usual'. The mandate for the new Programme was to provide leadership on the global response and policy, and to ensure coordination and coherence across the UN system in responding to the AIDS epidemic. It was seen as essential to maximize the collective effectiveness of the cosponsoring agencies.

---

[11] WHO (2007).

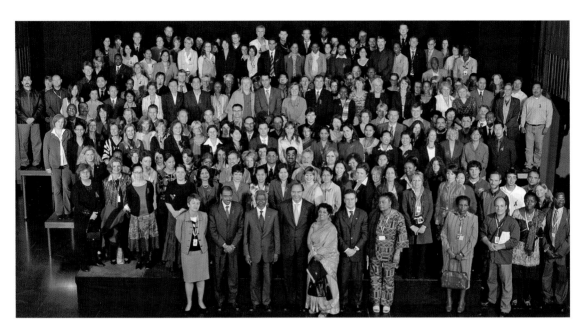

UN Secretary-General Kofi Annan with UNAIDS staff, Geneva, 2005.
UNAIDS

Indeed, since its creation in 1996, several international development agencies have referred to UNAIDS as an example for UN reform as a whole. On 30 October 1997, almost two years after the Joint Programme was born, then UN Secretary-General Kofi Annan made a speech in which he called UNAIDS "an experiment in interagency coordination"[12]. He also said, "I expect the UNAIDS experience to show us how to reap the full benefits of a genuinely collective effort which will be greater than the sum of its parts. We cannot afford to fail. The issue addressed by the programme is too crucial, the experiment it represents in interagency coordination too important"[13].

In a recent interview for this book, Annan said he was proud of "the creation of UNAIDS, pulling together the various parts of the UN and getting them to make a major contribution which hopefully is much larger than the sum of its parts". He also said that "working cooperatively the way we did was also a message for the governments themselves that they also need to work with the various ministries, with civil society, [and] community organizations. I think that was an innovation that has worked well".

The UNAIDS Secretariat and Cosponsors have worked to achieve more coherence. The new Joint UN Teams on AIDS, established in 2007, should achieve this at country level, though it may be a slow process in some countries. Another important initiative for improving AIDS coordination among donors is the Global Task Team. Now there is a country-level common system and indicators for monitoring and evaluation. Globally, there is increasing coherence in policy, budget setting and advocacy. These experiences of UNAIDS are informing the next stages of the UN reform process.

---

[12] UNAIDS (1997). Press Release, Secretary-General Appeals to United Nations Agencies for Coordinated Response in Fight against HIV/AIDS', 30 October. Geneva, UNAIDS.
[13] Ibid.

United Nations collaboration and Cosponsors

The bitter disagreements about the establishment of UNAIDS, and between Cosponsors and the Secretariat for many years afterwards, were a barrier to the much-needed collaboration between agencies – the reason for setting up UNAIDS in the first place. However, there have been significant improvements at all levels in recent years.

Individually and in collaboration, cosponsoring organizations work on many different areas, and have been at the forefront of setting the global agenda on AIDS.

Hansen explained: "[UNAIDS] began to create a space in which the agencies could sort out their comparative advantages and see what unique role each of them could play. Nobody should be trying to duplicate WHO's role or take it away; no one should be trying to horn in on what UNICEF alone can do, or what UNICEF does best, and, obviously, the Bank had certain roles, skills and access that the rest of the UN family did not. And this helped each of us to see how that would contribute and give us a comfort level that, even if we weren't worrying about some aspect of the epidemics, one of the other agencies was covering that".

"And, of course, success is mixed so far, but I think it is a much more cohesive and better organized response – certainly than it would have been without UNAIDS".

The former UN Deputy Secretary-General, Mark Malloch Brown, noted the constraints UNAIDS has faced in terms of collaboration: "I would argue that UNAIDS is probably the best success we have [in terms] of coordinated action across different agencies, but it is not a gold standard. We have a huge way to go, I think, and in this history of the first 10 years, too much time has been spent trying to get Country Teams to work together, trying to get them to act strategically from the base of what needs to be done, rather than from the base of dividing up the spoils of AIDS money between them, and I think it's been an issue that's led to a fair amount of reform, but it's also been an issue that shows the limits of reform so far".

Piot agreed: "We wasted a lot of energy and time on bureaucratic processes because of turf wars and entrenchment, the unwillingness of UN agencies to give up territory. There was also the competition for funds. The recent openness to reform is helping us greatly".

Stephen Lewis, the former Special Envoy of the UN Secretary-General for HIV/AIDS in Africa, is strongly critical of the UN response: "I think that the absence of leadership, which UNAIDS could not overcome, at the centre of the UN system has resulted in far less progress than should otherwise have been the case. There is no question in my mind that, when history is written, when the significant history of the pandemic is written, the inability of the UN to orchestrate a response far more vigorous, far more effective, far more searching than the response we've had thus far, that that will be seen as one of the sad components of the pandemic. That is not – I don't really believe that's a commentary on UNAIDS. I think it goes much further than that; I think it goes to the heads of agencies and to the Heads of the [UN] Secretariat".

"I would argue that UNAIDS is probably the best success we have [in terms] of coordinated action across different agencies, but it is not a gold standard".

Stigma, human rights and the greater involvement of people living with HIV

Eradicating the stigma experienced by people living with HIV has been an essential part of UNAIDS' strategy from its inception, but it is an uphill task in many countries. In both the 2001 Declaration of Commitment on HIV/AIDS and the 2007 Political Declaration on HIV/AIDS, governments committed themselves to taking action to address stigma and discrimination, recognizing that such a step is a 'critical element in combating the global HIV/AIDS pandemic'.

However the stigma experienced by specific groups such as sex workers and injecting drug users is such that these groups are still not named in the 2007 Political Declaration.

There is sound, research-based evidence of the significant amount of stigma experienced by people living with HIV, with women experiencing it more than men and of the personal suffering caused by stigma. Edwin Cameron, the South African judge who is HIV-positive, has written movingly that[14] 'stigma is perhaps the greatest dread of those who live with AIDS and HIV... Stigma's irrational force springs not only from the prejudiced, bigoted, fearful reactions others have to AIDS – it lies in the fears and self-loathing, the self-undermining and ultimately self-destroying inner sense of self-blame that all too many people with AIDS or HIV experience themselves'.

Involving positive people in work at all levels has been an important aspect of UNAIDS' work to combat stigma, whether through supporting the establishment and work of networks of people living with HIV or negotiating with governments to free positive people from jail.

With UNAIDS' support over six years, for example, the All-Ukrainian Network of People Living with HIV helped to found, in 2005, the Union of People Living with HIV in Eastern and Central Europe. The network has united associations in 10 countries to mobilize resources for underfinanced networks in the region. People living with HIV were supported in various ways; for example, a photo exhibition of positive people was organized, and this included pictures of people who had not shared their status with the family before. The Ukrainian network is very strong in its support for people who decide to 'come out' and in reaching out to those who don't yet feel comfortable about doing so.

However, in many countries there are no legal and policy frameworks for establishing networks of people living with HIV.

Natashya Ong, a Singaporean woman living with HIV and a member of the Programme Coordinating Board, welcomed the involvement of positive people but explained the

[14] Cameron E (2005). *Witness to AIDS*. New York, I B Taurus.

challenges they face. Groups and networks of positive people want to be included in decision-making and implementation, but often lack the support and capacity to do so. "[Often] we're not [given] enough time and space to be able to communicate amongst ourselves or to caucus prior to a meeting we're expected to attend … sometimes networks are expected to be more participatory in meetings but don't have the capacity to do that". She also highlights the problem of sustainable finances; most funders support periodic projects or those of their own interest, but not core funding.

Mary Balikungeri of the Rwanda Women's Network is also a member of the PCB. She commented: "I assure you, this is an empowering tool for civil society. The process addresses the challenges of the 'disconnect' between global and local levels. The civil society model of participating in the high-level meeting was also important because it is the only channel to bring issues of communities to the table".

At a global level, UNAIDS is working closely with the Office of the High Commissioner for Human Rights to help integrate the issue of HIV stigma and discrimination into the work of national human rights institutions and the UN human rights treaty bodies and special procedures. UNAIDS has always worked with governments to establish and/or improve legislation and to ensure that their AIDS response has a clear human rights perspective. However, 10 years on, human rights frameworks are either non-existent or extremely weak in many countries[15]. As the UN Secretary-General's 2007 report revealed, half the countries reporting noted existing policies that prevent stigmatized groups such as sex workers and injecting drug users from accessing prevention programmes[16]. UNAIDS has intensified its support to countries to address the vulnerability of these specific groups.

Another of UNAIDS' key priorities has been to work in partnership with a wide range of players in recognition of the fact that AIDS is more than just a health problem.

UNAIDS advocacy led to Panama enacting legislation to eradicate the sexual and commercial exploitation of children and adolescents, Cambodia's official adoption of harm-reduction programmes for drug users and formal steps by Ukraine to increase the access of drug users to antiretroviral treatment. The United Nations Development Programme has formulated draft model legislation for countries in West Africa to protect and promote the rights of people living with HIV.

---

[15] UNAIDS (2005). *Executive Director's Report to the 17th Meeting of the UNAIDS PCB*, June. Geneva, UNAIDS.
[16] UNAIDS (2007). *UN Secretary-General's Report, 2007*. Geneva, UNAIDS.

Coalition building

As this account has shown, another of UNAIDS' key priorities has been to work in partnership with a wide range of players in recognition of the fact that AIDS is more than just a health problem.

In 1997, UNAIDS stimulated the establishment of the Global Business Coalition on AIDS (formerly the Global Business Council on AIDS) which has grown to a membership of more than 200 companies. The UNAIDS Secretariat and the International Labour Organization have encouraged the business sector to recognize the impact of AIDS; it is now on the agenda of the World Economic Forum through its Global Health Initiative. In countries where adult HIV prevalence exceeds 20%, a majority of companies (58%) do have a written HIV policy. ILO has provided technical assistance on workplace policies and programmes in more than 25 countries in Africa, Asia, Eastern Europe and the Caribbean[17]. UNAIDS has also supported the launching of national business AIDS coalitions in numerous countries and regional business coalitions in most regions such as the Pan-Caribbean Business Forum on AIDS.

ILO and the World AIDS Campaign also work closely with trade unions on AIDS issues; for example, with UNDP it brought together trade unions in Ukraine to devise strategies that would mobilize workers in promoting workplace programmes.

Religious and faith-based organizations have been closely involved in the AIDS response since the early days of the epidemic. UNAIDS has, over the past 10 years, worked with many faith-based organizations, religious leaders and theologians – Buddhist, Christian, Hindu and Muslim. Although there are clearly differences in attitude – one of the most obvious being the use of condoms – careful diplomacy and attention to theological discourse, as well as practical actions, have led to good working relationships. In many countries, religious leaders are closely involved in policy and programmatic work.

In 2003, for example, Calle Almedal, UNAIDS Senior Adviser on Partnerships Development, organized a workshop for Christian academic theologians in Windhoek, Namibia. He worked with them to produce a document that sets out a Christian perspective on HIV related stigma and discrimination and thousands of copies were eventually distributed – in English, French, Spanish and Russian.

The former Deputy Secretary-General of the UN, Louise Fréchette, commended UNAIDS for being "an innovative organization that has not hesitated to reach out to a variety

---

[17] UNAIDS (2005).

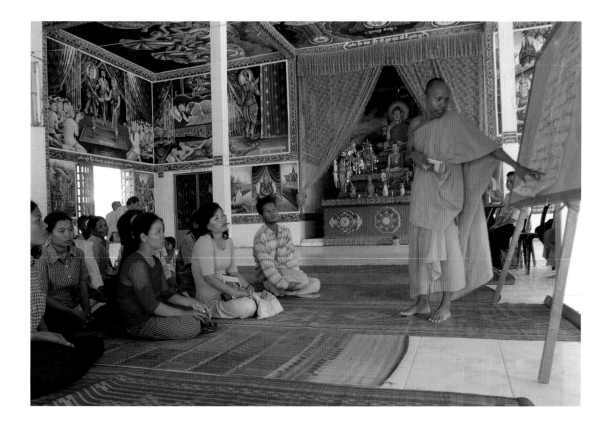

of stakeholders. I think UNAIDS has been particularly successful in reaching out to the nongovernmental organization community, to the local communities, to the business community, and I find it has been very agile in doing that".

Ambassador Randall Tobias, former United States Global AIDS Coordinator and former Director of United States Foreign Assistance and Administrator of the United States Agency for International Development (USAID), commented: "I think UNAIDS has played a very important role in bringing others to the table and doing so in a way that is not political and makes every effort to keep people focused on the fact that the enemy is intolerance and indifference and lack of resources and those kinds of things; the enemy is not each other".

Religious and faith-based organizations have been closely involved in the AIDS response since the early days of the epidemic.
UNAIDS/
O.O'Hanlon

The challenges: the need for an exceptional response to AIDS

It is only too clear that despite the significant increase in political engagement, the huge hike in funding for the AIDS response and the work of UNAIDS and so many others, the powerful human immunodeficiency virus is still spreading.

Piot has argued strongly and forthrightly that AIDS is an exceptional threat to the world – and that it therefore demands an exceptional response.

The impact of AIDS is exceptional because of its impact now and the future threats it poses. It primarily kills adults in their prime, those who drive economic growth and provide care for the very young and the elderly. Too many countries, especially in sub-Saharan Africa, are being stripped of this generation; the labour force is being steadily wiped out, and in severely affected countries, the result could, over another two generations or so, be "the unravelling of economic and social development. ... The key factor here would be the cumulative weakening from generation to generation of human and social capital ... Within the next five years, every sixth or seventh child in the worst-affected sub-Saharan countries will be an orphan, largely because of AIDS. ... Apart from chronic armed conflicts, such as in the Democratic Republic of Congo ... there is arguably no other cause today of such utter economic and social regress"[18].

Piot has written[19] that the AIDS epidemic has 'continually outstripped the worst-case global scenarios ... national HIV prevalence has risen far beyond what we thought possible ... we are witnessing multiple waves of HIV spread even in countries where incidence has peaked'.

The UNDP's *Human Development Report* in 2005 concluded that 'the HIV/AIDS pandemic has inflicted the single greatest reversal in human development'.

However, unlike most health problems, and probably because it is transmitted largely through sex, AIDS affects all social classes. In that sense, it is not a classic 'disease of poverty'.

Another exceptional aspect of AIDS is its link to issues that are taboo in most, if not all, cultures – sex, homosexuality, sex work and injecting drug use. If HIV were transmitted in some other way, through some 'innocuous means', the world might well not be experiencing today's pandemic. But prejudice leading to stigma has silenced politicians and other leaders for too long, and everywhere action has come too late.

The result of such stigma and discrimination is that AIDS has always been treated differently from other diseases. Strong emphasis was placed on clinical confidentiality, informed consent for HIV testing and surveillance systems that preserved people's anonymity[20].

---

[18] Piot P (2005). *Why AIDS is Exceptional.* Address given at the London School of Economics, London, 8 February.
[19] Piot P (2007). 'AIDS: from crisis management to sustained strategic response'. *The Lancet*, 368.
[20] De Cock K M, Johnson A M (1998). 'From exceptionalism to normalisation: a reappraisal of attitudes and practices around HIV testing'. *British Medical Journal*, 316.

A number of developments, in particular the increased accessibility of antiretroviral therapy, has raised a debate about the need to 'normalize' the way medical professionals and health-care workers deal with people living with HIV, or those deemed to be at risk. If people are not offered testing (and many now promote routine offers of testing), they will not receive life-saving treatment. As Cameron has argued[21], the extra attention and 'hullabaloo' with which doctors approach the disease can reinforce the internal stigma that prevents 'AIDS-literate people' from being tested.

Both Paul Bekkers, the Dutch AIDS Ambassador, and Kazatchkine believe that AIDS should be integrated into a health system offering a complete range of services. "It is not acceptable that a patient should have access to antiretroviral drugs but not to an aspirin", said Kazatchkine.

However, Piot argues that it would be a gross mistake to match the reasonable need for "medical normalization" with a "normalization" or "medicalization" of the response to AIDS, and thus abandon the need for an exceptional response in terms of specific leadership, financing and policies. A recent backlash has seen several journalists and public health specialists disputing that too much money is spent on AIDS compared with other diseases, and that AIDS has produced large vertical programmes, quite separate from the treatment of other diseases[22].

But, says Piot, because this exceptional epidemic calls for an exceptional response, "AIDS should be the top priority for policy-makers and budgets". AIDS should be placed in the broader context of development and security, and not in competition with other diseases. Without an exceptional response, if AIDS is treated as one of many diseases, there will be insufficient protected funding for antiretroviral treatment, thus resulting immediately in millions of deaths and lack of support for harm-reduction programmes, general HIV prevention programmes, the Global Fund, PEPFAR and other AIDS funding mechanisms.

Furthermore, as Paul De Lay, from the UNAIDS Secretariat Evaluation Department, argues[23], HIV funding 'should provide an opportunity and entry point for strengthening health and social services systems if it is used appropriately. For example, large amounts have been spent on laboratory networks, universal precautions, blood bank safety, and safe injections, as well as focusing on the wellbeing and training of health workers, doctors and nurses and not only those working in AIDS'.

---

[21] Cameron E (2005). *Legal and Human Rights Responses to the HIV/AIDS Epidemic.* University of Stellenbosch, Matieland, South Africa.
[22] For example, see England R (2007). 'Are we spending too much on HIV?' *British Medical Journal*, 334:344; Garrett L (2007). 'The challenge of global health'. *Foreign Affairs*, January/February.
[23] Ibid.

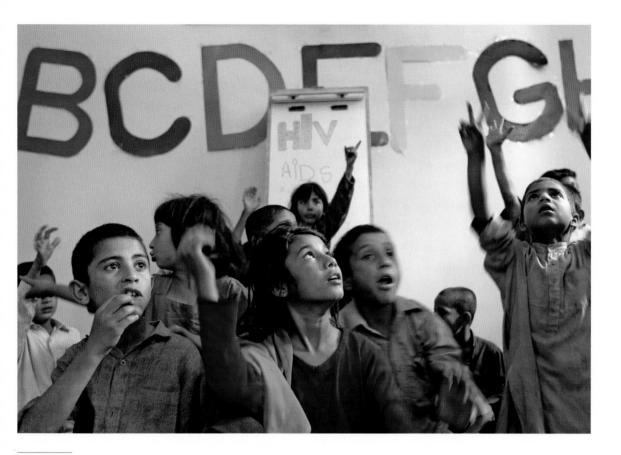

The challenges: making the money work

A major challenge – now and in the future – is to use the funding for AIDS effectively,
if both comprehensive HIV prevention and treatment programmes are to meet the scale
of the need in many countries, and certainly if there is to be any chance of achieving
universal access. The Global Task Team (see Chapter 7) was established in 2005 partly
to strengthen national responses through improved coordination, harmonization and
tackling technical bottlenecks that hinder the response.

'Making the money work', and thus achieving universal access to prevention and
treatment, also calls for a coherent response from all players and the implementation
of the "Three Ones". There has to be a focus on coordination among all the players –
government, civil society, donors, etc. Some countries still have to develop a single,
costed, evidence-based and inclusive national AIDS plan, nor have they ensured the
necessary link between AIDS activities and broader development frameworks.

The Global Task Team also encourages all donors to align their support to countries'
needs and priorities; these must come first. Programmes must be adapted to local needs
and social and cultural contexts and serious investment in capacity is needed – of health
workers in particular. A number of commitments and initiatives came from the Global

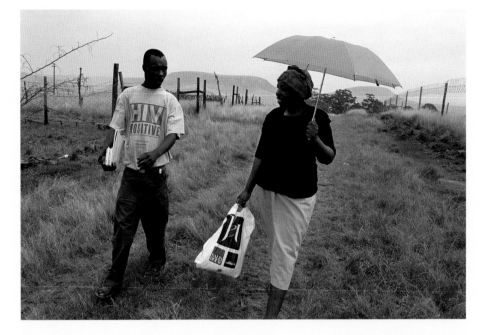

*Bavuyise Mbebe is
walking with his mother
to the local HIV treatment
centre to collect his first
antiretroviral drugs, in
Palmerton, Eastern Cape,
South Africa
Corbis/Gideon Mendel*

Task Team. The AIDS Strategy and Action Plan service, run by the World Bank for
UNAIDS, seeks to support national aids authorities in assessing the quality of their plan
and provides technical support to improve it so it can more effectively translate resources
into services and permit alignment by external funds. The Global Implementation
Support Team[24] was established to solve problems in the implementation of programmes,
such as the procurement of drugs and other commodities – the major bottleneck for
implementing major grants and projects at country level. The Country Harmonization
and Alignment Tool aims to improve the transparency and accountability of partner
engagement at country level. It encourages the national AIDS authority to ask questions
of its partners in the AIDS response relating to the *quality* of aid: how engaged is civil
society in policy, strategy, and resourcing decisions; how well are the international
partners adhering to the commitments of the "Three Ones", the Global Task Team and
the Paris Declaration on Aid Effectiveness. Only by helping ensure these commitments
are applied in country responses, will any real progress be made.

Countries are being encouraged by UNAIDS to 'know your epidemic' through an
understanding of the key populations most likely to be exposed to HIV, and of the
behaviour that leads to transmission (for example, people having sexual relationships with
a number of partners and without using condoms). 'Knowing your epidemic' provides
the basis for countries to 'know your response', by recognizing the organizations and
communities that are, or could be, contributing to the response, and by critically assessing
the extent to which the existing response is meeting the needs of those most vulnerable

---

[24] Originally composed of the Global Fund to Fight AIDS, Tuberculosis and Malaria, the World Bank, WHO,
UNDP, the United Nations Children's Fund (UNICEF) and the United Nations Population Fund (UNFPA),
GIST was subsequently expanded to include the US Government, the United Kingdom Department for
International Development (DFID), the German development agency Deutsche Gesellschaft für Technische
Zusammenarbeit(GTZ), the International HIV/AIDS Alliance, the International Council of AIDS Service Organi-
zations (ICASO) and the Asia Pacific Council of AIDS Service Organizations.

to HIV infection. Thus countries can review, plan, match and prioritize their national responses. A challenge in many countries is the reluctance by national AIDS bodies to involve civil society fully – often specifically those people living with HIV. Their voices must be heard; their experiences and actions are invaluable to an effective response.

The challenges: a long-term response to AIDS

Unlike so many tragedies, such as the tsunami in 2007 or severe droughts, AIDS is a continuing crisis. The fundamental challenge for everyone working to combat this epidemic is to sustain a full-scale response to AIDS over at least another generation. UNAIDS must continue its advocacy to ensure that leaders do not lose sight of the exceptional nature – and threat – of the AIDS epidemic. Building and retaining popular support for the AIDS cause in both low and high-income countries will be key, as will be the achievement of results in the fight against AIDS. Thus, UNAIDS and others have to show returns on the investments of billions of dollars made, so that the latter are commensurate with the numbers of averted infections, illness and deaths.

Activist Zackie Achmat explained: "Everybody said to me why did you not go to Toronto [the 16th International AIDS conference]? I said, Sweetie Dear, there [will] be AIDS conferences for another 100 years and I hope to be around for another 50 of them, not for the conference but for those years … the epidemic is going to last a long, long time and we have to pace ourselves. The biggest problem we face is how we focus political leadership on AIDS as an emergency and on AIDS as a long-term issue. And to maintain that interest in that".

In order to ensure a sustained response, there is a **need to retain and develop exceptional leadership**. An exceptional response calls for exceptional leadership to ensure sustainability and long-term, funded strategies but political commitment is by definition fragile. Politicians' horizons are often short, sometimes only as far as the next election or two rather than for decades to come; there are so many immediate issues competing for their attention.

Despite the considerable growth of political engagement with AIDS since UNGASS in 2001, governments are not doing enough. As the UN Secretary-General's report for the 2007 High-Level Meeting revealed[25], '… five years after the Special Session, the available evidence underscores the great diversity among countries and regions in implementing the response envisioned in the Declaration of Commitment on HIV/AIDS. While certain countries have reached key targets and milestones for 2005 as set out in the declaration, many countries have failed to fulfil the pledges'.

As well as retaining and increasing the engagement of political leaders and elected representatives at every level, **sustained activism** is essential to hold governments and other actors accountable. Engaging the broad coalition of public and private sectors, of

[25] UNAIDS (2007). *Declaration of Commitment on HIV/AIDS: Five Years Later. Report of the Secretary-General.* Geneva, UNAIDS.

business and nongovernmental organizations, for example, is vital. As US Ambassador Richard Holbrooke, President and Chief Executive Officer of the Global Business Coalition on HIV/AIDS, called for[26], many companies should offer support, not just donations but also by 'enhancing their own activities in offering education, testing, counselling, treatment and a pledge of non-discrimination to employees and their families'. There is also still a serious lack of meaningful participation of people living with HIV. UNAIDS is now providing support to embark on a re-mobilization of HIV-positive communities worldwide.

There is a need for increased and sustainable funding. Although funding has greatly increased over the past decade, there is still a major gap between what is needed for a sustained response and what is actually being provided. At the 2007 UN General Assembly High-Level Meeting on AIDS, UN Member States recognized that by 2010, US$ 20–23 billion will be needed annually for developing countries to scale up towards universal access to antiretrovirals. But existing pledges, commitments and trends suggest that the rate of increase might be declining, as indicated by the fact that available funds were US$ 9 billion in 2007 and will be around US$ 10 billion in 2007.

UNAIDS has advocated for funding to be more predictable and guaranteed for the long term. Volatile funding makes it hard for countries to make long-term plans. As more treatment programmes are rolled out, and treatment keeps more people alive longer, the need for funding is also increased. So for some time the financing needs will increase.

The epidemic will be halted only if AIDS is placed firmly in mainstream development work.

Many developing countries are able to spend more on their AIDS response, but whether they do so depends on the political will to reallocate resources. However, this is not true for many of the poorest African countries. 'Fulfilling promises on official development assistance, and a continued ring-fencing of AIDS funding by governments, donor agencies and the World Bank, will be essential for many years to come … The world needs nothing less than fiscal commitments for universal access to HIV prevention and treatment services covering at least 10 years'[27].

Existing funding mechanisms such as the Global Fund to Fight AIDS, Tuberculosis and Malaria need to be supported and strengthened. From its early days, the Fund has had to endure an almost 'stop-start' policy of funding flows from donors; this does not guarantee a sustained response. Developing mechanisms for not only increased but also sustained and predictable financing should be a priority – as it is for development in general.

Getting the relationship right between the Global Fund and UNAIDS will be crucial for more effective multilateral support to the AIDS response in developing countries. As both organizations are entirely complementary, in theory creating greater institutional synergy should not be so difficult, as long as the will is there in the boards and management of both.

---

[26] Jack A (2007). 'Between hope and despair: why the fight against AIDS is at a turning point'. *Financial Times*, 31 May.
[27] Piot (2007).

The challenges:
need to tackle the major 'drivers' of the epidemic

"We live in a world that must be changed to survive".

The epidemic will be halted only if AIDS is placed firmly in mainstream development work. Major drivers of the epidemic such as poverty, inequality—especially of women in most societies—and stigma have to be tackled.

Jim Yong Kim, former Director of WHO's HIV/AIDS Department, and Paul Farmer, both co-founders of Partners in Health, a non-profit organization working for international health and social justice, have written[28]: '... poverty is far and away the greatest barrier to comply with ART [antiretroviral therapy] ... far and away the greatest barrier to the scale-up of treatment and prevention programmes. Our experience in Haiti and Rwanda has shown us that it is possible to remove many of the social and economic barriers to adherence but only with what are sometimes termed "wrap-around services": food supplements for the hungry, help with transportation to clinics, child care and housing ... Coordination among initiatives such as PEPFAR, the GF [Global Fund] and WFP [World Food Programme] can help in the short term; fair-trade agreements and support of African farmers will help in the long run'.

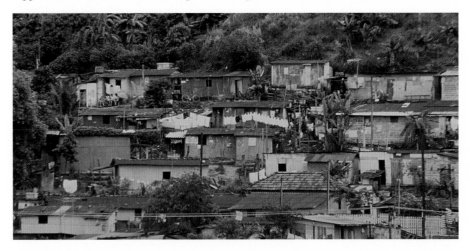

A major challenge to combating the epidemic is poverty and the conditions in which people live – in Brazilian favelas, for example UNAIDS/J.Maillard

'AIDS flourishes in poor societies because illiteracy and penury make people vulnerable; success against the virus depends partly on broader progress'. As President Paul Kagame of Rwanda told the *Washington Post*, 'there's no use in giving someone antiretroviral drugs if he has no food'[29].

Achmat put it very simply when addressing a conference: "We live in a world that must be changed to survive"[30].

[28] Kim JY, Farmer P (2007). 'AIDS in 2007 – moving towards one world, one hope?' *New England Journal of Medicine*, 355.

[29] Interview (2007). 'Another $10 billion. The world has only begun to wake up to the AIDS challenge'. *Washington Post*, 2 June.

[30] Achmat Z (2007). *Make Truth Powerful: Leadership in Science, Prevention and the Treatment of HIV/AIDS.* Address at the Microbicides 2007 conference, Cape Town, 26 April.

The challenges:
the need for scientific and technological innovation

The development of antiretroviral treatment has been a major breakthrough but treatment is not a cure, it is a life-long commitment and it will take decades to stop the spread of HIV. Thus another major challenge is to achieve more scientific and technological breakthroughs – such as vaccines and unobtrusive technologies including microbicides for women.

Scientists have been searching for a vaccine against HIV since the early days of the epidemic and numerous vaccine candidates are in various stages of development across the globe. But despite the dedication of many scientists and considerable funding, there are complex scientific problems that hinder progress such as the variability of the virus in different parts of the world.

With over 600 000 children contracting HIV infection each year, mostly through mother-to-child transmission, access to affordable HIV treatment represents an urgent challenge and global health priority; similarly, accurate diagnosis of HIV infection in children can be difficult and expensive in resource-limited settings. Procedures and formulations of antiretrovirals suitable for use in children remain rare and tend to be more expensive and difficult to administer than adult regimens. To overcome these obstacles, a new method for diagnosis has been developed (dried spot testing), which may help to reduce the cost and facilitate HIV diagnosis in children. With regard to treatment, some manufacturers have piloted the production of mini-pills, which are particularly suitable for young children. However, all new products need to be properly tested, prequalified and licensed for use, and this takes time.

Recently, the scientific community has confirmed that an age-old practice can help to reduce the risk of HIV transmission. Research evidence demonstrates that male circumcision may help to protect against HIV infection by removing cells in the inner foreskin that serve as entry points for the virus. Three trials[31,32,33] have revealed an approximate halving of risk of HIV infection in men who were circumcised. Although these results demonstrate that male circumcision reduces the risk of men becoming infected with HIV, the UN agencies emphasize that it does not provide complete protection against HIV infection. Male circumcision should never replace other known effective prevention methods and should always be considered as part of a comprehensive prevention package, which includes correct and consistent use of male or female condoms, reduction in the number of sexual partners, delaying the onset of sexual relations and HIV testing and counselling.

[31] Bailey C, Moses S, Parker CB et al. (2007) 'Male circumcision for HIV prevention in young men in Kisumu, Kenya: a randomized controlled trial'. *The Lancet*, 369: 643-56.

[32] Gray H, Kigozi G, Serwadda D et al. (2007) 'Male circumcision for HIV prevention in young men in Rakai, Uganda: a randomized trial'. *The Lancet*, 369:657-66.

[33] Auvert B, Taljaard D, Lagarde E et al. (2005) 'Randomized, controlled intervention trial of male circumcision for reduction of HIV infection risk: the ANRS 1265 Trial'. *PLoS Medicine*, 2(11):e298.

Conclusion

Given the many challenges to the global and national responses to AIDS, UNAIDS will continue to play a vital role in the response to AIDS for many years to come. Progress has undoubtedly been made in its first decade but HIV infections and AIDS deaths continue to rise.

Thus the organization must play an important role in the AIDS response. UNAIDS will continue to engage the United Nations system to assist countries in developing and maintaining effective response to the AIDS epidemic.

UNAIDS' immediate objective for the next few years is clear: supporting countries to move towards the goal of universal access to HIV prevention programmes, treatment, care and support. However, the ever-present challenge for UNAIDS – and its many partners– is to promote continuing change in many areas; in working within the UN system and alongside other partners in development to overturn poverty and inequality, to combat stigma and injustice and defend human rights, to enable people living with HIV to claim their rights and to thus give voice to the voiceless and powerless. At the same time, UNAIDS must fight for a response in terms of political commitment, funding and policy that is both sustained and flexible enough to adapt to the as yet unforeseen challenges ahead. The response to AIDS has to be as complex as the epidemic itself; the ability to respond to changes in the epidemic is essential if it is ever to be overcome.

Abbreviations

AAI	Accelerating Access Initiative
ABC	abstain, be faithful and use condoms
ACT UP	AIDS Coalition to Unleash Power
AIDS	acquired immunodeficiency syndrome
CARICOM	Caribbean Community
CCM	Country Coordinating Mechanism
CCO	Committee of Cosponsoring Organizations
CDC	Centers for Disease Control and Prevention
CEO	Chief Executive Officer
CIPLA	Chemical, Industrial and Pharmaceutical Laboratories
CPA	Country Programme Adviser
CRIS	Country Response Information System
CRN+	Caribbean Regional Network of People living with HIV/AIDS
DFID	Department for International Development
ECOSOC	Economic and Social Council
G8	Group of Eight
GCWA	Global Coalition on Women and AIDS
GHESKIO	Haitian Study Group on Kaposi's Sarcoma and Opportunistic Infections
GIPA	Greater Involvement of People living with HIV/AIDS
GMAI	Global Media AIDS Initiative
GNP+	Global Network of People living with HIV/AIDS
GPA	Global Programme on AIDS
HIV	human immunodeficiency virus
ICASA	International Conference on AIDS and STIs in Africa
ICASO	International Council of AIDS Service Organizations
ICPD	International Conference on Population and Development
ILO	International Labour Organization
IPAA	International Partnership against AIDS in Africa
JAPR	Joint HIV/AIDS Programme Review
MAP	Multi-Country HIV/AIDS Programme for Africa

NACC	National AIDS Control Council
NGO	nongovernmental organization
NIH	National Institutes of Health
OAFLA	Organisation of African First Ladies against HIV/AIDS
OECD	Organisation for Economic Co-operation and Development
PAF	Programme Acceleration Funds
PANCAP	Pan Caribbean Partnership against HIV/AIDS
PCB	Programme Coordinating Board
PEPFAR	U.S. President's Emergency Plan for AIDS Relief
TAC	Treatment Action Campaign
TASO	The AIDS Support Organisation
TRIPS	WTO Agreement on Trade-Related Aspects of Intellectual Property Rights
UK	United Kingdom
UN	United Nations
UNAIDS	Joint United Nations Programme on HIV/AIDS
UNDCP	United Nations Drug Control Programme
UNDP	United Nations Development Programme
UNESCO	United Nations Educational, Scientific and Cultural Organization
UNFPA	United Nations Population Fund
UNGASS	United Nations General Assembly Special Session
UNHCR	United Nations High Commissioner for Refugees
UNICEF	United Nations Children's Fund
UNODC	United Nations Office on Drugs and Crime
UNV	United Nations Volunteers
US	United States
USA	United States of America
USAID	United States Agency for International Development
WFP	World Food Programme
WHO	World Health Organization
WTO	World Trade Organization

Index

A